Case Studies in Neurology

Case Studies in Neurology

Editor: Brody Jenkins

AMERICAN
MEDICAL PUBLISHERS
www.americanmedicalpublishers.com

AMERICAN
MEDICAL PUBLISHERS
www.americanmedicalpublishers.com

Cataloging-in-Publication Data

Case studies in neurology / edited by Brody Jenkins.
p. cm.
Includes bibliographical references and index.
ISBN 979-8-88740-608-4
1. Neurology. 2. Nervous system--Diseases. I. Jenkins, Brody.
RC346 .N48 2023
616.8--dc23

American Medical Publishers,
41 Flatbush Avenue,
1st Floor, New York,
NY 11217, USA

ISBN 979-8-88740-608-4 (Hardback)

Contents

Preface

Neurology is a specialized branch of medicine that focuses on the study, diagnosis and treatment of disorders and diseases affecting the nervous system. The nervous system is a complex network of cells, tissues and organs that coordinate and control the functions of the body. It consists of the central nervous system, which is made up of the brain and spinal cord, and the peripheral nervous system, which comprises nerves and ganglia outside the brain and spinal cord. A few of the neurological conditions which are diagnosed and treated within this field include stroke, epilepsy, multiple sclerosis, Parkinson's disease, Alzheimer's disease, migraine and neuropathies. This book explores all the important aspects of neurology in the present day scenario. It will serve as a valuable source of reference for graduate and postgraduate students.

This book has been the outcome of endless efforts put in by authors and researchers on various issues and topics within the field. The book is a comprehensive collection of significant researches that are addressed in a variety of chapters. It will surely enhance the knowledge of the field among readers across the globe.

It gives us an immense pleasure to thank our researchers and authors for their efforts to submit their piece of writing before the deadlines. Finally in the end, I would like to thank my family and colleagues who have been a great source of inspiration and support.

Editor

1

Extraneural Metastasis of Primary Glioma Occurring in a Setting of Occupational Ionizing Radiation Exposure

Nitya Prabhakaran,[1] Douglas C. Miller,[1] N. Scott Litofsky,[2] and Shellaine R. Frazier[1]

[1]*Department of Pathology and Anatomical Sciences, University of Missouri School of Medicine, Columbia, MO 65212, USA*
[2]*Division of Neurological Surgery, Department of Surgery, University of Missouri School of Medicine, Columbia, MO 65212, USA*

Correspondence should be addressed to Nitya Prabhakaran; drnityaprabhakaran14@gmail.com

Academic Editor: Hidetoshi Ikeda

Malignant gliomas account for 60% of all primary brain tumors in adults. Glioblastoma Multiforme (GBM) is the most common primary glial tumor with a dismal prognosis and a median survival of approximately 14 months. Extra-neural metastases from primary brain tumors are unusual with an incidence rate of less than 2%. This has been attributed to factors such as short survival, lack of true lymphatics in the CNS, and physical barriers provided by the dura, extracellular matrix, and basement membrane. Although most GBMs occur sporadically, there is a known association with therapeutic radiation exposure and with work in nuclear disaster cleanup. To our knowledge, no case of GBM with metastasis occurring in a patient with occupational radiation exposure currently exists in the literature. In this article, we present a case of GBM with lung metastasis occurring in a 51-year-old Caucasian male, whose history is significant for occupational exposure to ionizing radiation, and review the literature on GBM risk factors and potential mechanisms of metastasis.

1. Introduction

Glioblastomas (GBMs) are the most common and yet the most aggressive primary intraparenchymal brain tumors in adults [1–9]. They occur throughout the central nervous system (CNS) but are most common in the brain [1, 5]. Primary malignant brain tumors are thought to develop through accumulations of genetic alterations that permit cells to evade normal regulatory mechanisms and escape destruction by the immune system [1]. Factors that have positive and negative associations with GBM development have been described. While allergies or atopic disease(s) have been reported by some to decrease the risk, an increased risk has been shown with exposure to ionizing radiation (IR) [3, 10, 11]. An association with high-dose IR and all brain tumors has been observed in atomic bomb survivor studies, nuclear-test fallout data, therapeutic radiation for cancer or for benign conditions, and occupational and environmental studies [1, 10–12]. Like all primary brain tumors, extraneural metastasis of GBM is very rare, reported in less than 2% of all GBM cases [4, 7–9, 13–19]. The exact mechanisms of spread outside of the CNS of gliomas are not completely understood. The rarity of this phenomenon has been attributed to the usually short survival of affected patients and also due to intrinsic biological obstacles that prevent the tumor cells from infiltrating and surviving beyond the CNS environment [4, 7–9, 13–19]. Furthermore, we present a unique case of a middle-aged Caucasian man with a history of occupational IR exposure who developed a GBM with subsequent metastasis to the left lung.

2. Material and Methods

2.1. Presentation and Clinical Course. A 50-year-old Caucasian man nuclear power plant worker with an unremarkable medical history presented with complaints of recurrent headaches, nausea, and vomiting with left sided facial droop and personality changes, all occurring for 3-4 weeks. A computerized tomography (CT) scan of the brain showed a right frontal mass. Subsequently a pre- and postcontrast magnetic resonance imaging (MRI) was performed that showed a right frontal mass [Figures 1(a) and 1(b)]. A

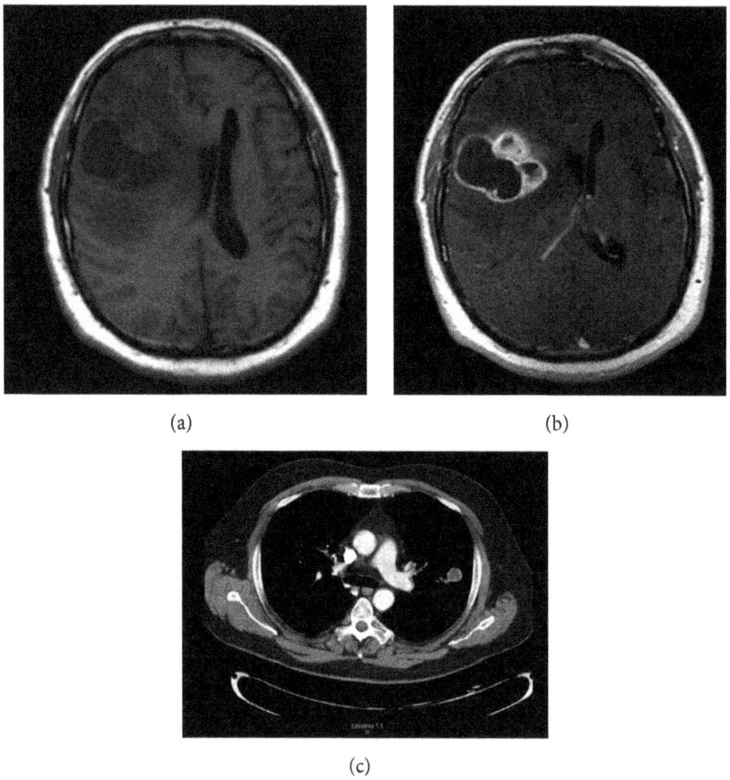

FIGURE 1: (a) and (b): pre- and postcontrast MRI demonstrating large right frontal ring-enhancing mass, October 2008. (c) Chest CT with mass in the left lung, May 2009.

right frontal craniotomy with gross total excision of the tumor was performed, after which the patient was treated with chemoradiation. Despite this, the patient continued to have frequent headaches and tremor with occasional gait imbalance. He also suffered multiple episodes of abdominal pain and diarrhea that was attributed to increased dosage of Temozolomide. The patient came back with increased frequency of headaches. This prompted a magnetic resonance imaging (MRI) scan which showed a large recurrent tumor. He subsequently underwent a right frontotemporal craniotomy with gross total excision of the recurrent mass, followed by Temozolomide and radiation therapy. Six months later, chest imaging performed in preparation for insertion of a central catheter showed a left upper lobe lung lesion which was suspicious for malignancy [Figure 1(c)]. This was removed as a wedge resection and was found to contain a malignant tumor which was morphologically and immunohistochemically identical to the primary brain tumor. The patient died 16 months after his initial presentation.

2.2. Pathology Findings. Histologically, the initial resection specimen of the right frontal lobe mass was a high-grade glioma that infiltrated the adjacent brain tissue [Figure 2]. The tumor had combined features of a high-grade glioma, WHO grade IV. There were foci of necrosis surrounded by palisades of tumor cells, extensive vascular hyperplasia, and a high mitotic rate. The tumor was composed of a mixture of small to medium sized cells and some very large, often multinucleated, giant cells [Figures 2(a)–2(c)]. The cytoplasm of the large cells was brightly eosinophilic. The background of smaller cells included a mixture of cells with round nuclei centrally placed in clear to pale cell bodies. Immunostains revealed nearly 100% tumor cell immunopositivity for vimentin, with the large cell population also immunopositive for glial fibrillary acidic protein (GFAP). The smaller cell population was negative for GFAP. An immunostain for Ki-67 showed up to 50% tumor cell nuclear immunopositivity in the most labeled areas. An immunostain for the protein product of the isocitrate dehydrogenase-1 R132H mutation (IDH1 R132H) showed no immunoreactivity in tumor cells.

The resection of the recurrent brain tumor yielded a high-grade infiltrating glioma with predominantly astrocytic features in that the predominant cell population had elongated bipolar processes. The tumor again had vascular hyperplasia. There was also extensive radiation induced necrosis.

The left lower lobe lung tumor was a metastatic glioma characterized by nests and sheets of cells with moderate to abundant amounts of eosinophilic to pale cytoplasm [Figure 3(a)]. Individual cells had eccentrically placed nuclei with moderate to marked pleomorphism. The markedly enlarged and hyperchromatic nuclei had prominent nucleoli, and, occasionally, nuclear pseudoinclusions. Mitotic figures were easily identifiable, and there were areas of necrosis [Figure 3(b)]. Immunostains revealed tumor cells with cytoplasmic immunoreactivity for vimentin, GFAP [Figure 3(c)], and S100 protein along with rare cells immunopositive

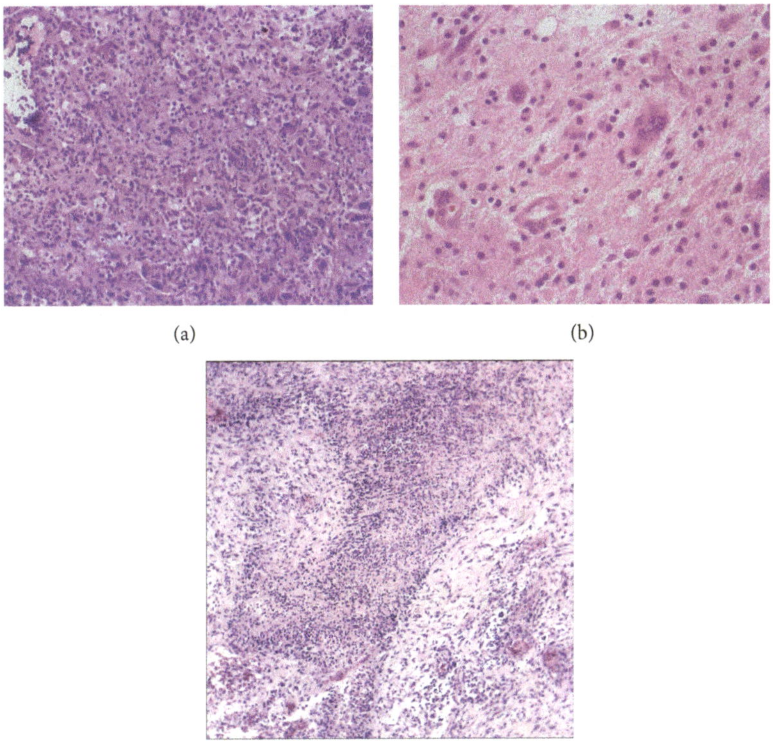

(a) (b) (c)

FIGURE 2: Brain tumor. (a) The tumor is composed of large and small cells (LFB/H&E, 100x). (b) The tumor contains many multinucleated giant cells (LFB/H&E, 400x). (c) The tumor displaying necrosis with palisade (H&E, 100x).

for epithelial membrane antigen (EMA). These EMA-immunopositive cells were consistent with entrapped normal lung epithelial cells. There was no immunoreactivity for cytokeratin (CK), epithelial membrane antigen (EMA), thyroid transcription factor 1 (TTF1), synaptophysin, HMB45, or Melan A/MART1 (antibody A103) in the neoplastic cells.

3. Discussion

Historically, the glial origin of GBMs was first recognized by Virchow in 1863. The erstwhile term "glioblastoma multiforme" was coined by Mallory in 1914 [2]. In 1926 Bailey and Cushing definitively changed the name from spongioblastoma multiforme to GBM and also went on to state that distant metastases from primary brain tumors do not occur [2, 7, 19, 20]. Scherer and Kernohan each recognized that GBMs may sometimes develop from the progression of a low-grade lesion, an observation that has since been confirmed by molecular studies [2]. The first case of extraneural metastases from a GBM was reported in 1928. In 1955, Weiss suggested diagnostic criteria for extraneural metastases from primary CNS tumors, which included a documented history of a primary CNS tumor, and histologic similarity between the primary tumor and presumed metastatic lesion [9]. More recently immunohistochemical similarities have also been important in such diagnoses.

Incidence rates of gliomas vary significantly by histologic type, age at diagnosis, sex, race, and country [1, 3, 10, 11]. Many factors have been postulated as potential risk factors for gliomas, including both heritable and acquired factors. Although numerous familial cancer syndromes are associated with an increased glioma risk, monogenic Mendelian disorders account for only a small proportion of adult glioma incidence at the population level [1].

Several epidemiologic risk factors have also been examined as potential contributors to glioma risk. Amongst these factors, those which seem to have a significant association include a decrease in risk by history of allergies or atopic disease(s) and an increase in risk by exposure to IR [1, 3, 10, 11].

Certain forms and doses of IR are generally accepted as having the potential to cause brain tumors. Atomic bomb studies, nuclear test fall-out data, studies of survivors of therapeutic radiation for cancer and for benign conditions, and occupational and environmental studies have connected IR to glioma genesis [11]. Nuclear facility employees and nuclear material production workers may have an elevated relative risk for brain tumors. Loomis and Wolf followed workers exposed to nuclear radiation between 1947 and 1974. They found that deaths from brain cancer and lymphopoietic malignancies were increased in white men so exposed [20]. Though several studies have been done in the past to demonstrate a heightened risk of development of glioma in patients exposed to IR [21–28], conflicting opinions exist in the scientific literature.

The data showing the association between radiation and gliomas is limited but data in adults show heightened greater

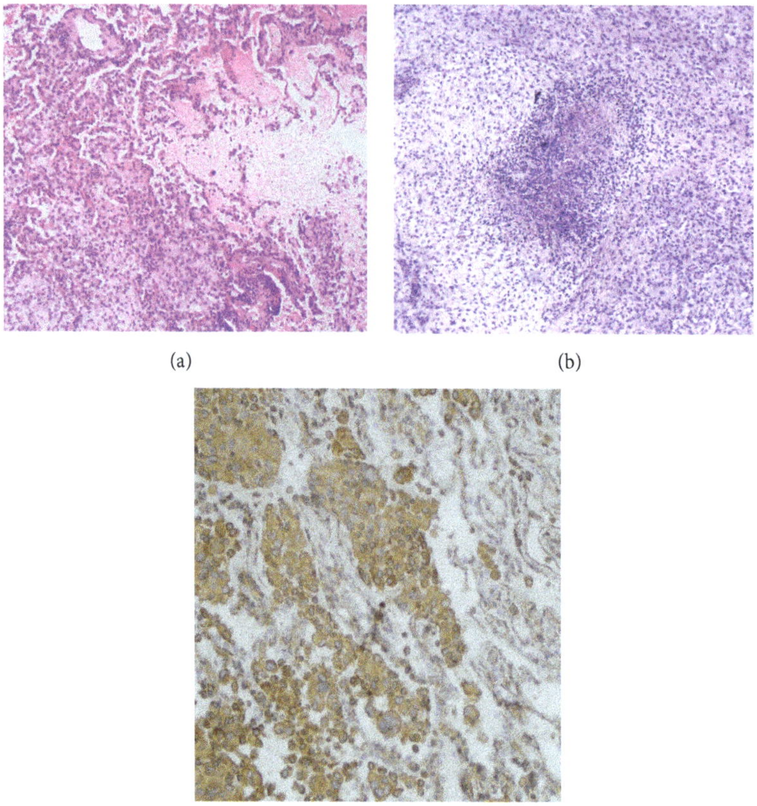

(a) (b)

(c)

Figure 3: Lung tumor. (a) The tumor forms a solid mass (left side) with bordering alveoli (right side) (H&E, 100x). (b) Necrosis in the lung tumor (H&E, 100x). (c) GFAP immunostain demonstrating immunopositive tumor cells in the lung with immunonegative pulmonary cells (right side) (GFAP immunostain, 100x).

risk in certain groups exposed to radiation. Two cohorts from Latvia and Estonia that consisted of approximately 10,000 individuals exposed to nuclear radiation showed a statistically significant increase in brain cancers [29]. Cardis *et al.* reviewed 95,673 workers who were exposed to IR for six months or longer across three countries. They found that mortality from leukemia, excluding chronic lymphocytic leukemia (CLL), was most strongly and consistently related to low dose IR exposure [30]. In a review of ten carefully conducted cohort mortality studies of U.S. workers in the nuclear industry published during the past decade, Alexander mentions that there is a significantly increased brain cancer risk. Further, these index studies of more than 78,000 workers followed for an average of 21 years, with more than 1.6 million person years of observation, establish that there is a statistically significant 15% increased risk of brain cancer for workers in the U.S. nuclear industry who have low-dose average cumulative radiation exposures [31]. Our patient had a history of working as a reactor operator in a nuclear power plant. The duration and dose of exposure were not available which makes it difficult to assess whether the IR exposure could have been a contributory factor in his GBM.

Morphologically GBMs are composed of cells that resemble astrocytes with irregular, ovoid, or elongated but mostly round nuclei that tend to lie toward one side or edge of the cell body. The *sine qua non* for this diagnosis is tumor necrosis. Often this necrosis is surrounded or outlined by a "palisade" of small poorly differentiated tumor cells with negligible eosinophilic cytoplasm and elongate hyperchromatic nuclei. Other features include vascular hyperplasia, mitotic figures in tumor cells, and pleomorphism [32].

Metastatic spread of GBM outside the CNS is unusual, reported to occur in less than 2% of all GBMs [4, 7–9, 13–19]. Pasquier *et al.* reviewed the reported cases of extraneural spread of GBM and documented 72 case reports published between 1928 and 1980 [33].

The most common sites of metastatic spread are the lungs and pleurae followed by lymph nodes, bone, and liver [34]. Patients with lung metastases are known to have the worst prognosis [13].

Several theories have been proposed as possible routes and mechanisms of such metastatic spread but, despite all the theories and evidence, such metastasis by gliomas is still a poorly understood process. Historically, it has been postulated that the lack of lymphatic vessels in the CNS constitutes a barrier to tumor spread [4, 7, 8, 13, 15, 18, 19]. However studies done in the last few years have highlighted the presence of a robust surrogate for a lymphatic system within the CNS.

Functional lymphatic vessels lining the dural sinuses have been demonstrated. These structures express all the molecular hallmarks of lymphatic endothelial cells (LYVE1, PROX1, and vascular endothelial growth factor receptor 3 (VEGFR3)) and are able to carry both fluid and immune cells from the CSF and drain to the deep cervical lymph nodes [35, 36]. Two types of afferent lymphatic vessels are known to exist. These are of the initial and collecting types. They differ anatomically in the expression pattern of adhesion molecules and in their permissiveness to fluid and cell entry. In contrast to the dural venous sinuses, the meningeal lymphatic vessels are devoid of smooth muscle cells. In addition, the meningeal lymphatic vessels are immunopositive for the immune-cell chemoattractant protein, CCL21 [35].

In 2014, a study done by Muller *et al.* identified the presence of circulating tumor cells (CTC) in the peripheral blood in 29 of 141 patients with GBM by immunostaining of enriched mononuclear cells with antibodies directed against GFAP, thus demonstrating hematogenous dissemination of glioma cells [15]. The concept of CTCs has also been mentioned in a few other studies [8, 13, 14]. The hematogenous route is the main pathway for metastases to lung, bone, and spleen [7]. In 2014, Ray *et al.* reviewed three case reports of systemic metastasis of GBMs and stated that the majority of metastases occur through the leptomeninges or intramedullary dissemination to the spinal cord [4].

Patients with GBM typically respond initially to therapy but ultimately relapse within the high-dose irradiation field, suggesting the presence of a subpopulation of resistant cells. While heterogeneity of tumors in different patients can in part explain varied patient responses to therapy, *intratumoral* heterogeneity is now recognized as a critical factor in determining therapeutic response. GBM initiating cells (GICs) are a subgroup of cancer stem cells that exhibit the ability to self-renew and express putative stem cell markers such as CD133, SSEA-1 (CD15), L1CAM, and CD44. GICs are defined functionally by their ability to repopulate the tumor upon serial transplantation [6].

In 2000, Park *et al.* reported the molecular genetic findings in six cases of extraneural metastasis of GBM. Four of these cases had TP53 mutations, but remarkably two different TP53 alterations were observed in paired primary and metastatic tumors [37]. This would suggest the emergence of subclones which were not dominant in the original GBM arising in the brain [4, 7]. A meta-analysis done by Elena *et al.* supports the idea that prolonged survival of GBM patients is associated with a greater risk of extraneural dissemination [14].

The standard therapy for newly diagnosed GBM is the "Stupp regimen" that uses Temozolomide and radiation. Our patient failed this regimen and in fact developed a metastatic lesion that we have described in this case report [38].

4. Conclusion

While gliomas occurring in the setting of occupational IR exposure may not represent a distinct clinical entity, it has been shown that certain forms of IR exposure do impart an increased risk of GBM development. The occurrence of a metastatic glioma in our patient with a history of occupational radiation exposure is both unique and intriguing as to what role might have been played by his occupational IR exposure. If the dose and duration of exposure were known in our patient it would have contributed to a better understanding of the association between low dose and high dose IR with primary brain tumors such as gliomas. This perhaps warrants more focused studies exploring the effects of IR on specific tumor subtypes and their relationship to specific dosage and duration of exposure. As innovative therapeutic interventions such as targeted therapies become increasingly available, longer GBM survival rates and subsequently more cases of dissemination of GBMs outside the CNS can be expected. For this reason, it is essential that physicians be cognizant of the potential for such metastatic disease in patients with GBMs.

Disclosure

All the authors have no financial disclosures to declare.

References

[1] Q. T. Ostrom, L. Bauchet, F. G. Davis et al., "The epidemiology of glioma in adults: a "state of the science" review," *Neuro-Oncology*, vol. 16, no. 7, pp. 896–913, 2014.

[2] G. Iacob and E. B. Dinca, "Current data and strategy in glioblastoma multiforme," *Journal of Medicine and Life*, vol. 2, no. 4, pp. 386–393, 2009.

[3] J. P. Thakkar, T. A. Dolecek, C. Horbinski et al., "Epidemiologic and molecular prognostic review of glioblastoma," *Cancer Epidemiology, Biomarkers & Prevention*, vol. 23, no. 10, pp. 1985–1996, 2014.

[4] A. Ray, S. Manjila, A. Hdeib et al., "Extracranial metastasis of gliobastoma: three illustrative cases and current review of the molecular pathology and management strategies," *Molecular and Clinical Oncology*, vol. 3, no. 3, pp. 479–486, 2015.

[5] K. K. Karipidis, G. Benke, M. R. Sim, T. Kauppinen, and G. Giles, "Occupational exposure to ionizing and non-ionizing radiation and risk of glioma," *Occupational Medicine*, vol. 57, no. 7, pp. 518–524, 2007.

[6] M. Rivera, K. Sukhdeo, and J. Yu, "Ionizing radiation in glioblastoma initiating cells," *Frontiers in Oncology*, vol. 3, 2013.

[7] P. Beauchesne, "Extra-neural metastases of malignant gliomas: myth or reality?" *Cancers*, vol. 3, no. 1, pp. 461–477, 2011.

[8] W. Harrison, C. Hulette, C. Guy, T. Sporn, and T. Cummings, "Metastatic glioblastoma: a case report and review of the literature," *Journal of Medical & Surgical Pathology*, vol. 1, article 115, 2016.

[9] M. D. Johansen, P. Rochat, I. Law et al., "Presentation of two cases with early extracranial metastases from glioblastoma and review of the literature," *Case Reports in Oncological Medicine*, vol. 2016, Article ID 8190950, 5 pages, 2016.

[10] M. Wrensch, Y. Minn, T. Chew, M. Bondy, and M. S. Berger, "Epidemiology of primary brain tumors: current concepts and review of the literature," *Neuro-Oncology*, vol. 4, no. 4, pp. 278–299, 2002.

[11] M. L. Bondy, M. E. Scheurer, B. Malmer et al., "Brain tumor epidemiology: consensus from the brain tumor epidemiology consortium," *Cancer*, vol. 113, no. 7, pp. 1953–1968, 2008.

[12] M. Z. Braganza, C. M. Kitahara, A. Berrington De González, P.

D. Inskip, K. J. Johnson, and P. Rajaraman, "Ionizing radiation and the risk of brain and central nervous system tumors: a systematic review," *Neuro-Oncology*, vol. 14, no. 11, pp. 1316–1324, 2012.

[13] M. Lun, E. Lok, S. Gautam, E. Wu, and E. T. Wong, "The natural history of extracranial metastasis from glioblastoma multiforme," *Journal of Neuro-Oncology*, vol. 105, no. 2, pp. 261–273, 2011.

[14] A. Elena, C. Melina, N. Raffaele et al., "Extraneural metastases in glioblastoma patients: two cases with YKL-40-positive glioblastomas and a meta-analysis of the literature," *Neurosurgical Review*, vol. 39, no. 1, pp. 37–46, 2016.

[15] C. Muller, J. Holtschmidt, M. Auer et al., "Hematogenous dissemination of glioblastoma multiforme," *Science Translational Medicine*, vol. 6, no. 247, Article ID 247ra101, 2014.

[16] K. Yokosuka, R. Ishii, Y. Suzuki et al., "Extraneural metastasis of high grade glioma without simultaneous central nervous system recurrence - Case report," *Neurologia medico-chirurgica*, vol. 47, no. 6, pp. 273–277, 2007.

[17] Q. Sun, R. Xu, H. Xu, G. Wang, X. Shen, and H. Jiang, "Extracranial metastases of high-grade glioma: The clinical characteristics and mechanism," *World Journal of Surgical Oncology*, vol. 15, article 181, 2017.

[18] J. D. Hamilton, M. Rapp, T. M. Schneiderhan et al., "Glioblastoma multiforme metastasis outside the CNS: three case reports and possible mechanisms of escape," *Journal of Clinical Oncology*, vol. 32, no. 22, pp. e80–e84, 2014.

[19] A. Mujic, A. Hunn, A. B. Taylor, and R. M. Lowenthal, "Extracranial metastases of a glioblastoma multiforme to the pleura, small bowel and pancreas," *Journal of Clinical Neuroscience*, vol. 13, no. 6, pp. 677–681, 2006.

[20] P. Bailey and H. Cushing, *A Classification of the Tumors of the Glioma Group on a Histogenetic Basis with a Correlated Study of Prognosis*, J. B. Lippincott & Co., Philadelphia, Pa, USA, 1928.

[21] B. H. Liwnicz, T. S. Berger, R. G. Liwnicz, and B. S. Aron, "Radiation-associated gliomas: a report of four cases and analysis of postradiation tumors of the central nervous system," *Neurosurgery*, vol. 17, no. 3, pp. 436–445, 1985.

[22] G. Marus, C. V. Levin, and G. S. Rutherfoord, "Malignant glioma following radiotherapy for unrelated primary tumors," *Cancer*, vol. 58, no. 4, pp. 886–894, 1986.

[23] S. Shapiro, J. Mealey, and C. Sartorius, "Radiation-induced intracranial malignant gliomas," *Journal of Neurosurgery*, vol. 71, no. 1, pp. 77–82, 1989.

[24] C. K. Chung, J. A. Stryker, R. Cruse, R. Vannuci, and J. Towfighi, "Glioblastoma multiforme following prophylactic cranial irradiation and intrathecal methotrexate in a child with acute lymphocytic leukemia," *Cancer*, vol. 47, no. 11, pp. 2563–2566, 1981.

[25] J. R. Anderson and C. S. Treip, "Radiation-induced intracranial neoplasms: a report of three possible cases," *Cancer*, vol. 53, no. 3, pp. 426–429, 1984.

[26] M. Malone, H. Lumley, and M. Erdohazi, "Astrocytoma as a second malignancy in patients with acute lymphoblastic leukemia," *Cancer*, vol. 57, no. 10, pp. 1979–1985, 1986.

[27] M. Fontana, C. Stanton, A. Pompili et al., "Late multifocal gliomas in adolescents previously treated for acute lymphoblastic leukemia," *Cancer*, vol. 60, no. 7, pp. 1510–1518, 1987.

[28] I. J. Rimm, F. C. Li, N. J. Tarbell, K. R. Winston, and S. E. Sallan, "Brain tumors after cranial irradiation for childhood acute lymphoblastic leukemia. A 13-year experience from the Dana-Farber cancer institute and the children's hospital," *Cancer*, vol. 59, no. 8, pp. 1506–1508, 1987.

[29] G. Prasad and D. A. Haas-Kogan, "Radiation-induced gliomas," *Expert Review of Neurotherapeutics*, vol. 9, no. 10, pp. 1511–1517, 2009.

[30] E. Cardis, E. S. Gilbert, L. Carpenter et al., "Effects of low doses and low dose rates of external ionizing radiation: cancer mortality among nuclear industry workers in three countries," *Journal of Radiation Research*, vol. 142, no. 2, pp. 117–132, 1995.

[31] V. Alexander, "Brain tumor risk among united states nuclear workers," *Occupational medicine (Philadelphia, Pa.)*, vol. 6, no. 4, pp. 695–714, 1991.

[32] D. Miller, *Modern Surgical Neuropathology*, Cambridge University Press, Cambridge, UK, 2009.

[33] B. Pasquier, D. Pasquier, A. N'golet, M. H. Panh, and P. Couderc, "Extraneural metastases of astrocytomas and glioblastomas clinicopathological study of two cases and review of literature," *Cancer*, vol. 45, no. 1, pp. 112–125, 1980.

[34] A. Cervio, F. Piedimonte, J. Salaberry et al., "Bone metastases from secondary glioblastoma multiforme: a case report," *Journal of Neuro-Oncology*, vol. 52, no. 2, pp. 141–148, 2001.

[35] A. Louveau, I. Smirnov, T. J. Keyes et al., "Erratum: Structural and functional features of central nervous system lymphatic vessels," *Nature*, vol. 523, pp. 337–341, 2015.

[36] A. Aspelund, S. Antila, S. T. Proulx et al., "A dural lymphatic vascular system that drains brain interstitial fluid and macromolecules," *The Journal of Experimental Medicine*, vol. 212, no. 7, pp. 991–999, 2015.

[37] C. C. Park, C. Hartmann, R. Folkerth et al., "Systemic metastasis in glioblastoma may represent the emergence of neoplastic subclones," *Journal of Neuropathology & Experimental Neurology*, vol. 59, no. 12, pp. 1044–1050, 2000.

[38] R. Stupp, W. P. Mason, M. J. van den Bent et al., "Radiotherapy plus concomitant and adjuvant temozolomide for glioblastoma," *The New England Journal of Medicine*, vol. 352, pp. 987–996, 2005.

2

Ominous Occurrence of Spinal Intradural Primary Malignant Peripheral Nerve Sheath Tumor Four Decades following Radiation Therapy for Testicular Seminoma

Osmond C. Wu,[1] Berje H. Shammassian,[1] Arunit J. S. Chugh,[1] Aparna Harbhajanka,[2] and Manish K. Kasliwal[1]

[1]*Department of Neurological Surgery, University Hospitals Cleveland Medical Center, Cleveland, OH, USA*
[2]*Department of Pathology, University Hospitals Cleveland Medical Center, Cleveland, OH, USA*

Correspondence should be addressed to Arunit J. S. Chugh; arunit.chugh@uhhospitals.org

Academic Editor: Dominic B. Fee

Primary intradural malignant peripheral nerve sheath tumor (MPNST) is an extremely rare diagnosis and is associated with an extremely poor prognosis. A 77-year-old man diagnosed with an intradural MPNST, more than 40 years after radiation for a testicular seminoma, is reported. Intradural MPNSTs of the spine outside the setting of neurofibromatosis is extremely rare and can masquerade as common benign nerve sheath tumors, on imaging. An older age at presentation with short duration of symptoms and prior regional radiation treatment encompassing the spine in the treatment field regardless of remoteness should alert the oncologists and neurosurgeons to the possible existence of this rare and aggressive tumor, as the management, and overall prognosis of this tumor is distinctly different compared to the usual intradural spinal tumors.

1. Introduction

Malignant peripheral nerve sheath tumors (MPNSTs) are aggressive, locally invasive rare soft tissue sarcomas arising from peripheral nerves that originate from Schwann cells or pluripotent cells of neural crest origin [1, 2]. MPNSTs represent 3–10% of all soft tissue sarcomas, with an overall incidence of 0.001% in the general population that peaks in the seventh decade [2–4]. In patients with neurofibromatosis type 1 (NF1), the annual incidence is 1.6 per 1000 with a lifetime risk of 8–13% [5]. Prior radiation exposure is another important risk factor, with a reported incidence of radiation induced MPNST ranging from 5.5–11% of patients [6]. MPNSTs are usually located in the extremities, trunk, and head, and neck. Spinal MPNSTs, however, are exceedingly rare. Table 1 comprises a list of the spinal MPNSTs in the literature. While there are a few instances of spinal and paraspinal MPNST following radiation for testicular seminomas, all the cases reported occurred within 7–10 years following radiation and were mainly extradural in location [7–10]. An intradural spinal MPNST with subsequent intracranial leptomeningeal metastasis diagnosed forty years after radiation is presented in this report with a pertinent review of the literature.

2. Case Report

2.1. History and Presentation. A 77-year-old man with past medical history significant for esophageal adenocarcinoma as well as testicular seminoma that was treated with conventional external bean radiation therapy (EBRT) almost 40 years back presented with three months of left hip and buttock pain in addition to left foot weakness. He had no history or clinical stigmata of neurofibromatosis.

A magnetic resonance imaging (MRI) of the lumbar spine with and without gadolinium demonstrated a homogenously enhancing, well demarcated intradural extramedullary neoplasm (Figure 1). An initial MRI of the cervical and thoracic spine with and without gadolinium was negative for additional lesions. While a diagnosis of benign nerve sheath tumor was suspected given typical radiological appearance, a metastatic lesion was also considered in the differential because of prior

Table 1: Primary spinal malignant peripheral nerve sheath tumors (MPNST) reported in the literature.

Author & year	Age (yrs), sex	Location	Presentation	NF history	Radiation history	Extent of resection	Radiation therapy	Chemotherapy	Recurrence	Metastasis	Outcome
Thomeer et al., 1981 [12]	42, M	Cauda equina	Low back pain for 9 yrs with occasional L radiculopathy, impotence for 4 wks, leg weakness for 3 wks		Not specified	Total	T11-S4 2.5 Gy 4x/wk for 6 wks		Yes, 3 yrs T9-11	No	Alive at 3 yrs
Valdueza et al., 1991 [13]	40, F	Thoracic	Thoracic pain, R leg weakness		Not specified	Partial	Total 12 Gy after initial operation, total 40 Gy after spinal metastasis	No	Yes, 2 mo	Chest, pelvis, spine	Alive at 4 yrs
	43, F	Thoracic	Low back pain for 1 mo, leg weakness for 2 wks		Not specified	Partial	Total 24 Gy after first operation, total 32 Gy after second operation for recurrence	No	Yes, 8 yrs	No	Alive at 10 yrs
	47, M	Cervical	Neck pain radiating to R shoulder for 9 mo, R arm weakness for 1 mo	NF1	Not specified	Total	Total 10 Gy	No	Yes, 3 mos	Brain, lumbar	Dead at 18 mos
	18, M	Cervical	*L* shoulder and arm pain for 4 mos		Not specified	Total	No	No	No	No	Alive at 8 mos
	70, F	Cervical	Neck pain radiating to R shoulder for 6 mos		Not specified	Total	No	No	No	No	Alive at 7 mos
Seppälä et al., 1993	13, M	Lumbar	Paraparesis	NF1	12 yrs ago for Wilm's tumor	Partial	Not specified	Not specified	Yes	Brain, systemic	Dead at 2 mos
	13, M	Lumbar	Paraparesis		Not specified	Total	Not specified	Not specified	Yes	Systemic	Dead at 7 mos
	45, F	Sacral	Not specified	NF1	Not specified	Partial	Not specified	Not specified	Yes	Systemic	Dead at 2 mos
	35, M	Lumbar	Radiculopathy	NF2	Not specified	Total	Not specified	Not specified	Yes	Systemic	Dead at 18 mos
	23, F	Thoracic	Not specified		Not specified	Total	Not specified	Not specified	Yes	Systemic	Dead at 8 mos
	37, F	Cervical	Radiculopathy		Not specified	Total	Yes	No	Yes, 2 yrs	Systemic	Dead at 6 yrs

Table 1: Continued.

Author & year	Age (yrs), sex	Location	Presentation	NF history	Radiation history	Extent of resection	Radiation therapy	Chemotherapy	Recurrence	Metastasis	Outcome
	52, F	Thoracic	Pain for 8 mos, weakness		Not specified	Total	No	No	No	No	Alive at 6 yrs
	68, F	Lumbar	Pain for 9 mos, weakness		Not specified	Total	No	No	No	No	Alive at 2 yrs
Celli et al., 1995 [15]	43, M	Lumbar	Pain for 3 mos		Not specified	Total	No	No	No	No	Alive at 6 yrs
	36, F	Thoracic	Pain for 5 mos		Not specified	Total	Yes	No	Yes	No	Alive at 4 yrs
	22, F	Cervical	Pain for 2 yrs, weakess, incontinence	NF1	Not specified	Total	Yes	No	Yes	Lung	Dead at 6 mos
	30, M	Thoracic	Pain for 3 yrs, weakness		Not specified	Total	Yes	No	Yes	Lung	Dead at 14 mos
West et al., 1997 [7]	40, M	Sacral	Radiculopathy		8 yrs ago for testicular seminoma, 30.6 Gy	Total	No	No	Yes, 7 mos	No	Not specified
	11, F	Lumbar, sacral	Not specified	NF1	Not specified	Partial	Yes	Yes	Yes, 0.5 mos	Yes, location not specified	Dead at 5 mos
	25, F	Lumbar	Not specified	NF1	Not specified	Partial	Yes	Yes	No	No	Alive at 18 yrs
	33, F	Lumbar	Not specified	NF1	Not specified	Partial	No	No	No	Yes, location not specified	Dead at 2 mos
	33, M	Lumbar	Not specified	NF1	Not specified	Partial	Yes	Yes	Yes, 3 mos	Yes, location not specified	Dead at 22 mos
	31, F	Lumbar	Not specified	NF1	Not specified	partial	yes	Yes	yes, 6 mos	yes, location not specified	dead at 10 mos
Kourea et al., 1998 [8]	37, F	Lumbar	Incidental		Not specified	Partial	No	Yes	Yes, 3 mos	No	Dead at 4 mos
	40, M	Sacral	Not specified		For testicular seminoma	Total	No	No	Yes, 9 mos	Yes, location not specified	Alive at 14 mos
	17, M	Thoracic	Not specified	NF1	Not specified	Partial	No	Yes	Yes	Yes, location not specified	Dead at 11 mos
	19, F	Thoracic	Incidental	NF1	Not specified	Total	No	No	No	No	Alive at 35 mos
	53, F	Thoracic	Not specified		For breast carcinoma	Partial	No	No	Yes, 6 mos	Yes, location not specified	Dead at 7 mo
	26, M	Thoracic	Not specified		For Hodgkin's lymphoma	Partial	Yes	No	Yes, 13 mos	Yes, location not specified	Dead at 27 mo

Table 1: Continued.

Author & year	Age (yrs), sex	Location	Presentation	NF history	Radiation history	Extent of resection	Radiation therapy	Chemotherapy	Recurrence	Metastasis	Outcome
Acharya et al., 2001 [20]	32, M	Cauda equina	Back pain, leg weakness, bowel and bladder dysfunction		Not specified	Partial	Yes	No	No	No	Alive at 18 mos
Yone et al., 2004 [16]	4, M	Cauda equina	Low back pain, radiculopathy, bladder dysfunction		Not specified	Total	Yes	Yes	Yes	Brain, spine	Dead at 21 mos
Adamson et al., 2004 [17]	37, M	Cervical	L C6 radiculopathy		6 yrs ago for Hodgkin's lymphoma	Partial	Yes	No	Not specified	No	Dead after 1 yr
	30, F	Cervical	R Horner syndrome, R C6 radiculopathy, R tricep and wrist extensor weakness		5 yrs ago for Hodgkin's lymphoma	Partial	No	No	Not specified	No	Dead after 1 yr
Amin et al., 2004 [9]	38, M	Cauda equina	Back pain, leg weakness, bowel and bladder dysfunction		10 yrs ago for testicular seminoma, 30 Gy/15 fractions over 3 wks	Biopsy	No	Yes, palliative	Yes, 7 mos	Not specified	Not specified
Albayrak et al., 2006 [18]	25, M	Thoracic	Paraparesis, bladder dysfunction	NF1	Not specified	Total	No	No	Yes, 7 wks	Lung	Alive at 7 wks
Chamoun et al., 2009 [14]	5, F	Cervical	Pain, gait disturbance		Not specified	Partial	Yes	Yes	Yes	Brain, thoracic and lumbar spine	Alive at 4 mos
Xu et al., 2012	8, M	Lumbar	Pain		Not specified	Total	Yes	No	Yes	Brain	Dead at 16 mos
Mitsuhara et al., 2013	47, F	Cauda equina	Back pain, R leg weakness, bowel and bladder dysfunction, altered mental status	NF2	15 yrs ago for uterine and cervical cancer, 22 Gy	Partial	Yes, 36 Gy brain and spine, additional 14.4 Gy to lumbosacral lesion/28 fractions	No	Not specified	No	Not specified

Table 1: Continued.

Author & year	Age (yrs), sex	Location	Presentation	NF history	Radiation history	Extent of resection	Radiation therapy	Chemotherapy	Recurrence	Metastasis	Outcome
Stark et al., 2013	56, F	Sacral	L leg radiculopathy, L foot paresis		15 yrs ago for non-Hodgkin's lymphoma	Not specified	No	Yes	Yes	Brainstem, spine	Dead at 24 mos
Wu et al., 2014	9, F	Thoracic, lumbar, sacral	R hip pain, bilateral leg weakness	NF2	Not specified	Partial	No	No	Yes	Brain	Dead at 9 mos
Li et al., 2014	33, F	Low thoracic, upper lumbar	Low back pain, R leg radiculopathy, hydrocephalus		Not specified	Partial	Yes, 28 Gy/19 fractions	No	Yes	Brain, diffuse spine	Dead at 29 mos
Lau et al., 2014 [10]	43, M	Cauda equina	Low back pain, L leg radiculopathy for 5 mos		10 yrs ago for testicular seminoma	Total	No	Yes, alternating between ifosfamide/ doxorubicin and ifosfamide/ etoposide	Yes, about 60 mos	Brainstem, cervical spine, renal	Dead at 5 yrs
Thomas et al., 2014	49, M	Cauda equina	Low back pain, paraparesis		Not specified	Partial	No	No	No	Brain and spine	Not specified
Baharvahdat et al., 2016	3, F	Cervical, upper thoracic	Paraplegia, bladder and bowel dysfunction		Not specified	Partial	No	No	No	Brain and spine	Dead shortly after surgery
Chou et al., 2017[a]	5–74 (mean 40)						76% had adjuvant therapy		38% over 2 yrs		59% alive at 2 yrs
Samancia et al., 2017	27, M	Cervical, upper thoracic	Hydrocephalus		Not specified	Partial	Yes	Yes	No	No	Not specified
Present study	77, M	Lumbar	Left hip and buttock pain for 3 mos		About 45 yrs ago for testicular cancer	Partial	No	No	No	Intracranial leptomeningeal disease	Dead at 2 mos

F: Female, Gy: gray, L: left, M: male, mos: months, NF1: neurofibromatosis type 1, NF2: neurofibromatosis type 2, R: right, wks: weeks, yrs: years. [a] Multicenter series ($N = 29$), individual patient data not available.

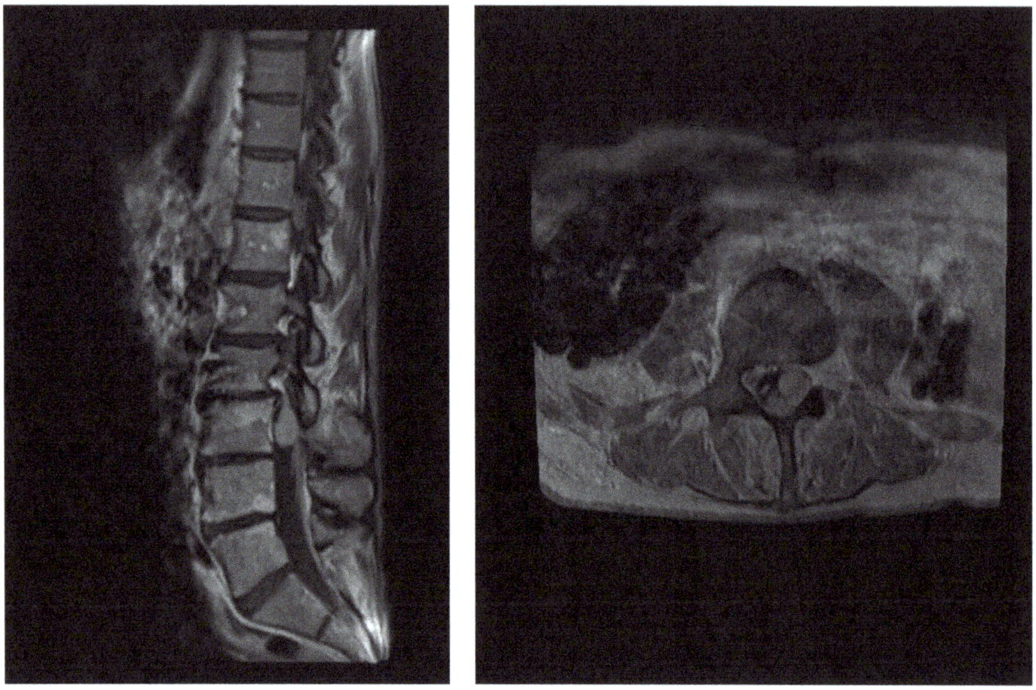

(a) (b)

FIGURE 1: (a) Magnetic resonance imaging (MRI) T1-weighted sagittal image of the lumbar spine with gadolinium demonstrates a well demarcated intradural extramedullary mass. (b) Corresponding axial image.

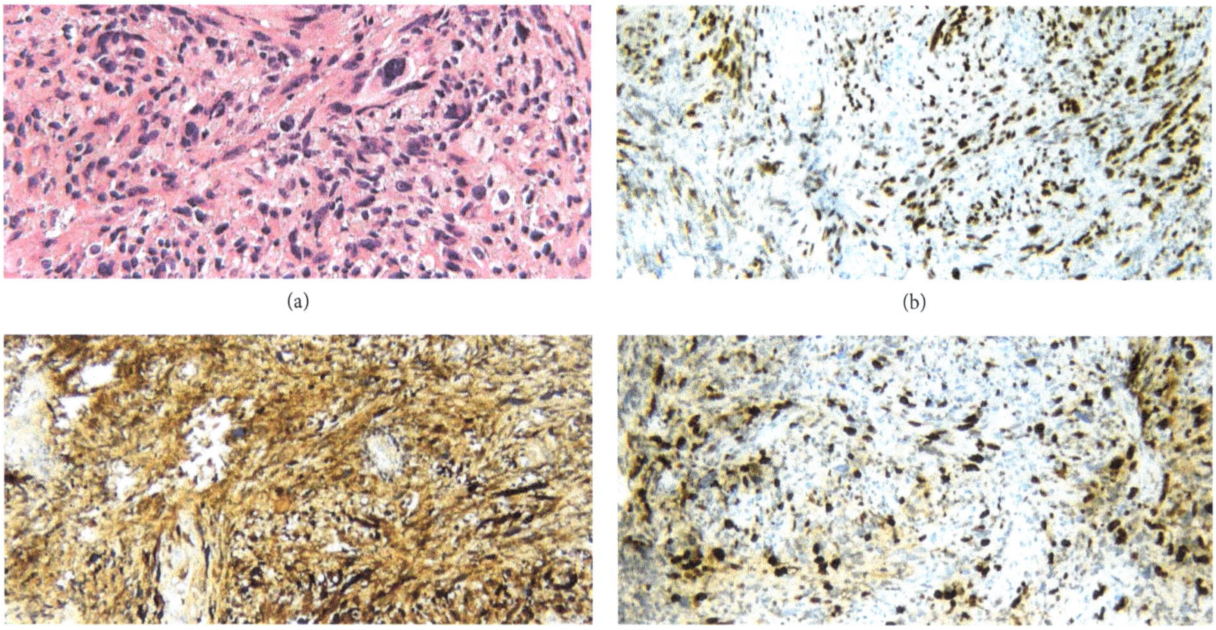

(a) (b) (c) (d)

FIGURE 2: (a) Hematoxylin and eosin (H&E) staining showed high cellular density with marked pleomorphism and spindle cells arranged in fascicles (200x). (b) Immunohistochemistry was positive for SOX 10 (100x) and (c) S-100 (100x). (d) Ki-67 labeling revealed a high proliferative index (100x).

history of cancer. A metastatic work up performed to look for any additional lesions was negative.

2.2. Operative Course. A partial L2 and complete L3 laminectomy was performed and a midline durotomy was made. A greyish mass was found in the intradural space arising from the left L3 nerve root with obvious enlargement and involvement of the nerve root. A frozen specimen was sent early for pathological evaluation that was diagnosed as MPNST. The nerve root of interest was clearly identified both proximally and distally, which on stimulation resulted in robust electrophysiological response suggestive of origin

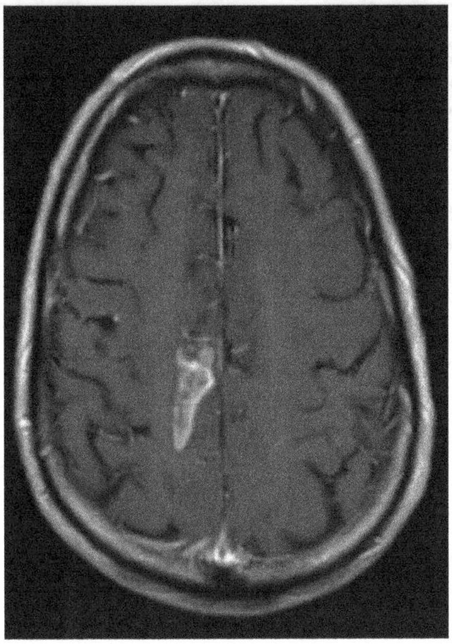

(a)

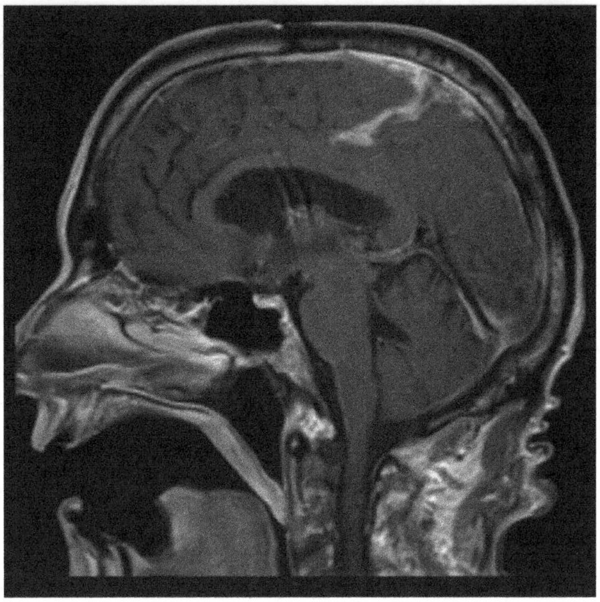

(b)

FIGURE 3: (a) Magnetic resonance imaging (MRI) T1-weighted axial image of the brain with gadolinium demonstrates leptomeningeal metastasis. (b) Corresponding sagittal image.

from a motor nerve root. No obvious plane was found between the tumor and the nerve root. Given the risk of motor deficit, the nerve root was preserved with partial resection of the tumor. Final pathology confirmed the diagnosis of MPNST (Figure 2).

2.3. Post-Operative Course. Given the initial pathologic diagnosis on frozen section, subsequent management including reoperation with extensive resection was discussed. Given his preoperative status, the patient, and family elected to observe in the short term with consideration of further treatment options following final pathology. The patient did well initially and was discharged to a skilled nursing facility. Two weeks post-operatively, however, the patient was readmitted with encephalopathy. An MRI brain with and without gadolinium demonstrated leptomeningeal metastasis (Figure 3) with cerebral spinal fluid (CSF) cytology positive for malignant cells. Given the extent of disseminated disease and his progressive worsening mental status, the family elected to pursue palliative care, and the patient died two months after his initial surgery.

3. Discussion

MPNSTs are rare entities with an incidence of 0.001%, with 20–50% of cases arising in patients with NF-1. The most common locations include the trunk, extremities, and head, and neck [2]. Primary spinal MPNSTs are extremely rare. Primary MPNSTs of the spine that are exclusively intradural extramedullary without extension into the extradural compartment are exceptionally rare. Outside the setting of NF-1, prior radiation treatment is a risk factor for development of MPNSTs. There have been few reports of MPNST following prior radiation for testicular seminomas. Most occurred after a short latent period and in an extradural location, with a purely intradural occurrence being exceptionally rare [7–10].

The present case developed almost four decades after being treated with EBRT for testicular seminoma, which is a significantly longer latency period as compared to other cases previously reported. Also, the imaging features were fairly characteristic of a benign intradural extramedullary neoplasm unlike a MPNST, which is typically an irregularly-bordered heterogeneously enhancing mass often with destruction of surrounding osseous structures. Similarly, the presence of leptomeningeal spread is also rare in primary intradural MPNSTs and as illustrated in this case, portends an ominous prognosis [11]. Unique to this case, however, is the rapid development of disseminated disease two weeks after surgery. Patients in other reported cases of intradural MPNSTs with leptomeningeal spread were diagnosed with dissemination ranging from present on presentation to 24 months following initial surgery [10–19]. The authors advocate that regardless of imaging characteristics or the duration since radiation, surgeons should retain a high index of suspicion for a MPSNT. Lumbar puncture may be considered to obtain CSF to identify potential malignant cells.

4. Conclusion

A rare case of an intradural MPNST diagnosed more than 40 years after radiation for a testicular seminoma is reported. Intradural MPNSTs of the spine outside the setting of neurofibromatosis are extremely rare and can masquerade common benign nerve sheath tumors on imaging. Short duration of symptoms and prior regional radiation treatment encompassing the spine in the treatment field regardless of remoteness should alert the physician to the possible existence of this rare and aggressive tumor. Being cognizant of this rare pathology can help initiate appropriate work up and evaluation, allow preoperative counselling, and alter overall surgical strategy.

Abbreviations

CSF: Cerebral spinal fluid
CT: Computer tomography
EBRT: External bean radiation therapy
H&E: Hematoxylin and eosin
MPNST: Malignant peripheral nerve sheath tumor
MRI: Magnetic resonance imaging
NF1: Neurofibromatosis type 1.

References

[1] A. N. D'Agostino, E. H. Soule, and R. H. Miller, "Sarcomas of the peripheral nerves and somatic soft tissues associated with multiple neurofibromatosis (Von Recklinghausen's disease)," *Cancer*, vol. 16, no. 8, pp. 1015–1027, 1963.

[2] B. S. Ducatman, B. W. Scheithauer, D. G. Piepgras, H. M. Reiman, and D. M. Ilstrup, "Malignant peripheral nerve sheath tumors. A clinicopathologic study of 120 cases," *Cancer*, vol. 57, no. 10, pp. 2006–2021, 1986.

[3] S. I. Hajdu, "Peripheral nerve sheath tumors histogenesis, classification, and prognosis," *Cancer*, vol. 72, no. 12, pp. 3549–3552, 1993.

[4] B. Zhu, X. Liu, Z. Liu et al., "Malignant peripheral nerve sheath tumours of the spine: clinical manifestations, classification, treatment, and prognostic factors," *European Spine Journal*, vol. 21, no. 5, pp. 897–904, 2012.

[5] D. G. Evans, M. E. Baser, J. McGaughran, S. Sharif, E. Howard, and A. Moran, "Malignant peripheral nerve sheath tumours in neurofibromatosis 1," *Journal of Medical Genetics*, vol. 39, no. 5, pp. 311–314, 2002.

[6] G. Gupta and A. Maniker, "Malignant peripheral nerve sheath tumors," *Neurosurgical Focus*, vol. 22, no. 6, pp. 1–8, 2007.

[7] D. A. West, R. O. Parra, A. Manepalli, R. J. Bernardi, and J. M. Cummings, "Development of a malignant peripheral nerve sheath tumor following treatment for testicular seminoma," *Urology*, vol. 50, no. 2, pp. 292–294, 1997.

[8] H. P. Kourea, M. H. Bilsky, D. H. Leung, J. J. Lewis, and J. M. Woodruff, "Subdiaphragmatic and intrathoracic paraspinal malignant peripheral nerve sheath tumors: a clinicopathologic study of 25 patients and 26 tumors," *Cancer*, vol. 82, no. 11, pp. 2191–2203, 1998.

[9] A. Amin, A. Saifuddin, A. Flanagan, D. Patterson, and J. Lehovsky, "Radiotherapy-induced malignant peripheral nerve sheath tumor of the cauda equina," *Spine*, vol. 29, no. 21, pp. E506–E509, 2004.

[10] D. Lau, D. H. Moon, P. Park, S. Hervey-Jumper, P. E. McKeever, and D. A. Orringer, "Radiation-induced intradural malignant peripheral nerve sheath tumor of the cauda equina with diffuse leptomeningeal metastasis," *Journal of Neurosurgery: Spine*, vol. 21, no. 5, pp. 719–726, 2014.

[11] A. M. Stark and H. M. Mehdorn, "Leptomeningeal metastasis of an intradural malignant peripheral nerve sheath tumor," *Journal of Clinical Neuroscience*, vol. 20, no. 8, pp. 1181–1183, 2013.

[12] J. M. Valdueza, C. Hagel, M. Westphal, M. Hänsel, and H. D. Herrmann, "Primary spinal malignant schwannoma: clinical, histological and cytogenetic findings," *Neurosurgical Review*, vol. 14, no. 4, pp. 283–291, 1991.

[13] K. Yone, K. Ijiri, K. Hayashi et al., "Primary malignant peripheral nerve sheath tumor of the cauda equina in a child case report," *Spinal Cord*, vol. 42, no. 3, pp. 199–203, 2004.

[14] R. B. Chamoun, W. E. Whitehead, R. C. Dauser et al., "Primary disseminated intradural malignant peripheral nerve sheath tumor of the spine in a child: case report and review of the literature," *Pediatric Neurosurgery*, vol. 45, no. 3, pp. 230–236, 2009.

[15] Q. Xu, B. Xing, X. Huang, R. Wang, Y. Li, and Z. Yang, "Primary malignant peripheral nerve sheath tumor of the cauda equina with metastasis to the brain in a child: case report and literature review," *The Spine Journal*, vol. 12, no. 4, pp. e7–e13, 2012.

[16] L. Wu, X. Deng, C. Yang, and Y. Xu, "Spinal intradural malignant peripheral nerve sheath tumor in a child with neurofibromatosis type 2: the first reported case and literature review," *Turkish Neurosurgery*, vol. 24, no. 1, pp. 135–139, 2014.

[17] Y. Li, F. Fan, J. Xu, J. An, and W. Zhang, "Primary malignant peripheral nerve sheath tumor of the spine with acute hydrocephalus: a rare clinical entity," *Journal of Neurosurgery: Spine*, vol. 21, no. 3, pp. 367–371, 2014.

[18] J. G. Thomas, C. Lincoln, J. C. Goodman, and S. P. Gopinath, "Malignant peripheral nerve sheath tumor of the cauda equina with craniospinal metastasis," *Journal of Clinical Neuroscience*, vol. 21, no. 12, pp. 2239–2242, 2014.

[19] H. Baharvahdat, B. Ganjeifar, N. Mohamadian Roshan, and A. Baradaran, "Spinal intradural primary malignant peripheral nerve sheath tumor with leptomeningeal seeding: case report and literature review," *Turkish Neurosurgery*, vol. 28, no. 2, pp. 317–322, 2018.

[20] R. Acharya, S. Bhalla, and A. Sehgal, "Malignant peripheral nerve sheath tumor of the cauda equina," Neurological Sciences, vol. 22, no. 3, pp. 267–270, 2001.

3

Reversible MR Findings in Marchiafava-Bignami Disease

Carmine Franco Muccio,[1] Luca De Lipsis ,[2] Rossella Belmonte,[2] and Alfonso Cerase[3]

[1]*Neuroradiology Unit, Neuroscience Department, "G. Rummo" Hospital, Benevento, Italy*
[2]*Anesthesia Department, "Sacred Heart of Jesus" Hospital, Benevento, Italy*
[3]*Neuroimaging and Neurointervention Unit, NHS and University Hospital "Saint Mary alle Scotte", Siena, Italy*

Correspondence should be addressed to Luca De Lipsis; codelip@libero.it

Academic Editor: Peter Berlit

Marchiafava-Bignami Disease (MBD) is a toxic demyelinating disease often diagnosed in chronic alcoholics. The disease process typically involves the corpus callosum and clinically presents with various manifestations resulting in MBD type A and type B on the basis of clinical condition, extent of callosal involvement and extracallosal involvement at brain magnetic resonance imaging (MRI), and prognosis. The death rate is high. We report a patient affected by MBD type B, who presented an isolated reversible splenial lesion at brain MRI and achieved a favorable recovery.

1. Introduction

Marchiafava-Bignami disease (MBD) is a rare neurological disease characterized by primary degeneration of the corpus callosum associated with chronic consumption of ethanol. MBD occasionally occurs in chronically malnourished, despite nonalcoholics. Clinical manifestation of MBD is nonspecific with a wide variation, including split-brain syndrome, difficult walking, para- or tetraparesis, altered mental status, seizure, and even coma or death. A deficiency of group B vitamins is the main etiopathogenic hypothesis, and many patients improve after the administration of these compounds. Magnetic resonance imaging (MRI) is generally used to support the diagnosis.

2. Case Presentation

A 51-year-old man was admitted to the Emergency Room in a state of altered sensorium, with motor deficit of the lower limbs. The patient had been suffering from chronic alcohol abuse for 30 years, with an average daily intake of 700 mL/die. Physical examination revealed a Glasgow Coma Scale score of 9 (E2V3M4). No meningeal signs were present. Pupils showed normal size and were reactive to light. The patient did not suffer from diabetes, hypertension, seizure nor other significant diseases. Routine blood test and cerebrospinal fluid studies were negative. Electroencephalographic examination was normal. Brain MRI showed an area of high signal on fast-spin-echo (FSE) T2-weighted images and high signal on diffusion weighted imaging (DWI) with a decreased apparent diffusion coefficient (ADC) value of 670 x10-3 mm^2/sec, observed with a region of interest size of 19 mm^2, in the splenium of the corpus callosum (Figures 1(a)–1(c)). On the basis of history, findings on physical examination, and MR imaging features, the diagnosis of MBD was hypothesized. He was transferred to the intensive care unit where he required noninvasive ventilation and was treated with thiamine 400 mg/day [1] hydration and parenteral nutrition with vitamin supplement, so the electrolyte balance was quickly restored. We did not use steroid therapy. He showed improvement of symptoms with a good recovery in twenty days. Thirty-day follow-up brain MRI showed resolution of the abnormal callosal finding on both T2-weighted images and DWI-ADC maps (Figures 1(d)–1(f)).

3. Discussion

MBD is a rare disorder of unknown etiology characterized by demyelination of the corpus callosum with various clinical manifestations which is often mismanaged and mistreated [2]. It mainly affects the male population, in the age group between 40 and 60 years. Chronic alcohol abuse plays

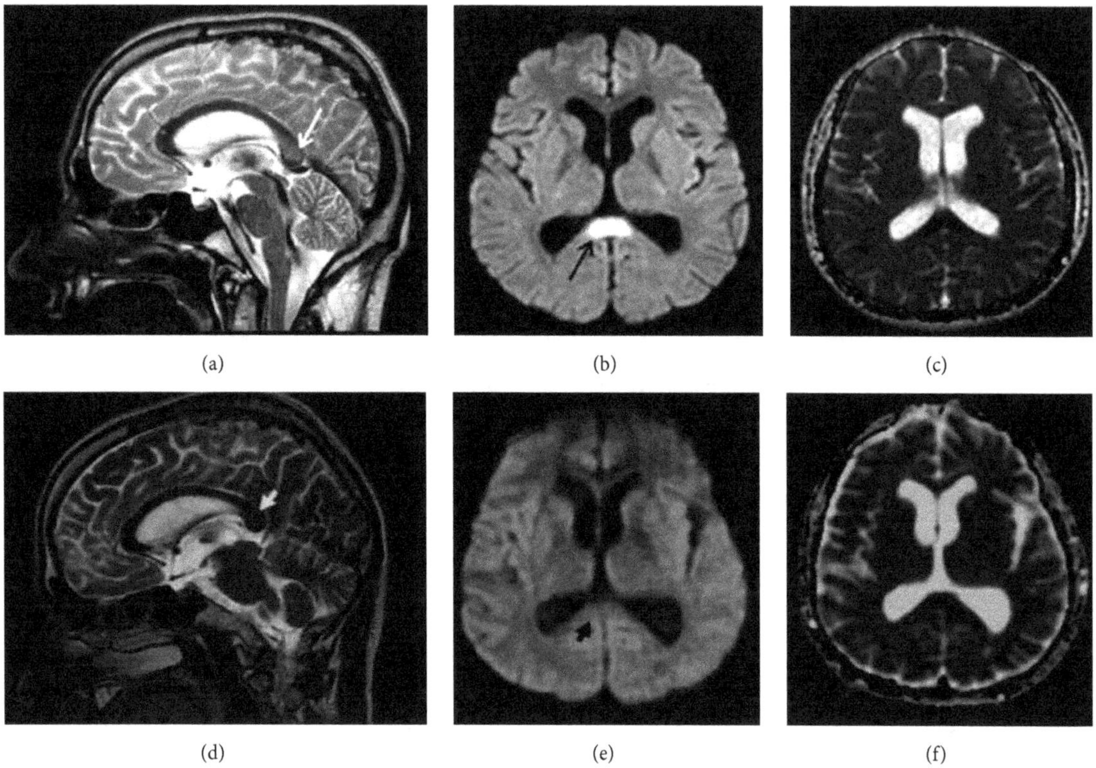

FIGURE 1: MRI studies at onset (a-c) and 1-month follow-up (d-f). Sagittal FSE-T2 image (a) demonstrating hyperintense regions in the splenium of the corpus callosum (*white arrow*). DWI (b) image shows its hyperintense signal (*black arrow*) and ADC map (c) shows its reduced diffusivity. Corresponding sagittal FSE-T2 image (d) and DWI images (e) showing normal signal in the splenium of the corpus callosum (*white arrow head* and *black arrow head*, respectively) where the ADC map (f) shows normalization of water diffusivity.

an important role in its development, even though MBD has been occasionally diagnosed in nonalcoholic patients as well [3]. These cases might have been diagnosed as a mild encephalitis/encephalopathy with a reversible splenial lesion, a recently described condition semiotically similar to MBD for the specific callosal localization, restricted water diffusivity, and reversibility at MRI [4].

Differential diagnosis includes other conditions which can present as splenial hyperintensity on T2/FLAIR like epilepsy, antiepileptic drug withdrawal, acute disseminated encephalomyelitis, infarction, viral and bacterial infections, especially influenza, HIV, and hypoglycaemia, other demyelinating diseases [5]. These conditions can be differentiated on the basis of clinical and laboratory analyses [6], such as occurred in the patient reported herein. Wernicke's encephalopathy was ruled out on the basis of clinical presentation and site of brain MRI lesion.

Despite several authors have postulated possible mechanism behind MBD, its pathophysiology still remains unclear. Nutritional deficiencies in newborns and in alcoholics and the use of some categories of drugs including benzodiazepines and antidepressants may be conditions predisposing the onset of the disease. Some authors believe to a genetic predisposition. Possible mechanisms include cytotoxic edema, blood-brain barrier breakdown, demyelination, and necrosis. Pathologically, MBD is characterized by symmetrical demyelination and necrosis of the central part of the corpus callosum, with relative sparing of thin upper and lower edges. Subsequently, necrosis leads to cavitation and atrophy of the corpus callosum in chronic stages [7]. Occasionally, similar lesions can involve other areas out of corpus callosum, such as anterior and posterior commissures, brachium pontis, optic chiasm, putamen, and frontal cortex [8, 9]. Few reports of partial damage to the corpus callosum and associated cortical lesions with good outcome are described.

Notably, a clinical and neuroradiological classification describes two subtypes of MBD.

(i) Type A is characterized by acute to subacute onset of altered state of level or state of consciousness, cognitive deterioration and language deficiencies (dysarthria, aphasia, etc.), hypertonia of the limbs, focal neurological deficits seizures, and pyramidal tract signs including hemiparesis or hemihypoesthesia, edema, and swelling of the entire corpus callosum at MRI, frequently with extracallosal lesions, resulting in an unfavourable and poorer prognosis.

(ii) Type B is characterized by an insidious clinical onset and progression, resulting in normal or slightly impaired level of consciousness, gait disturbance, dysarthria, signs of interhemispheric disconnection, high-signal intensity lesions on T2-weighted MR images partially involving the corpus callosum [10, 11], and less frequent extracallosal lesions associated with favorable prognosis including less severe and disabling clinical symptoms and less long-term disabilities.

Thus, diagnosis is made on the basis of clinical findings in combination with MRI features, such as that occurring in the patient reported herein. Therapy with thiamine and vitamine B complex, steroid, and antiepileptic is indicated [8]. A prompt therapy likely breaks the intramyelinic edema process and, subsequently, the disease progression [12, 13].

4. Conclusions

MBD diagnosis has been made possible as a result of recent advance in neuroimaging including DWI and ADC maps. Recognition of the neuroradiologic features is crucial in order to establish a proper diagnosis. Considering the complete reversibility of restricted diffusion in our patient, the lesion was probably the result of intramyelinic edema rather than cytotoxic edema or demyelination.

Acknowledgments

We thank the patient for providing his consent to process clinical data for publication. We also thank Raffaella Pastore (M.S.) for translating the manuscript.

References

[1] G. Pinter, K. Borbely, and L. Peter, "Marchiafava-Bignami disease (Case-report)," *Neuropsychopharmacol Hung International Journal*, vol. 18, no. 2, pp. 115–118, 2016.

[2] J. Marjama, M. T. Yoshino, and C. Reese, "Marchiafava-Bignami Disease," *Journal of Neurogenetics*, vol. 4, no. 2, pp. 106–109, 1994.

[3] M. Caulo, C. Briganti, F. Notturno et al., "Non-Alcoholic Partially Reversible Marchiafava-Bignami Disease: Review and Relation with Reversible Splenial Lesions," *The Neuroradiology Journal*, vol. 22, no. 1, pp. 35–40, 2009.

[4] J.-I. Takanashi, A. Imamura, F. Hayakawa, and H. Terada, "Differences in the time course of splenial and white matter lesions in clinically mild encephalitis/encephalopathy with a reversible splenial lesion (MERS)," *Journal of the Neurological Sciences*, vol. 292, no. 1-2, pp. 24–27, 2010.

[5] C. Kakkar, K. Prakashini, and A. Polnaya, "Acute Marchiafava-Bignami disease: Clinical and serial MRI correlation," *BMJ Case Reports*, 2014.

[6] P. Singh, D. Gogoi, S. Vyas, and N. Khandelwal, "Transient splenial lesion: Further experience with two cases," *Indian Journal of Radiology and Imaging*, vol. 20, no. 4, pp. 254–257, 2010.

[7] M. Victor, R. D. Adams, and G. H. Collins, "The Wernicke-Korsakoff Syndrome and related neurologic disorders due to alcoholism and malnutrition," *Journal of Neurology, Neurosurgery, and Psychiatry*, vol. 52, pp. 1217-1218, 1989.

[8] M. Hillbom, P. Saloheimo, S. Fujioka, Z. K. Wszolek, S. Juvela, and M. A. Leone, "Diagnosis and management of Marchiafava-Bignami disease: A review of CT/MRI confirmed cases," *Journal of Neurology, Neurosurgery & Psychiatry*, vol. 85, no. 2, pp. 168–173, 2014.

[9] C. G. Kohler, B. M. Ances, A. R. Coleman, J. D. Ragland, M. Lazarev, and R. C. Gur, "Marchiafava-Bignami disease: Literature review and case report," *Cognitive and behavioral neurology*, vol. 13, no. 1, pp. 67–76, 2000.

[10] A. Heinrich, U. Runge, and A. V. Khaw, "Clinicoradiologic subtypes, of Marchiafava-Bignami disease," *Journal of Neurology*, vol. 251, no. 9, pp. 1050–1059, 2004.

[11] P. E. M. Carrilho, M. B. M. Dos Santos, L. Piasecki, and A. C. Jorge, "Marchiafava-Bignami disease: A rare entity with a poor outcome," *Revista Brasileira de Terapia Intensiva*, vol. 25, no. 1, pp. 68–72, 2013.

[12] J. Ruiz-Martinez, A. Martinez Perez-Balsa, M. Ruibal, M. Urtasun, J. Villanua, and J. F. Marti Masso, "Marchiafava-Bignami disease with widespread extracallosal lesions and favourable course," *Neuroradiology*, vol. 41, no. 1, pp. 40–43, 1999.

[13] S. Bano, S. Mehra, S. N. Yadav, and V. Chaudhary, "Marchiafava-Bignami disease: Role of neuroimaging in the diagnosis and management of acute disease," *Neurology India*, vol. 57, no. 5, pp. 649–652, 2009.

4

Conversion Disorder: Early Diagnosis and Personalized Therapy Plan is the Key

Lauren Miller, Robert L. Archer, and Nidhi Kapoor

Department of Neurology, University of Arkansas for Medical Sciences, Little Rock, AR, USA

Correspondence should be addressed to Nidhi Kapoor; nkapoor@uams.edu

Academic Editor: Samuel T. Gontkovsky

Conversion disorder is characterized by one or more symptoms of altered voluntary motor or sensory functions that cannot be explained by a neurological disease (Keynejad, 2019; Samuels et al., 2019). We present a patient with conversion disorder and discuss her process in overcoming this disorder. Additionally, we review the literature about this specific disorder. A 15-year-old white female was diagnosed with conversion disorder and has shown significant recovery with physical therapy and group therapy since. It is essential to recognize this disorder early to lessen the financial burden on families and to speed up the recovery process for these patients.

1. Introduction

Conversion disorder, formerly known as hysteria, can be defined as one or more symptoms of altered voluntary motor or sensory functions that cannot be explained by a neurological disease [1, 2]. Conversion disorder is usually seen in women and younger aged people, but rare before age 10 and often clinical based [3]. Often this disorder is caused by childhood trauma, a stressful event, physical and sexual abuse, and depression/anxiety [4].

2. Case Report

A 15-year-old white female presented with flu-like symptoms, progressed 2 days later to throwing up blood. She was sent to the Emergency Room where she was diagnosed with possible appendicitis and was discharged the next day. That weekend, she was still vomiting, unable to hold food down, and nauseated. The patient was admitted to Arkansas Children's Hospital (ACH) for 1–2 weeks where she received extensive workup including MRI, CT scan, gastrointestinal imaging, and a spinal tap, and all the results came back normal. She was also evaluated by an ophthalmologist and a cardiologist, and no organic etiology was found for her symptoms. She was discharged home with an unknown diagnosis and started on symptomatic medical management to help relieve some of the symptoms. Soon after discharged from ACH, her legs started getting weak, and it was discussed that she may be having some neurological disorders and would need to be evaluated further. Presenting with symptoms of throwing up, unable to keep food down, leg numbness, and a constant migraine, she was readmitted at ACH for another two weeks where even more extensive workup was done again, including CT and MRI scans of the brain. All results came back normal, and she was sent home without a true diagnosis and was treated for depression and anxiety.

She was referred to a neurologist at the University of Arkansas for Medical Sciences (UAMS) 2–3 weeks later where she was evaluated and admitted to the hospital for one day to treat migraine. With no evidence of any organic etiology found on the extensive workup and no sign of relief with continued treatment, she was diagnosed with conversion disorder. She was discharged to receive physical therapy (3x a week) and cognitive behavioral therapy (1x a week) and also seen by a therapist. The therapist uncovered that from the age of 6–12 years, the patient experienced two active addicted parents, and she received physical and mental abuse from her father. During that time, she was required to become the head of the household to ensure bills were being paid and that her parents were being taken care of. At the age of 12, her mom received de-addiction treatment for 3–4 months and has been clean and sober for the past 5 years. Between the ages of 12 and 13, her parents got divorced, and she moved with her mom. She attended high school for one year but then transferred to another city. Growing up in an environment where she was in a constant fight-or-flight mode, she found a sense of security at this new city and was able to relax. The February of her sophomore year, she started gradually showing signs of weakness on the right side, seizures (nonepileptic spells), tingling, and numbness in her legs. Seven months later, she was referred and accepted into Mayo Clinic as outpatient for further management. At Mayo Clinic, she went to group therapy everyday from 8 am to 4 pm for 4 weeks with people who were experiencing other neurological disorders not just conversion disorder. During the group therapy at Mayo Clinic, she not only went through physical therapy and occupational therapy but also learned how to stay on a schedule, how to live a normal life with conversion disorder, and how to manage and tolerate the pain. She believes that the group therapy at Mayo helped her the best in her recovery.

The patient states that there were no real triggers that caused this disorder, but her history could have been an underlying cause. The patient is now still in recovery, all symptoms have improved but not completely gone away. The patient still experiences numbness and weakness on the right side, headaches, nausea, and pain in the right leg. She learned, at Mayo Clinic, how to tolerate and deal with the pain, which she believes helps her. The patient is currently on Topamax, iron, vitamin D3, and calcium. The patient plans to graduate high school this year and plans to attend college as premedical.

3. Discussion

3.1. Diagnosis. Conversion disorder is hard to diagnose due to symptoms being similar to other disorders. One key factor in identifying conversion disorder is its sudden onset of symptoms including nonepileptic seizure, weakness, and paralysis; abnormal movement; visual, speech, and sensory loss; or finally globus sensation [5]. Several tests can be done to ensure that the diagnosis of conversion disorder is correct [5]. Those tests include Hoover sign, fingertip test, signature test, menace reflect, tearing reflex, optokinetic test, cocontracting sign, and finally sternocleidomastoid test [5].

3.2. Misdiagnosis. Since there is little research on conversion disorder, it can often go misdiagnosed, which can lead to patients spending even more money for tests and treatment that might not relieve symptoms. Some common misdiagnoses are multiple sclerosis (MS), stroke or a spinal disorder, myasthenia gravis, movement disorder, epilepsy, laryngeal dystonia, factitious disorder, or malingering [6]. People with these disorders, when compared to people with conversion disorder, have different outcomes. For instance, a person with myasthenia gravis will show bulbar symptoms, diplopia, ptosis, and may have autoantibodies while a patient with conversion disorder will not have these symptoms instead they will have definite evidence of inconsistent movement without fatigue [6].

3.3. Prognosis. In patients with conversion disorder, early diagnosis often leads to good prognosis and is crucial to having a successful outcome. Once a physician confirms that a patient's symptoms do not conform anatomically and are atypical or do not correlate with physical examination or neurological finding, they should immediately be referred to a psychiatrist or psychologist for further assessment including an assessment regarding psychiatric comorbidities [7]. Furthermore, the patient should be given a treatment plan designed personally for them based on their symptoms and prognosis of the disorder [7].

3.4. Treatment. When presenting a treatment plan to someone with conversion disorder, four levels can make the process easier. First is to educate the patient; provide a diagnosis, discuss why you made that decision, and emphasize that the patient does not have a neurological disease [8]. Secondly, a physician needs to focus on what type of therapy would be best in relieving their symptoms [8]. Some of the most common therapies seen to help people with conversion disorder are physical therapy, group therapy, or family therapy, or even in some cases, a placebo effect was seen useful [8]. Thirdly, if standard therapy still does not relieve symptoms, they can be treated with psychotherapies, which include pharmacotherapy, psychodynamic psychotherapy, hypnosis, and so forth [8]. Lastly, when all other resources have been exerted, you can treat a patient with transcranial magnetic stimulation (TMS), sedation, and biofeedback [8].

4. Conclusion

Conversion disorder is more common than people think, but due to lack of research and knowledge of how to properly diagnose a patient, it oftentimes gets misdiagnosed. This disorder is debilitating to the patient and can be extremely costly if not diagnosed early. Therefore, prompt recognition and treatment stand to help significantly reduce patient morbidity and the health care cost.

References

[1] R. C. Keynejad, T. Frodl, R. Kanaan, C. Pariante, M. Reuber, and T. R. Nicholson, "Stress and functional neurological disorders: mechanistic insights," *Journal of Neurology, Neurosurgery & Psychiatry*, vol. 90, no. 7, pp. 813–821, 2019.

[2] A. Samuels, T. Tuvia, D. Patterson, O. Briklin, S. Shaffer, and A. Walker, "Characteristics of conversion disorder in an urban academic children's medical center," *Clinical Pediatrics*, vol. 58, no. 11-12, pp. 1250–1254, 2019.

[3] J. F. Stone and M. Sharpe, "Conversion disorder in adults: epidemiology, pathogenesis, and prognosis," 2017, https://www-uptodate-com.libproxy.uams.edu/contents/conversion-disorder-in-adults-epidemiology-pathogenesis-and-prognosis?

search=conversion%20disorder&source=search_result&selectedTitle=4~54&usage_type=default&display_rank=4.
[4] Mayo Clinic, Functional neurologic disorders/conversion disorder, https://www.mayoclinic.org/diseases-conditions/conversion-disorder/symptoms-causes/syc-20355197.
[5] J. Stone and M. Sharpe, *Conversion Disorder in Adults: Clinical Features, Assessment, and Comorbidity*, UpToDate, Waltham, MA, USA, 2018, https://www.uptodate.com/contents/conversion-disorder-in-adults-clinical-features-assessment-and-comorbidity#H13157790.
[6] J. Stone, PhD. FRCP, M. Sharpe, and M. D., *Conversion Disorder in Adults: Terminology, Diagnosis, and Differential Diagnosis*, UpToDate, Waltham, MA, USA, 2019, https://www.uptodate.com/contents/conversion-disorder-in-adults-terminology-diagnosis-and-differential-diagnosis?sectionName=Neurologic%20and%20general%20medical%20disorders&topicRef=85765&anchor=H2516698&source=see_link#H2516698.
[7] Consultant360, "Sudden vision loss: a case report and overview of conversion disorder," *Consultant360*, vol. 54, no. 8, 2014, https://www.consultant360.com/articles/sudden-vision-loss-case-report-and-overview-conversion-disorder.
[8] J. Stone and M. Sharpe, *Conversion Disorder in Adults: Treatment*, UpToDate, Waltham, MA, USA, 2018, https://www.uptodate.com/contents/conversion-disorder-in-adults-treatment?sectionName=Presenting%20the%20diagnosis&topicRef=85765&anchor=H1634982&source=see_link#H1634982.

5

Targeted Transforaminal Epidural Blood Patch for Postdural Puncture Headache in Patients with Postlaminectomy Syndrome

Yu Na Choi,[1] Sang Ji Kang,[2] Jin Deok Joo,[2] Yu Mi Kim,[2] Jang Hyeok In,[2] and Yoo Jung Park[2]

[1]*Department of Anesthesiology and Pain Medicine, Bucheon ST. Mary's Hospital, College of Medicine, The Catholic University of Korea, Bucheon 14647, Republic of Korea*
[2]*Department of Anesthesiology and Pain Medicine, Saint Vincent's Hospital, College of Medicine, The Catholic University of Korea, Suwon 16247, Republic of Korea*

Correspondence should be addressed to Yoo Jung Park; pyj@catholic.ac.kr

Academic Editor: Shahid Nimjee

Postdural puncture headache is a leak of cerebrospinal fluid that lowers intracranial pressure and usually presents as a positional headache. If conservative treatments are not successful, the epidural blood patch is the gold standard of the treatment for dural puncture. The interlaminar approach is the most commonly used technique for an epidural blood patch. This case report describes a patient who was treated with a transforaminal epidural blood patch for postdural puncture headache following an acupuncture procedure on his lower back after two epidural blood patches using an interlaminar approach had failed. The patient underwent an acupuncture therapy for management of chronic low back pain due to postlaminectomy syndrome. After the procedure, the patient had a severe headache and the conservative treatment was not effective. The two interlaminar epidural blood patches at the L2–3 level and at the L3–4 level were failed. We performed transforaminal epidural blood patch at the L3–4 and L4–5 levels on the left side, the site of leakage in the MRI myelogram. His symptoms finally subsided without complication. This case demonstrates that targeted transforaminal epidural blood patch is a therapeutic option for the treatment of postdural puncture headache when epidural blood patch using an interlaminar approach is ineffective.

1. Introduction

Postdural puncture headache (PDPH) is caused by reduced cerebrospinal fluid (CSF) pressure due to the loss of CSF from the epidural space through the dural puncture [1]. Typically, the postural headache worsens with sitting or standing and improves with lying down [2]. The headache can be accompanied by neck stiffness, tinnitus, and nausea and vomiting [3]. Risk factors include female sex, young age, pregnancy, repeated puncture, and low body mass index. Needle size, design, and the technique used also affect the risk [2].

Acupuncture, which is used to treat acute or chronic pain, can also cause PDPH. The depth of insertion of the acupuncture needle varies from a few millimeters to several centimeters, and the insertion direction varies from perpendicular to angled. Therefore, the tip of the needle can be placed in muscles or overlie other structures, such as nerves and the pleura [4].

Conservative therapies such as bed rest, hydration, caffeine, and acetaminophen are commonly used to treat PDPH. If conservative care is ineffective, an epidural blood patch (EBP) is often used. Traditionally, the interlaminar approach is the most common technique used for an EBP.

Here, we describe a patient who was treated with a transforaminal EBP for PDPH following an acupuncture procedure on his lower back after two EBPs using an interlaminar approach had failed.

2. Case

A 27-year-old man was referred to our pain clinic with an 8-day history of postural headache. He had undergone L4–5 laminectomy 7 years earlier to treat a herniated nucleus pulposus at the L4–5 level. He underwent acupuncture therapy 9 days before presenting to our clinic to manage chronic lower back pain caused by postlaminectomy syndrome. The acupuncture treatment involved the insertion of a needle 10 cm long from the center and laterally. After the procedure, the patient had a severe headache, which had a numeric rating scale of 7 to 9 out of 10. He felt pain upon sitting, together with fullness of the ears and neck stiffness. On assuming a supine position, his symptoms resolved within 5 min. The physical and neurological examinations were normal. He was diagnosed with PDPH and placed on bed rest. In the clinic, an EBP was performed via an interlaminar approach at the L2–3 level. However, his symptoms did not improve. Consequently, he was referred to our hospital.

In our clinic, under fluoroscopic guidance, we performed an interlaminar EBP using an 18-guage Tuohy needle (Tae-Chang Industrial, Seoul, Republic of Korea) at the L2–3 level. After successful loss of resistance, 15 mL sterile autologous blood was injected at the L2–3 level in the midline without a catheter. However, this failed to relieve the patient's symptoms, which still occurred within 5 min of standing or sitting up. The patient continued conservative care, including bed rest, hydration, and taking acetaminophen. Brain magnetic resonance imaging (MRI) looking for the site of CSF leakage was unremarkable, while a MRI myelogram showed an abnormal fluid signal intensity in the left lumbar area, along the left paraspinal muscle and soft tissues at the L3–4–5 level, probably due to CSF leakage. Because of the persistent symptoms, a repeat fluoroscopically guided interlaminar EBP was performed 4 days after the initial procedure using 15 mL autologous blood at the L4–5 level. The day after this procedure, the patient reported slight symptom relief but again experienced the same severe headache, posterior neck tenderness, and fullness of the ears after standing for 15 min. The conservative care was continued.

The patient's postural headaches persisted for 4 days, so we decided to perform a transforaminal EBP at the L3–4 and 4–5 levels on the left side, the site of leakage in the MRI myelogram (Figure 1). Under fluoroscopic guidance, a 22-gauge needle (Hakko, Japan) was inserted with a transforaminal approach and then contrast was injected at the left L3–4 and L4–5 levels (Figure 2). Then, after epidural spread was seen, 3 mL sterile autologous blood was injected into the transforaminal epidural space at each level. During injection, the patient's vital signs were monitored and the injection was stopped when the patient began to feel pressure in his lower back, but no pain or paresthesias were reported.

After the transforaminal EBP, his headache and other symptoms finally subsided without complications. The patient was symptom-free the next morning. After 4 days, the patient was discharged. At the 2-week follow-up, he reported being headache-free and his activities had returned to normal.

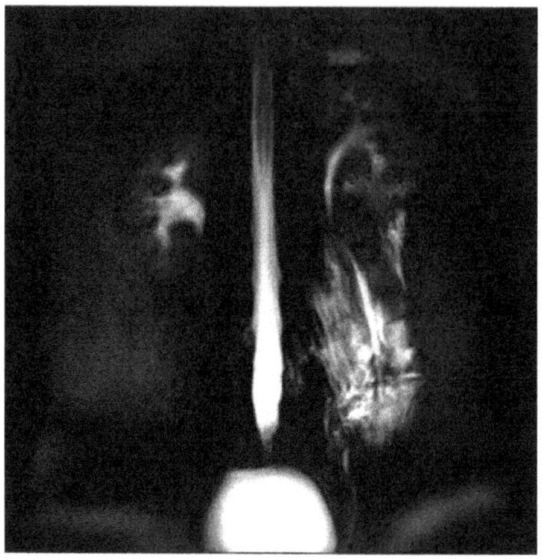

FIGURE 1: The MRI myelogram shows an abnormal fluid signal intensity in the left lumbar area, along the left paraspinal muscle and soft tissues at the L3–4–5 level, probably due to CSF leakage.

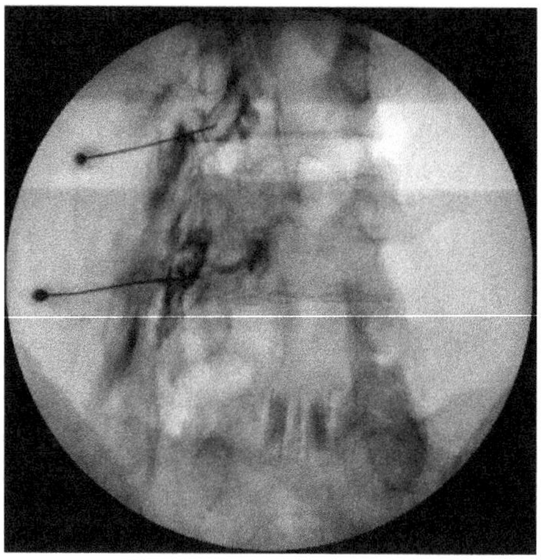

FIGURE 2: Fluoroscopic image of the epidural contrast injected through the left L3–4 and L4–5 foramens.

3. Discussion

August Bier first described spinal headache in 1898. One study found 10 cases in 453 patients who had 7,963 spinal injections. Although the exact mechanism of PDPH remains unknown, it might be caused by reduced CSF pressure due to the loss of CSF in the epidural space through the dural puncture site [1]. One possible cause of PDPH is that decreased CSF pressure leads to traction and tension across the pain-sensitive dural sinuses in the upright position [1, 5]. Therefore, the treatment is to seal the hole, which is how EBP works [6]. A second possible cause is vasodilation of the intracranial vessels. When the CSF pressure drops suddenly, the intracranial vessels vasodilate to maintain a constant intracranial volume [7]. Therefore, the use of a vasoconstrictor such as caffeine or theophylline is effective for treating PDPH. Both mechanisms likely have a role in the genesis of PDPH.

When PDPH occurs, several conservative treatments are commonly used, such as hydration, bed rest, and administration of acetaminophen or caffeine. For patients who do not respond to conservative treatment, EBP is the gold standard [5, 8]. The EBP is performed by injecting the patient's autologous blood into the epidural space around the site of suspected CSF leakage.

There are two theories about the mechanism by which EBP resolves PDPH. The "plug" theory for symptom resolution proposes that the injected autologous blood stops the loss of CSF by forming a clot over the defect in the meninges. In the absence of continued CSF loss, regeneration of CSF restores the CSF pressure and alleviates the PDPH [9]. The "pressure patch" theory posits that the injected blood or other fluid (crystalloid or colloid) elevates the subarachnoid CSF pressure by compressing the dura, which increases the pressure in the epidural space. According to this theory, PDPH is alleviated by reducing traction on pain-sensitive structures and decreasing vascular dilation. The relief of headache is not related to the hole in the dura, but persistent relief requires the elevated pressure to be maintained [9].

There is no consensus as to whether targeted or blind EBP is best. Although some studies have suggested that targeted EBP is more effective, targeted EBP in the cervical and thoracic regions has an increased risk for complications. Therefore, it is reasonable to try a blind approach first, followed by targeted EBP if the symptoms persist and the site of CSF leakage is identified [10].

Of the two approaches to the epidural space, an interlaminar approach is almost always used for the EBP [8, 11]. There are only a few reported cases using the transforaminal approach for EBP. In one report, transforaminal EBP was performed in a patient with a chronic headache secondary to spontaneous intracranial hypotension because it allowed the placement of blood at the exact site of the CSF leak when an interlaminar approach was impractical because of a previous laminectomy [12]. In another report, an 11-year-old boy underwent a transforaminal EBP to manage a refractory PDPH that was secondary to a ventral epidural CSF leak determined using radiological imaging. The PDPH resolved with the transforaminal EBP after three failures with an interlaminar EBP [13].

In our patient, fluoroscopically guided, blind interlaminar EBP at the L2–3 level failed. We hypothesized that the blind interlaminar EBP at the L2–3 level was likely ineffective because it failed to reach the site of the CSF leak. The targeted interlaminar EBP at the L4–5 level was also ineffective, possibly because the epidural blood did not spread due to adhesions caused by postoperative epidural fibrosis after the laminectomy. We believe that the targeted transforaminal EBP allowed us to inject blood directly at the site of the CSF leak seen on the MRI myelogram, while avoiding the epidural adhesions. We recommend the targeted transforaminal technique when the conventional interlaminar approach has failed or when a ventral or far-lateral CSF leak is identified with imaging studies.

4. Conclusion

The targeted interlaminar EBP in a patient who had laminectomy can be ineffective, possibly because the epidural blood did not spread due to adhesions caused by postoperative epidural fibrosis. This case demonstrates that targeted transforaminal EBP can be a therapeutic option for the treatment of PDPH in the patient with postlaminectomy syndrome when EBP using an interlaminar approach is ineffective. We suggest the targeted transforaminal technique when the conventional interlaminar approach has failed or when a ventral or far-lateral CSF leak is identified with imaging studies.

Disclosure

First author is Yu Na Choi. Coauthors are as follows: Sang Ji Kang, Jin Deok Joo, Yu Mi Kim, Jang Hyeok In. The English in this document has been checked by at least two professional editors, both native speakers of English. For a certificate, please see http://www.textcheck.com/certificate/NJWtDg.

References

[1] G. H. Morewood, "A rational approach to the cause, prevention and treatment of postdural puncture headache," *Canadian Medical Association Journal*, vol. 149, no. 8, pp. 1087–1093, 1993.

[2] R. R. Gaiser, "Postdural puncture headache: an evidence-based approach," *Anesthesiology Clinics*, vol. 35, no. 1, pp. 157–167, 2017.

[3] Headache Classification Committee of the International Headache Society, "The international classification of headache disorders," in *Cephalalgia*, vol. 24, 1, pp. 9–160, 2nd edition, 2004.

[4] D.-J. Jo, B. J. Lee, J. K. Sung, and J.-W. Yi, "Development of postdural puncture headache following therapeutic acupuncture using a long acupuncture needle," *Journal of Korean Neurosurgical Society*, vol. 47, no. 2, pp. 140–142, 2010.

[5] K. S. Olsen, "Epidural blood patch in the treatment of post-lumbar puncture headache," *PAIN*, vol. 30, no. 3, pp. 293–301, 1987.

[6] R. E. Willburger, H. Knorth, and R. Haaker, "Side effects and complications of injection therapy for degenerative spinal disorders," *Zeitschrift für Orthopädie und ihre Grenzgebiete*, vol. 143, no. 2, pp. 170–174, 2005.

[7] K.-H. Kwak, "Postdural puncture headache," *Korean Journal of Anesthesiology*, vol. 70, no. 2, pp. 136–143, 2017.

[8] G. Cooper, "Epidural blood patch," *European Journal of Anaesthesiology*, vol. 16, no. 4, pp. 211–215, 1999.

[9] B. Grant, B. Condon, I. Hart, and G. M. Teasdale, "Changes in intracranial CSF volume after lumbar puncture and their relationship to post-LP headache," *Journal of Neurology, Neurosurgery & Psychiatry*, vol. 54, no. 5, pp. 440–442, 1991.

[10] B. E. Harrington, "Postdural puncture headache and the development of the epidural blood patch," *Regional Anesthesia and Pain Medicine*, vol. 29, no. 2, pp. 136–163, 2004.

[11] P. J. Duffy and E. T. Crosby, "The epidural blood patch. Resolving the controversies," *Canadian Journal of Anesthesia*, vol. 46, no. 9, pp. 878–886, 1999.

[12] K. A. Smith, "Spontaneous intracranial hypotension: Targeted or blind blood patch," *Journal of Clinical Neuroscience*, vol. 25, pp. 10–12, 2016.

6

Paraplegia after Hypotension with Pneumothorax Episode during Thoracic Spine Tumor Surgery

Zhao-Quan Liu,[1] **Jen-Hsien Liao**,[2] **and Chih-Ju Chang**[1,3,4]

[1]*Department of Neurosurgery, Cathay General Hospital, Taipei City, Taiwan*
[2]*Department of Anesthesiology, Cathay General Hospital, Taipei City, Taiwan*
[3]*Department of Medicine, School of Medicine, Fu Jen Catholic University, New Taipei City, Taiwan*
[4]*Department of Mechanical Engineering, National Central University, Taoyuan City, Taiwan*

Correspondence should be addressed to Chih-Ju Chang; miklechang5639@gmail.com

Academic Editor: Dominic B. Fee

Paraplegia after spine surgery is a catastrophic complication. Here, we present a patient who, following laminectomy and fusion for decompression of metastatic tumor, developed paraplegia. We tried to find out the possible reason for the paraplegia. Due to prolonged hypotension during operation and new onset of pneumothorax, we think that intraoperative prolonged hypotension leads to the spinal cord ischemia which may cause neurological deterioration of paraplegia. Maintaining hemodynamic stability during spinal surgery is very important.

1. Introduction

Paraplegia after spine surgery is a severe complication. Hypotension (highly suspected to be caused by pneumothorax)-induced paraplegia is an uncommon situation. Here, we present a patient who, following laminectomy and fusion for decompression of metastatic tumor, developed paraplegia. We tried to find out the possible reasons for the paraplegia immediately after the operation and discovered that the patient had new-onset pneumothorax. Be that as it may, prolonged hypotension had caused ischemia condition for the spinal cord which might induce paraplegia.

2. Case History

The patient is a 62-year-old male who has right lung cancer with multiple metastasis, cT4N2M1c, stage 4B (Figure 1), after radiotherapy and chemotherapy. During the treatment protocol period, he complained about severe neck pain, bilateral arm numbness, and radiation to the subscapular area. He also had left upper limb muscle weakness. His lower limb had normal muscle power and no urine incontinence problems. The following T-spine MRI showed pathologic fracture at the T2 vertebral body (Figure 2). The patient's symptoms were related to pathologic fracture which was caused by the T2 vertebral body and T2 left-side pedicle tumor invasion. Therefore, radiculopathy and bone pain were chief symptoms instead of myelopathy.

The patient received adequate laminectomy and fusion surgery on purpose of decompression and stability of thoracic spine in order to relieve symptoms. During the operation, the patients' vital signs were stable, there was no excess blood loss, and the intraoperation somatosensory evoked potential (SSEP) revealed no special changes. Unfortunately, after 2 hours of surgery, just as we had removed the laminae to get well decompression (Figure 3), put all of pedicle screws, and prepared to fix the pedicle screws, sudden-onset blood pressure drop from 110/80 to 75/50 occurred and heart rate elevated to 120 bpm. Large amount of fluid challenge (2200 ml, including colloid and crystalloid fluid) and inotropic agent of norepinephrine (4 mg in 500 cc 5% glucose run 20 ml/hr) were given until the end of operation. According to the anesthesia record sheets, the patient's saturation was around 95~99% during the shock

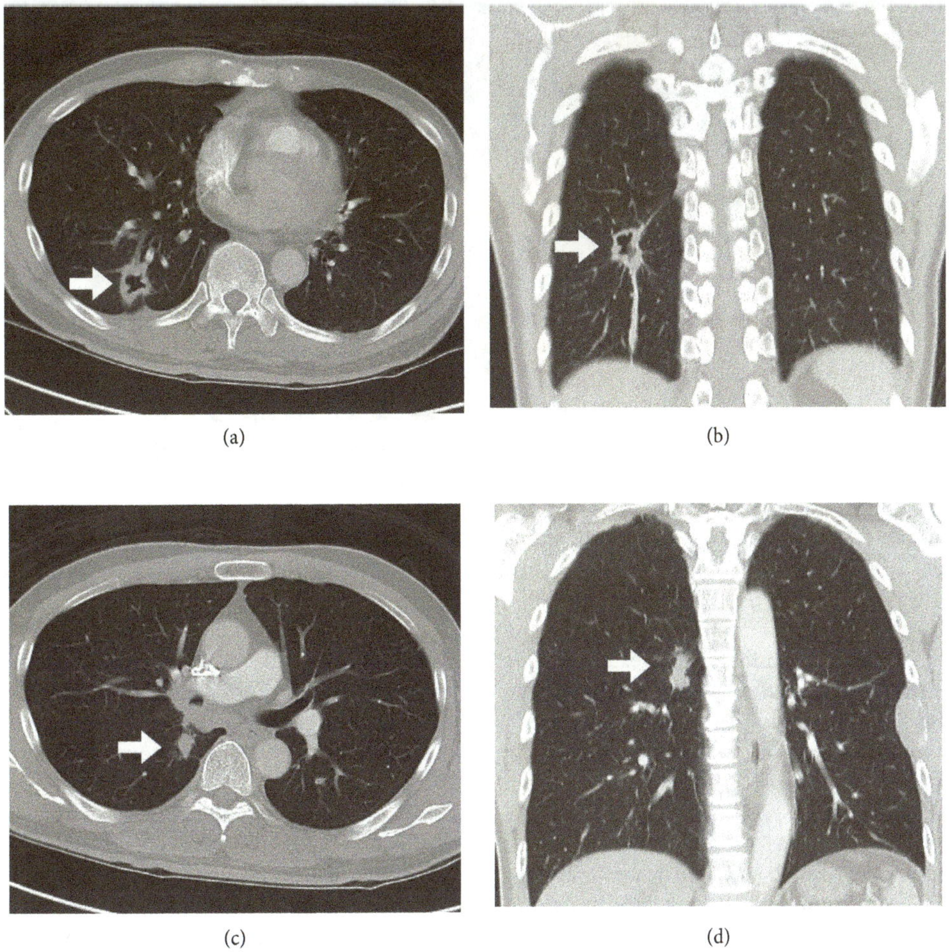

FIGURE 1: Low-dose lung CT demonstrated multiple right lung tumors (arrow).

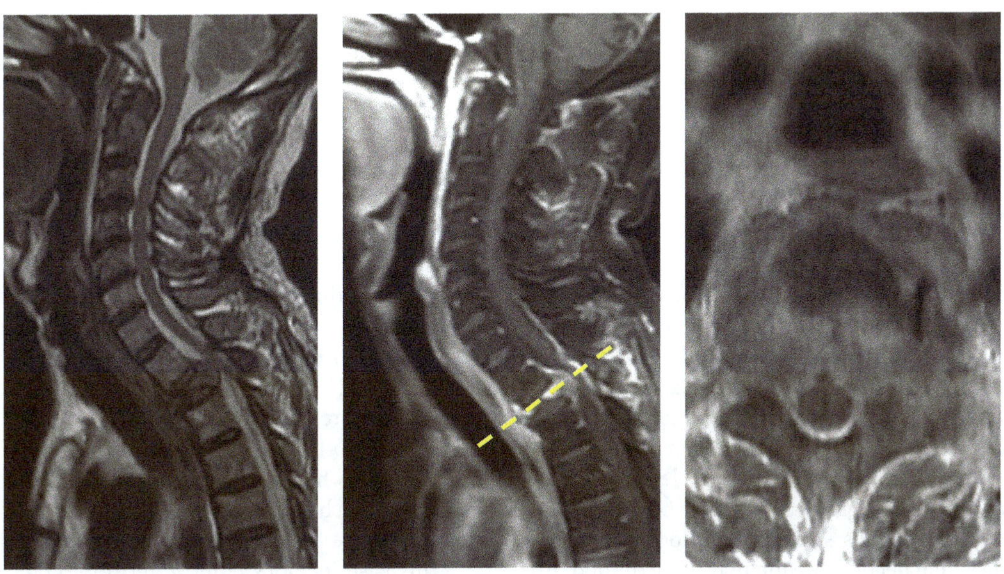

FIGURE 2: The patient presented spinal tumor at the T2 level with cord compression. (a) T2-weighted, (b) T1-weighted with a contrast sagittal view, and (c) T1-weighted with a contrast axial view.

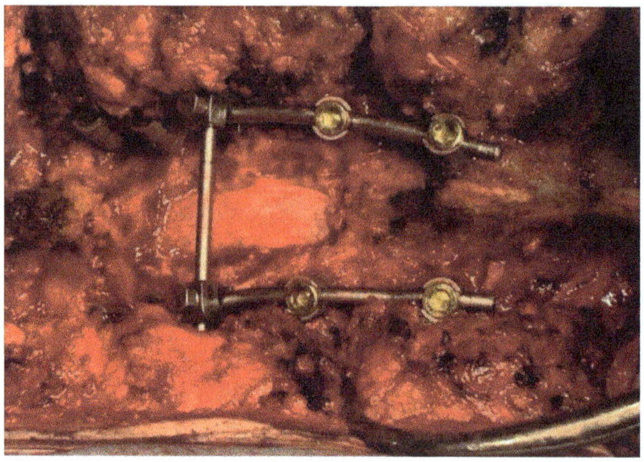

Figure 3: Intraoperative picture revealed the good decompression of the spinal cord.

condition. We completed the surgery as soon as possible. However, the shock status persisted for 1.5 hours in total even after surgery was completed. The estimated blood loss was about 250 ml, and total urine output was about 500 ml. The postoperation physical examination revealed muscle power score 0 at bilateral lower limbs. MRI would have been the best tool for assessing the epidural space and spinal cord condition. In our urgent condition, an immediate CT scan was performed instead to evaluate the condition, which showed all pedicle screws well positioned (Figure 4). The radiologist opined that there was no obvious compressive lesion around the spinal cord such as a hematoma or abscess between C1 and T9 but found right upper lung pneumothorax with obvious bullae (Figure 5). We then performed the needle thoracotomy at once; the following chest X-ray showed persistence of pneumothorax nevertheless.

When we wanted to arrange the further MRI examination, the patient's family hesitated and denied to receive the further examination or other aggressive treatment. The patient was managed with lower extremity physiotherapy and conservative treatment for terminal cancer; after 2 weeks of admission follow-up, however, no evidence of lower limbs' recovery was detected and the patient chose hospice management.

3. Discussion

Paraplegia is a catastrophic complication in spine surgery. There are various possible causes for paraplegia. However, the risk cannot be precisely quantified because of the lack of current data. In Delank et al.'s study [1], out of the 1194 patients surveyed, 7 (0.59%) experienced a postsurgical complete or incomplete paraplegia in scoliosis thoracic spine surgery [2].

Some studies report [3] that paraplegia may be caused by Adamkiewicz artery injury at the T3 to T6 level. Another possible cause of paraplegia was "white cord syndrome"(WCS) [4] which means sudden neurological deterioration following spinal decompression may be attributed to a reperfusion injury of the spinal cord. The spine cord edema extends to the cervical level or even the brain stem. Iatrogenic epidural hematoma-caused paraplegia also had been reported [5] as immediate postoperative period neurological deterioration. Furthermore, cord injury-caused paraplegia due to the pedicle screws malposition was also noted, especially at scoliosis patients [6].

Although the etiology of sudden-onset paraplegia remains obscure, the most important thing to prevent neurological deterioration such as paraplegia after posterior decompression surgery is to maintain the mean arterial pressure (MAP) during the spine surgery [7]. According to Kobrine et al.'s experimental study, spinal cord blood flow (SCBF) had autoregulation between MAP 50 to 135 mmHg. However, below 50 mmHg, further decreases in MAP effected corresponding decreases in the SCBF. The vessels were maximally dilated, vascular resistance was maximally reduced, and SCBF was a function of MAP [8].

In this respect, consensus [9] of preoperative optimization of volume status and aggressive maintenance of MAPs more than 110% of preoperative values in the procedure of spinal cord decompression were recommended in the surgical management of thoracic spine surgery.

The recommendation mentioned above contradicts the proper intraoperative MAP, as low blood pressure leads to spinal cord ischemia, whereas high pressure may cause excessive bleeding which could decrease the venous return [10] Therefore, the effective measures to prevent cord ischemia are to improve the surgical technique, shorten operation time, and pay more attention to hemostasis.

In hindsight, the blood supply of the thoracic spinal cord is much less collateralized than the cervical and lumbosacral regions, resulting in a greater risk of ischemia and infarction in conditions where blood flow is compromised [11]. The blood flow (I) is related to perfusion pressure (V) and resistance (R) ($I = V/R$). As tissue interstitial pressures secondary to pressure from the thoracic cavity (such as pneumothorax), spinal cord perfusion pressures decline. In an attempt to help mitigate the drop in blood flow, autoregulatory mechanisms result in a decrease in vascular resistance at the level of the penetrating arteriole.

This case includes clinical and radiological features related to hypotension-induced spinal cord ischemia change and paraplegia. We proposed the hypothesis that intraoperative hypotension might induce paraplegia and the pneumothorax could cause hypotension.

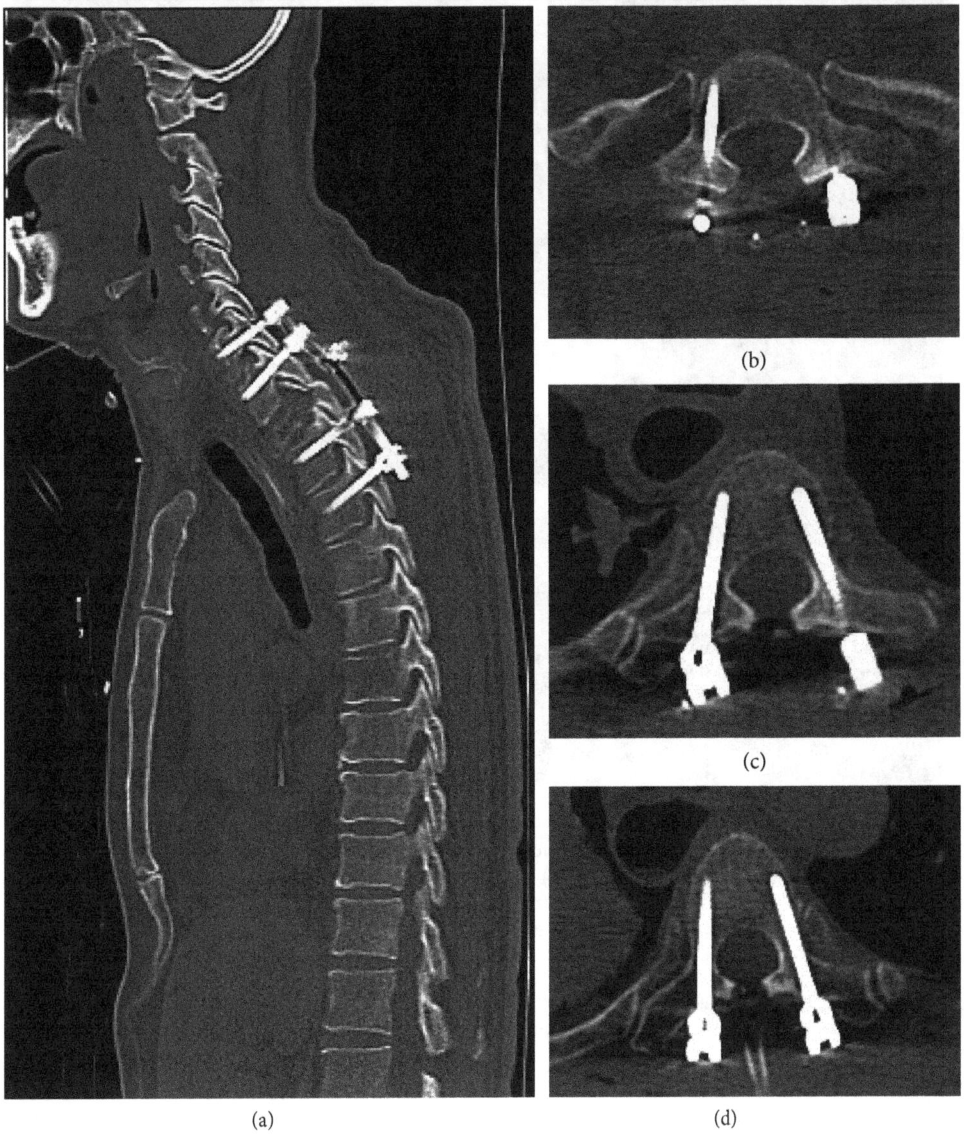

FIGURE 4: Postop immediate CT revealed all screws had good position: (a) sagittal view, (b) T1 level screws, (c) T3 screws, and (d) T4 screws.

The possible cause of pneumothorax during the procedure was tumor invaded to the pleura or pulmonary space. During the surgery by the posterior approach for decompression, the tension was released and pneumothorax was caused. The other possible reason may be primary lung lesion and prone position; both of them increased the aveolar positive end-expiratory pressure (PEEP) and induced pneumothorax. Intraoperative pneumothorax is a rare situation, but sometimes, it can potentially be life threatening [12]. The presence of emphysematous bullae or smaller blebs is a situation in which pneumothorax develops with positive pressure ventilation due to bullae or blebs rupture. On the other hand, an increase in central venous pressure can result in various situations such as distended neck veins and hypotension. Patients' clinical condition may have tachypnea, dyspnea, tachycardia, and hypoxia.

Moreover, some other reasons could cause unstable intraoperative hemodynamics including the impairment of spinal venous drainage, arterial thrombosis, inflammatory processes, or secondary injury processes. Inadvertent cord handling rarely causes the extension of edema more than two levels above the injured segment and should be evident in the immediate postoperative period.

Most of procedures were normal during the entire operation, except the unexplained shock condition. Also, after the operation, a newly occurring pneumothorax was found. We inferred that the patient's paraplegia is caused by shock which maybe induced by pneumothorax. In order to minimize the risk of paraplegia after thoracic spinal decompression, we strongly recommend that maintenance of hemodynamic stability and the carefulness about any possible reasons which may cause spinal cord ischemia. When the patient had hypotension status, pneumothorax may be the one of the possible reasons. Clinicians should be very careful of this devastating complication and include it during the informed consent-taking process preoperatively.

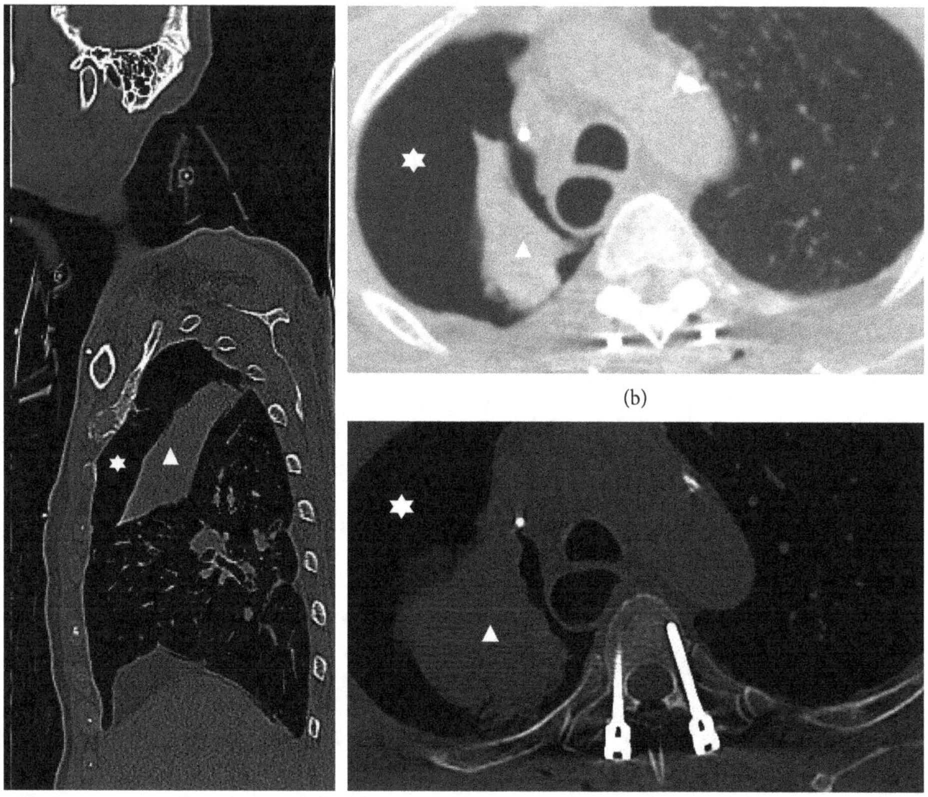

(a) (b) (c)

Figure 5: Postop immediate CT showed right apical lung pneumothorax (star) and consolidation at the right lung, leading to the radiologist's suspicion of tumor or collapsed lung (triangle): (a) sagittal view; (b) lung window.

References

[1] K. S. Delank, H. W. Delank, D. P. Konig, F. Popken, S. Furderer, and P. Eysel, "Iatrogenic paraplegia in spinal surgery," *Archives of Orthopaedic and Trauma Surgery*, vol. 125, no. 1, pp. 33–41, 2005.

[2] K. J. Noonan, T. Walker, J. R. Feinberg, M. Nagel, W. Didelot, and R. Lindseth, "Factors related to false- versus true-positive neuromonitoring changes in adolescent idiopathic scoliosis surgery," *Spine (Phila Pa 1976)*, vol. 27, pp. 825-830, 2002.

[3] J. L. Laratta, J. N. Shillingford, C. Saifi, and K. D. Riew, "Cervical disc arthroplasty: a comprehensive review of single-level, multilevel, and hybrid procedures," *Global Spine Journal*, vol. 8, no. 1, pp. 78–83, 2018.

[4] V. Vinodh, S. Rajapathy, P. Sellamuthu, and R. Kandasamy, "White cord syndrome: a devastating complication of spinal decompression surgery," *Surgical Neurology International*, vol. 9, no. 1, p. 136, 2018.

[5] I. Jusué-Torres, J. M. Ortega-Zufiria, M. Tamarit-Degenhardt et al., "Hematoma epidural cervical yatrogénico. Presentación de un caso clínico y revisión de la literatura," *Neurocirugía*, vol. 22, no. 4, pp. 332–336, 2011.

[6] J. M. Mac-Thiong, S. Parent, B. Poitras, J. Joncas, and L. Hubert, "Neurological outcome and management of pedicle screws misplaced totally within the spinal canal," *Spine (Phila Pa 1976)*, vol. 38, pp. 229–237, 2013.

[7] M. L. Marcus, D. D. Heistad, J. C. Ehrhardt, and F. M. Abboud, "Regulation of total and regional spinal cord blood flow," *Circulation Research*, vol. 41, no. 1, pp. 128–134, 1977.

[8] A. I. Kobrine, T. F. Doyle, and H. V. Rizzoli, "Spinal cord blood flow as affected by changes in systemic arterial blood pressure," *Journal of Neurosurgery*, vol. 44, no. 1, pp. 12–15, 1976.

[9] S. L. Zuckerman, J. A. Forbes, A. M. Mistry et al., "Electrophysiologic deterioration in surgery for thoracic disc herniation: impact of mean arterial pressures on surgical outcome," *European Spine Journal*, vol. 23, no. 11, pp. 2279–2290, 2014.

[10] H. Wang, L. Ma, R. Xue et al., "The incidence and risk factors of postoperative neurological deterioration after posterior decompression with or without instrumented fusion for thoracic myelopathy," *Medicine*, vol. 95, no. 49, Article ID e5519, 2016.

[11] N. L. Martirosyan, J. S. Feuerstein, N. Theodore, D. D. Cavalcanti, R. F. Spetzler, and M. C. Preul, "Blood supply and vascular reactivity of the spinal cord under normal and pathological conditions," *Journal of Neurosurgery: Spine*, vol. 15, no. 3, pp. 238–251, 2011.

[12] M. Heyba, A. Rashad, and A. A. Al-Fadhli, "Detection and management of intraoperative pneumothorax during laparoscopic cholecystectomy," *Case Reports in Anesthesiology*, vol. 2020, Article ID 9273903, 7 pages, 2020.

7

Bilateral Femoral Neuropathy: A Rare Complication of Drug Overdose due to Prolonged Posturing in Lithotomy Position

D. Tsiptsios,[1] D. Daud,[2] K. Tsamakis,[3] E. Rizos,[3] A. Anastadiadis,[4] and A. Cassidy[2]

[1]*Neurophysiology Department, Sunderland Royal Hospital, South Tyneside & Sunderland NHS Foundation Trust, Sunderland, UK*
[2]*Neurology Department, Sunderland Royal Hospital, South Tyneside & Sunderland NHS Foundation Trust, Sunderland, UK*
[3]*Second Department of Psychiatry, University General Hospital "Attikon", School of Medicine, Athens, Greece*
[4]*First Department of Urology, Aristotle University of Thessaloniki, School of Medicine, Thessaloniki, Greece*

Correspondence should be addressed to D. Tsiptsios; tsiptsios.dimitrios@yahoo.gr

Academic Editor: Norman S. Litofsky

Background. Bilateral femoral neuropathy is an uncommon complication of various surgical and nonsurgical procedures, such as pelvic/abdominal surgery or vaginal delivery. *Case Report.* We report a case of a 41-year-old male who was found unresponsive against the wall in a "lithotomy-type" position with both knees flexed at approximately 90 degrees and both hips flexed and externally rotated at approximately 90 and 60 degrees, respectively, 24–48 hours after a drug overdose (combination of dihydrocodeine, paracetamol, diazepam, and amitriptyline). During his recovery, he complained of severe bilateral proximal lower limb weakness and bilateral distal lower limb pain and allodynia. His symptoms were initially attributed to critical illness myopathy/neuropathy (CIMN). However, thorough clinical and neurophysiological evaluation revealed that his symptoms were due to severe bilateral femoral neuropathies. *Conclusions.* To our knowledge, this is the first reported case of bilateral femoral nerve palsy due to prolonged posturing in a "lithotomy-type" position in the context of a drug overdose.

1. Introduction

Bilateral femoral neuropathy is an uncommon complication of various surgical and nonsurgical procedures, such as pelvic/abdominal surgery or vaginal delivery, but rarely encountered in other scenarios or circumstances.

2. Case Presentation

We report the case of a 41-year-old male who was referred to our Neurophysiological Department with a suspected diagnosis of critical illness myopathy/neuropathy (CIMN) after he exhibited marked bilateral quadriceps muscle wasting with distal lower limb pain and allodynia following his recovery from coma due to a drug overdose.

Prominent fibrillations and positive sharp waves were EMGraphically recorded from the vastus medialis and vastus lateralis muscles bilaterally. Moreover, no motor unit action potentials (MUAPs) could be recruited from the aforementioned muscles. In the Intensive Care Unit (ICU) setting, such findings are usually encountered in cases of very severe critical illness myopathy.

However, tibial and peroneal motor nerve conduction studies and sural and superficial peroneal sensory nerve conduction studies were within normal limits bilaterally (Table 1). These findings were not suggestive of a large fibre peripheral neuropathy and led to a review of the clinical diagnosis of CIMN, and additional neurophysiological testing was undertaken. The findings on clinical examination were also hard to reconcile with a diagnosis of CIMN as, while the quadriceps muscles were severely wasted bilaterally, all other muscles including iliopsoas and hip adductors exhibited 5/5 motor strength. Moreover, the sensory loss was focal, with numbness and hypoesthesia over the anteromedial thighs and medial lower legs bilaterally. In addition, while the knee jerks were absent, the ankle jerks were present bilaterally.

Table 1: Neurophysiological findings.

Sensory nerve conduction studies							
Nerve and site	Onset latency	Peak latency	Amplitude	Segment	Latency difference	Distance	Conduction velocity
Peroneal R							
Ankle	2.0 ms	2.6 ms	15 μV	Dorsum of foot-ankle	2.0 ms	100 mm	49 m/s
Peroneal L							
Ankle	2.1 ms	2.9 ms	12 μV	Dorsum of foot-ankle	2.1 ms	95 mm	45 m/s
Sural R							
Lower leg	1.7 ms	2.6 ms	12 μV	Ankle-lower leg	1.7 ms	95 mm	55 m/s
Sural L							
Lower leg	1.7 ms	2.6 ms	12 μV	Ankle-lower leg	1.7 ms	95 mm	55 m/s
Saphenous R							
		No recording		Lower leg-ankle			
Saphenous L							
		No recording		Lower leg-ankle			

Motor nerve conduction studies							
Nerve and site	Latency	Amplitude	Segment	Latency difference	Distance	Conduction velocity	F-latency
Peroneal R							
Ankle	5.9 ms	2.7 mV	Extensor digitorum brevis-ankle	5.9 ms	mm	m/s	
Fibula (head)	13.0 ms	1.9 mV	Ankle-fibula (head)	7.1 ms	320 mm	45 m/s	
Tibial R							
Ankle	4.1 ms	20.0 mV	Abductor hallucis-ankle	4.1 ms	mm	m/s	53.9 msec
Tibial L							
Ankle	3.9 ms	20.7 mV	Abductor hallucis-ankle	3.9 ms	mm	m/s	53.3 msec

Electromyography							
	Spontaneous activity		MUAPs			Activation	Recruitment
	Fibrillations	PSWs	Amplitude	Duration	Phases		
Right vastus lateralis	+3	+3		No MUAPs could be recruited			
Right vastus medialis	+3	+3		No MUAPs could be recruited			
Left vastus lateralis	+3	+3		No MUAPs could be recruited			
Left vastus medialis	+3	+3		No MUAPs could be recruited			
Right iliopsoas	0	0	N	N	N	N	N
Left iliopsoas	0	0	N	N	N	N	N
Right adductor longus	0	0	N	N	N	N	N
Left adductor longus	0	0	N	N	N	N	N

PSWs, positive sharp waves; MUAPs, motor unit action potentials; N, normal.

Additional neurophysiological testing revealed that saphenous sensory nerve action potentials were absent bilaterally. Otherwise, EMG findings from iliopsoas and adductor longus muscles were unremarkable bilaterally (Table 1).

Thus, the clinical and neurophysiological findings were consistent with severe bilateral femoral neuropathies at the level of the inguinal region. It has to be stated that, while prominent abnormal spontaneous activity and unrecordable MUAPs from both quadriceps muscles are potentially suggestive of a severe underlying critical illness myopathy, it is important to realise that such EMGraphic findings can be seen in cases of severe underlying neuropathies, as in our case.

Due to the fact that a pelvic CT scan was unremarkable, with no evidence of an underlying hematoma or iliopsoas muscle swelling, and creatine phosphokinase value was within normal limits, thus excluding rhabdomyolysis and crush syndrome that could explain the patient's symptoms, his clinical history was reviewed. Interestingly, his mother had found him unresponsive 24–48 hours after a drug overdose (according to paramedics, empty packets of dihydrocodeine, paracetamol, diazepam, and amitriptyline were found around him) against the wall in a "lithotomy-type" position with both knees flexed at approximately 90 degrees and both hips flexed and externally rotated at approximately 90 and 60 degrees, respectively. This prolonged posturing seems to have resulted in severe bilateral femoral nerve palsies due to excessive nerve stretching and/or pressure under the inguinal ligament.

3. Discussion

Unilateral femoral neuropathy is an uncommon mononeuropathy and is usually caused by compression in the pelvis or inguinal region. Typical causes in the pelvis include compression by an iliacus or retroperitoneal hematoma, by a retractor blade during pelvic surgery, or by a pelvic mass. Typical causes in the inguinal region include compression by the inguinal ligament during the lithotomy position and by an inguinal hematoma or by other inguinal masses [1].

Bilateral simultaneous femoral neuropathy is even more uncommon. It is typically seen as a complication of either pelvic or abdominal surgery or vaginal delivery. In such instances, the proposed mechanisms of nerve injury are as follows:

(a) Stretching and/or prolonged compression of the nerve caused by the self-retaining retractors that can directly compress the nerve against the pelvic sidewall
(b) Compression of the iliac vessels causing direct ischemia of the nerve
(c) Prolonged compression of the femoral nerves under the inguinal ligament, or
(d) Excessive stretching due to excessive abduction and external rotation of the hips during lithotomy positioning [2–6]

In addition to the above iatrogenic causes, there are reports of rare cases of bilateral femoral nerve compression and ischemia due to iliopsoas hematomas [7–10] and iliopsoas swelling secondary to rhabdomyolysis [11, 12]. There are also individual reports of bilateral femoral neuropathy due to vasculitis in the context of disseminated intravascular coagulopathy [13] and due to blunt force trauma [14].

A single case of bilateral femoral neuropathy after drug overdose has also been reported [15]. On this occasion, a female had sat down on a chair with her legs stuck under a desk before then losing consciousness and falling backwards without any support for her head or arms. This prolonged hyperlordotic position resulted in a presumed stretch-induced ischemia of the nerve at the level of the iliopsoas groove.

Our case differs from the aforementioned in that our patient was found unresponsive in a different position, i.e., with both knees flexed at approximately 90 degrees and both hips flexed at approximately 90 degrees and externally rotated at approximately 60 degrees. Thus, to our knowledge, this is the first reported case of bilateral simultaneous femoral neuropathy due to prolonged posturing in a "lithotomy-type" position in the context of a drug overdose. The presumed mechanism of nerve injury is excessive nerve stretching and/or pressure under the inguinal ligament. More specifically, profound muscle relaxation due to lack of protective reflexes and muscle tone in the context of drug overdose might have resulted in excessive bilateral external hip rotation >45 degrees in a "lithotomy-type" position that also encompassed bilateral knee and hip flexion at approximately 90 degrees each. This position causes both femoral nerves to enter the thigh acutely angulated and twisted beneath the tough and inelastic inguinal ligament, leading to microvascular and/or local mechanical nerve injury. In case this position is kept for more than 4 hours, it may lead to permanent bilateral femoral nerve damage [6].

This case illustrates the importance of taking a thorough collateral history in those presenting with weakness following an admission to the ICU. A thorough neurological evaluation should always precede neurophysiological testing, as not all cases of acute or subacute lower limb weakness and sensory loss in this setting are due to CIMN. As we have described, rare neurological entities such as bilateral femoral neuropathies can also be encountered.

Acknowledgments

The author would like to thank the patient and the family.

References

[1] B. Katirji, "Compressive and entrapment neuropathies of the lower extremity," in *Neuromuscular Disorders in Clinical Practice*, H. Kaminksi and R. L. Ruff, Eds., pp. 933–937, Springer, Berlin, Germany, 2nd edition, 2014.
[2] V. Bono, V. La Bella, and R. Spataro, "Bilateral iatrogenic femoral neuropathy," *Journal of Clinical Neurology*, vol. 11, no. 4, pp. 398-399, 2015.
[3] J. A. Vanrell and J. Balasch, "Bilateral femoral neuropathy after microsurgical reversal of tubal sterilization: case report and analysis of contributing factors," *Human Reproduction*, vol. 2, no. 4, pp. 345–347, 1987.
[4] S.-P. Choi, B.-M. Oh, and W. Ahn, "Bilateral femoral neuropathy after vaginal delivery-a case report," *Korean Journal of Anesthesiology*, vol. 57, no. 2, pp. 228–232, 2009.
[5] M. A. Warner, D. O. Warner, C. M. Harper, D. R. Schroeder, and P. M. Maxson, "Lower extremity neuropathies associated with lithotomy positions," *Anesthesiology*, vol. 93, no. 4, pp. 938–942, 2000.
[6] L.-F. Hsieh, E.-S. Liaw, H.-Y. Cheng, and C.-Z. Hong, "Bilateral femoral neuropathy after vaginal hysterectomy," *Archives of Physical Medicine and Rehabilitation*, vol. 79, no. 8, pp. 1018–1021, 1998.
[7] P. Macauley, P. Soni, I. Akkad et al., "Bilateral femoral neuropathy following psoas muscle hematomas caused by enoxaparin therapy," *American Journal of Case Reports*, vol. 18, pp. 937–940, 2017.
[8] H. Podger and M. Kent, "Femoral nerve palsy associated with bilateral spontaneous iliopsoas haematomas: a complication of venous thromboembolism therapy," *Age and Ageing*, vol. 45, no. 1, pp. 175-176, 2016.
[9] S. Lamdhade, R. Dashti, A. Thussu, and R. Alroughani, "A young male presented with acute inguinal pain, bilateral quadriceps weakness and hyperesthesia of anterior thighs post-thrombolysis for acute myocardial infarction," *Annals of Saudi Medicine*, vol. 34, no. 3, pp. 265-266, 2014.
[10] X. Puéchal, F. Lioté, and D. Kuntz, "Bilateral femoral neuropathy caused by iliacus hematomas during anticoagulation after cardiac catheterization," *American Heart Journal*, vol. 123, no. 1, pp. 262-263, 1992.
[11] Y. Ng, H. Li, and C. Chan, "Bilateral femoral nerve compression and compartment syndrome resulting from influ-

enza A-induced rhabdomyolysis: a case report," *Journal of Orthopaedic Surgery*, vol. 16, no. 1, pp. 117–121, 2008.
[12] M. Nicolle, T. Doherty, and H. Algahtani, "Bilateral femoral neuropathy complicating rhabdomyolysis and acute renal failure," *Journal of Clinical Neuromuscular Disease*, vol. 6, no. 4, pp. 153–156, 2005.
[13] C. Y. Cheok, A. Merican, and W. M. Ng, "Bilateral femoral neuropathy associated with disseminated intravascular coagulopathy: a case report," *Medical Journal of Malaysia*, vol. 61, pp. 97–99, 2006.
[14] L. F. D'Amelio, D. J. Musser, and M. Rhodes, "Bilateral femoral nerve neuropathy following blunt trauma," *Journal of Neurosurgery*, vol. 73, no. 4, pp. 630–632, 1990.
[15] S. Mathis, F. d. Boisguéheneuc, G. Godenèche, S. Ansquer, and J.-P. Neau, "Bilateral femoral neuropathy after massive toxic ingestion in a suicide attempt," *The Neurologist*, vol. 18, no. 2, pp. 70–72, 2012.

8

A Case of Carbamazepine-Induced Aggravation of Self-Limited Epilepsy with Centrotemporal Spikes Epilepsy and Valproate-Induced Hyperammonemic Encephalopathy in a Child with Heterozygous Gene Variant of Carbomoyl Phosphatase Synthetase Deficiency

Imalke Kankananarachchi[1], **Eresha Jasinge**[2] **and Gemunu Hewawitharana**[3]

[1]*Department of Paediatrics, Faculty of Medicine, University of Ruhuna, Matara, Sri Lanka*
[2]*Lady Ridgeway Hospital, Colombo, Sri Lanka*
[3]*Teaching Hospital Karapitiya, University of Ruhana, Matara, Sri Lanka*

Correspondence should be addressed to Imalke Kankananarachchi; imalke@med.ruh.ac.lk

Academic Editor: Isabella Laura Simone

Antiepileptics drugs are the mainstay of the management of epilepsy in children. Sodium valproate (VPA) and carbamazepine (CBZ) are widely used medications in childhood epilepsy. Hyperammonemia has been described as a known side effect of valproate therapy. It is known that VPA-associated HA is common among patients who hold genetic mutations of the carbomoyl phosphatase synthase 1 gene (CPS1). Aggravation of self-limited epilepsy with centrotemporal spikes (SLECTS) is a rare side effect of CBZ. Here, we present a child who had CBZ-induced aggravation of rolandic epilepsy and VPA-induced HA encephalopathy in the background of an unrecognised heterozygous gene variant of CPS1. An 8-year-old boy with SLECTS presented with a history of abnormal behaviours and drowsiness. He was apparently well until six years when he developed seizures in favour of rolandic epilepsy. His electroencephalogram (EEG) showed bilateral predominantly on the right-sided central-temporal spikes and waves. The diagnosis of SLECTS was made, and he was commenced on CBZ. Though he showed some improvement at the beginning, his seizure frequency increased when the dose of CBZ was increased. His repeat EEG showed electrical status in slow-wave sleep, and CBZ was stopped. Subsequently, he was started on VPA, and with that, he developed features of encephalopathy. He had elevated serum ammonia with normal liver functions. VPA was stopped with the suspicion of VPA-induced hyperammonemia. Tandem mass spectrometry did not show significant abnormality in the amino acid profile. Specific genetic analysis revealed a c.2756 C > T.p (Ser919Leu) heterozygote genetic mutation of the CSP 1 gene. This is a classic example where side effects of treatment determine the choice of antiepileptics drugs (AEDs) in childhood epilepsy. It is essential to keep in mind that SLECTS can be aggravated with certain AEDs, and VPA-induced HA in the absence of live failure could be due to underlying inherited metabolic disorders.

1. Introduction

AEDs are the mainstay of the management of epilepsy in children. However, in 15% of the time, AEDs are withheld due to their adverse effects [1]. Sodium valproate has a wide range of indications in childhood epilepsy. Moreover, it is being used as a mood stabiliser and antimigraine treatment [1]. Hyperammonemia (HA) has been described as a known side effect of valproate therapy even in the absence of underlying liver disease [2, 3]. It has been described that valproate-associated HA is more common among patients who hold genetic mutations of the CPS1 gene [4, 5]. Carbamazepine (CBZ) is a widely used drug in both partial and generalised epilepsy. Neurological side effects are seen in

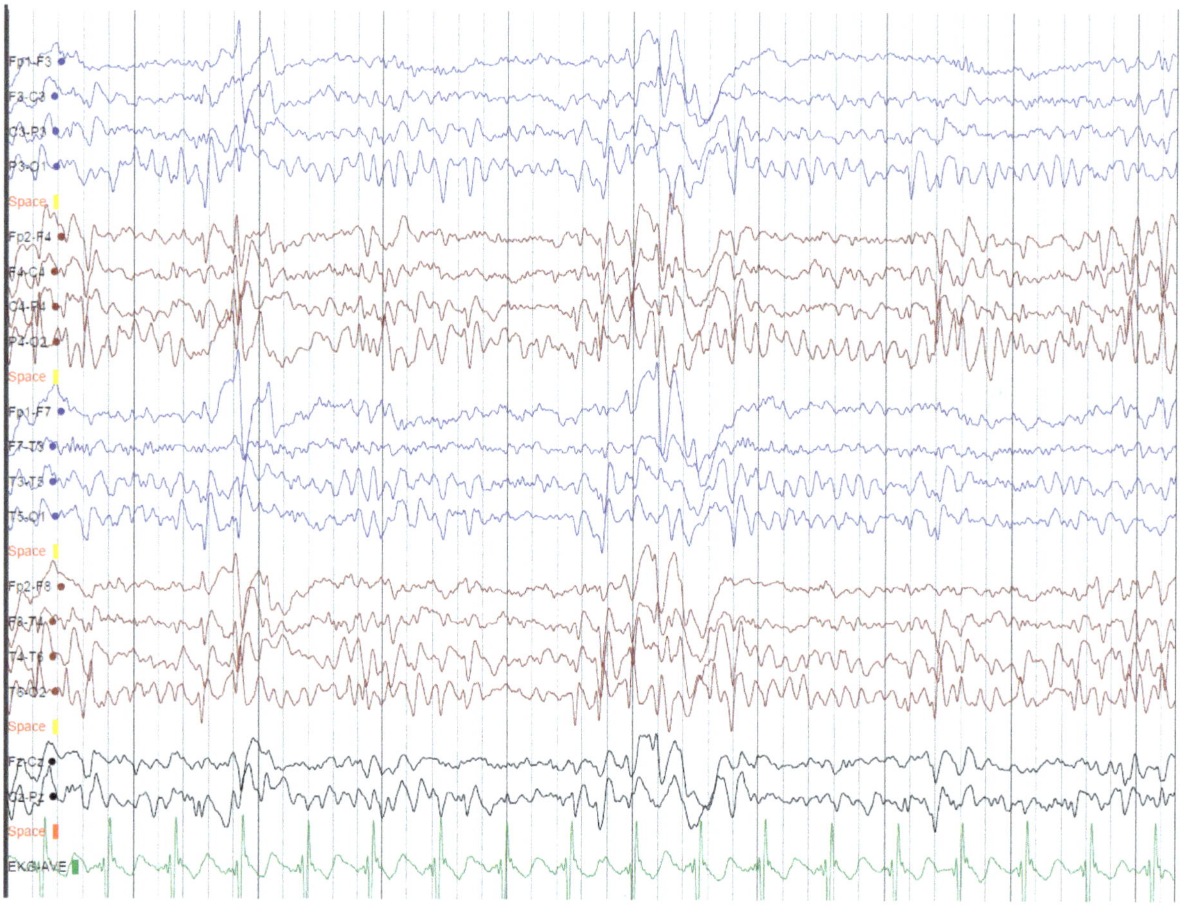

FIGURE 1: EEG showing predominant centrotemporal spikes and waves on the right side (voltage 70 mV/cm).

50% of patients receiving CBZ [6]. Aggravation of self-limited epilepsy with centrotemporal spikes (SLECTS) is a rare side effect of CBZ [7]. Here, we present a child who had carbamazepine-induced aggravation of rolandic epilepsy and valproate-induced hyperammonemic encephalopathy in the background of unrecognised heterozygous gene variant of carbomoyl phosphatase synthetase deficiency.

2. Case Presentation

An 8-year-old boy with self-limited epilepsy with centrotemporal spikes (SLECTS) was admitted to the paediatric ward for further evaluation of abnormal behaviours and drowsiness. He was the first child born to non-consanguineous healthy parents following an uneventful antenatal period. He was born at term via normal vaginal delivery with a birthweight of 3.1 kg. He did not require any resuscitation at birth. The child was well until six years of age when he developed seizures. The semiology of the seizures was predominantly focal motor hemifacial tonic-clonic movements with oropharyngo symptoms and associated with speech arrest and hypersalivation. Occasionally, he had bilateral tonic-clonic seizures as well.

His electroencephalogram (EEG) showed high voltage, diphasic spikes with slow activity predominantly on the right central-temporal region, creating a horizontal dipole with maximal electronegativity in the right centrotemporal region (Figure 1). The diagnosis of SLECTS was made based on the clinical and EEG features.

His brain MRI scan and basic biochemical tests were normal. Initially, the family was reassured about the prognosis of the condition, and the decision was taken to manage conservatively without starting AEDs. However, he continued to have at least one seizure fortnightly, and due to extreme parental concerns, he was commenced on CBZ 15 mg/kg/day. He had good seizure control for about one year after the commencement of CBZ. Subsequently, the CBZ dose was increased to 22 mg/kg/day since his seizure frequency increased. However, he had a poor response to CBZ where there was an increased seizure frequency to 1-2 seizures per week and behavioural changes such as violent and aggressive behaviour towards parents and peers. The repeat sleep EEG showed almost continuous spikes and wave activity suggestive of electrical status in slow-wave sleep, and the diagnosis of nonconvulsive status was established (Figure 2). However, there was no history of developmental regression.

Subsequently, he was started on sodium valproate (VPA) 10 mg/kg/day dose while tailing off CBZ. After a few weeks of staring VPA, his seizures were stopped, but the child became drowsy and encephalopathic. There was a significant change in his behaviour where he became very aggressive

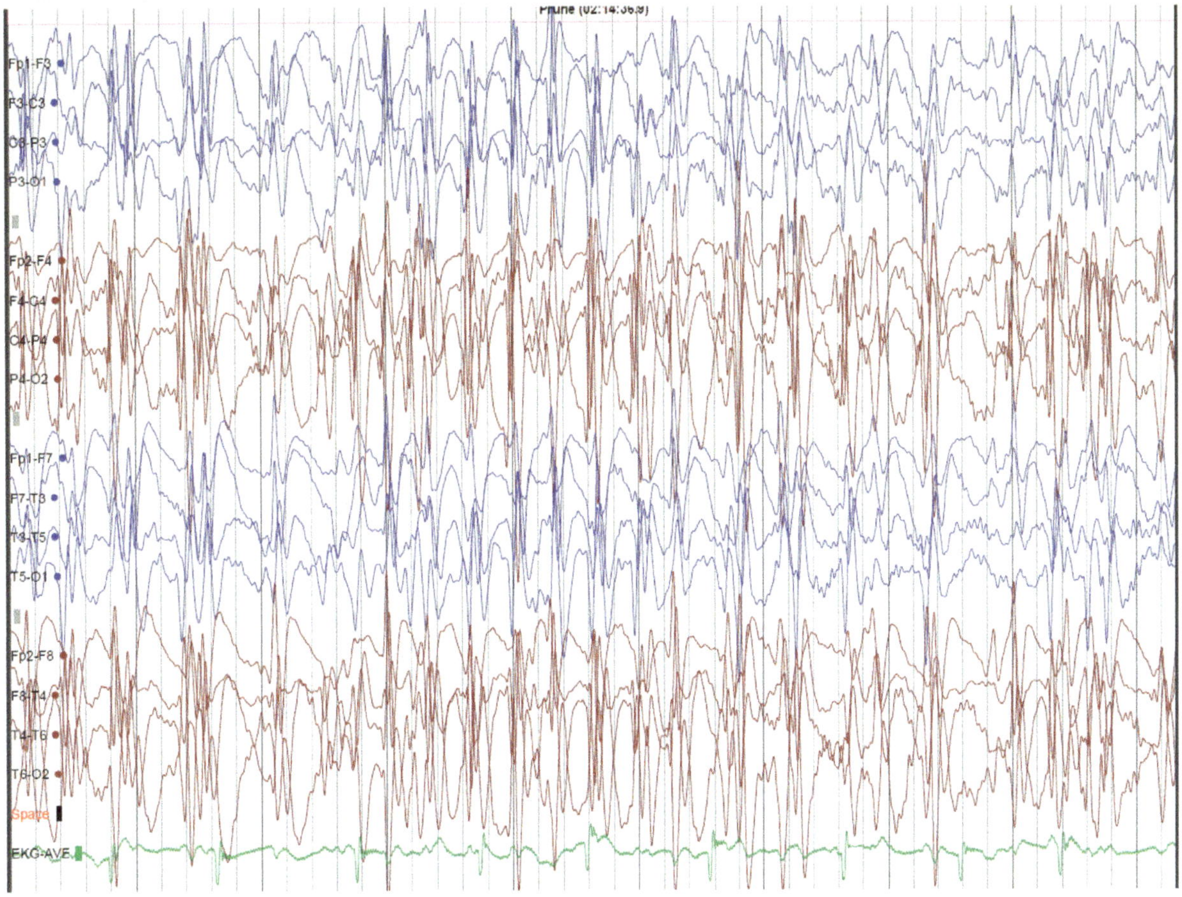

FIGURE 2: Abnormal EEG showing electrical status following increased carbamazepine dose (voltage 70 mV/cm).

and violent. Moreover, he was disoriented for time, place, and person. He had recurrent episodes of vomiting and ataxia but did not go into the level of coma. A repeat EEG was carried out during the drowsiness period and showed generalised high amplitude delta activity without frank evidence of epilepsy was in favour of evolving encephalopathy (Figure 3). His neurological examination was normal except for having a low Glasgow Coma Scale of 13. No abnormality was noted in the basic biochemical investigations, including liver enzymes and blood urea levels. A high degree of clinical suspicion of VPA-induced HA was there at this point, and he underwent second-line investigations. His serum ammonia level was 82.0. Plasma amino acid analysis was carried out using high-performance chromatography postcolumn derivatisation with ninhydrin. The analysis revealed mildly elevated arginine 167 μmol/L (6–140) and serine198 μmol/L (58–187). VPA-induced HA was diagnosed, and he was started on levetiracetam while tailing off VPA. Serum VPA level was not measured due to the unavailability of the test. He showed a marked improvement after stopping VPA. Specific genetic analysis revealed a c.2756 C > T.p (Ser919Leu) heterozygote genetic mutation of the CSP 1 gene. He was regularly followed up at the paediatric neurology clinic for more than a year, and he remained seizure-free while on levetiracetam.

3. Discussion

Though SLECTS carries an excellent prognosis, some clinicians start these children on AEDs depending on the clinical picture. However, a few antiepileptics such as CBZ and phenobarbitone result in electroclinical aggravation of the condition [7]. The increasing frequency of seizures, development of atypical absence seizures, speech difficulties, deterioration of school performances, and continuous spikes and waves during slow sleep are recognized as adverse effects of CBZ in SLECTS [7]. Furthermore, CBZ is known to exacerbate some cases of benign occipital epilepsy in childhood [8]. In this case, the child got worsen following the commencement of CBZ, but there were no other side effects noted. As the second-line therapy, the child was started on VPA while tailing off CBZ.

Carbomoyl phosphate synthetase-1 (CPS1) enzyme is responsible for the urea cycle's first and rate-limiting step. CPS1 deficiency (CPS1D) is a rare form of urea cycle defect (UCD), which has autosomal recessive inheritance [4]. The CPS1 gene, located in 2q35 consists of 4500 nucleotide coding sequences scattered through 38 exons, separated by 37 intervening introns [9]. Habre et al. in 2011 described 192 new gene changes of CPS1, amounting to 222 mutations altogether [10]. The CPS1 variant c.2756 C > T.p (Ser919Leu)

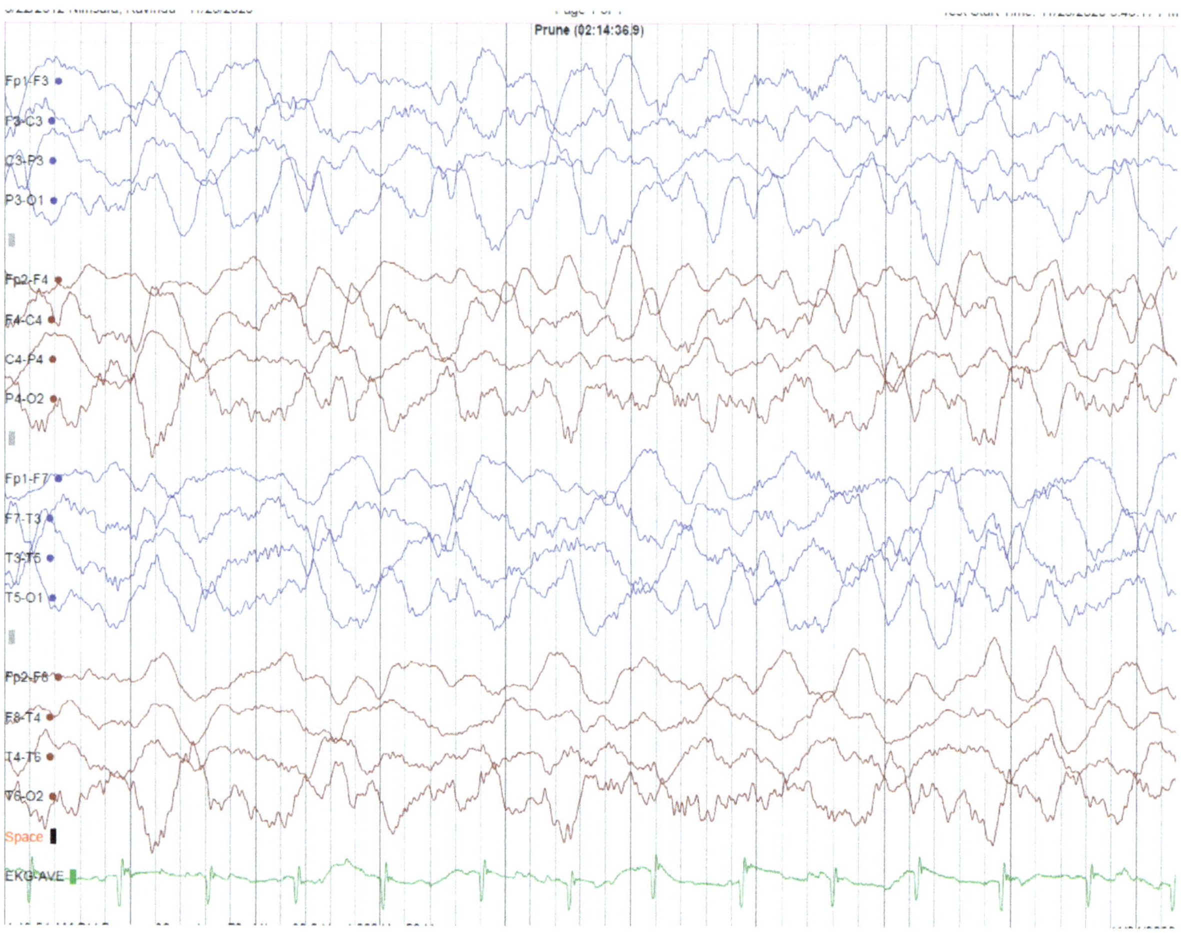

FIGURE 3: Abnormal EEG showing features of encephalopathy following sodium valproate (voltage 70 mV/cm).

has been identified as a cause for CPS1D in a few studies [10, 11]. This child was found to have the heterozygous CPS1 variant c.2756 C > T.p (Ser919Leu), and VPA-induced HA is likely to be secondary to the identified genetic mutation.

The precise mechanism of VPA-induced encephalopathy is not well known; however, the accumulation of toxic metabolites of VPA and HA is a possible explanation [2]. Moreover, VA-induced coma is more common when it is given in combination with other AEDs [2]. In this case, VPA was given while tailing off CBZ; therefore, the child was on two antiepileptics when he developed hyperammonemia (HA), which would have contributed to developing HA up to a certain degree. CPS1D has been identified as an underlying reason for VPA-induced encephalopathy in many case reports and series [5, 12]. Piotr et al., in 2013, did ammonia levels of 142 adults who were on VPA of more than 1-year duration and showed that 7.7% of them had elevated ammonia levels. Moreover, the study revealed that those who carry heterozygous T1405 N gene mutation of CPS1 have a higher incidence of HA [13]. In this child, the identified gene mutation was c.2756 C > T.p (Ser919Leu). This mutation was previously described by Harber et al. as one of 222 gene mutations of the CPS1 gene [10]. However, VPA-induced HA in the background of this gene mutation was not previously reported. Though urea cycle defects (UCD) can present with epilepsy, it is not known whether heterozygous individuals get epilepsy [14]. Furthermore, we could not find any association between SLECTS and UCD. Therefore, we do not believe whether there was a link between this identified gene mutation and the epilepsy of this child.

4. Conclusion

This is a classic example where the side effects of treatment determine the choice of AEDs in childhood epilepsy. It is essential to keep in mind that SLECTS can be aggravated with certain AEDs; therefore, the risk versus benefit of AEDs in SLECTS should be measured before starting on AEDs. Moreover, VPA-induced HA in the absence of live failure could be due to underlying diseases such as UCDs.

Abbreviations

VPA: Sodium valproate
CBZ: Carbamazepine
CPS: Carbomoyl phosphatase synthase
CPS1D: Carbomoyl phosphatase synthase-1 deficiency
SLECTS: Self-limited epilepsy with centrotemporal spikes
EEG: Electroencephalogram
AEDs: Antiepileptic drugs
UCD: Urea cycle defects.

Consent

Written informed consent was obtained from the father of the child for publication of this case report and accompanying EEG images.

Authors' Contributions

IK involved in managing the patient and manuscript writing. EJ involved with the biochemical and genetic diagnosis. GH managed the patient and arranged the follow-up.

Acknowledgments

The authors would like to thank Centogene for helping them with the genetic diagnosis.

References

[1] J. Lee, "Antiepileptic drugs in children: current concept," *Journal of Korean Neurosurgical Society*, vol. 62, no. 3, pp. 296–301, 2019.

[2] A. Chopra, B. P. Kolla, M. P. Mansukhani, P. Netzel, and M. A. Frye, "Valproate-induced hyperammonemic encephalopathy: an update on risk factors, clinical correlates and management," *General Hospital Psychiatry*, vol. 34, no. 3, pp. 290–298, 2012.

[3] V. Mittal, S. Muralee, and R. R. Tampi, "Valproic acid-induced hyperammonemia in the elderly: a review of the literature," *Case Reports in Medicine*, vol. 2009, Article ID 802121, 5 pages, 2009.

[4] A. I. Martínez, I. Pérez-Arellano, S. Pekkala, B. Barcelona, and J. Cervera, "Genetic, structural and biochemical basis of carbamoyl phosphate synthetase 1 deficiency," *Molecular Genetics and Metabolism*, vol. 101, no. 4, pp. 311–323, 2010.

[5] M. Yagi, T. Nakamura, Y. Okizuka et al., "Effect of CPS14217C > A genotype on valproic-acid-induced hyperammonemia," *Pediatrics International*, vol. 52, no. 5, pp. 744–748, 2010.

[6] M. N. Seetharam and J. M. Pellock, "Risk-benefit assessment of Carbamazepine in children," *Drug Safety*, vol. 6, no. 2, pp. 148–158, 1991.

[7] D. Corda, P. Gelisse, P. Genton, C. Dravet, and M. Baldy-Moulinier, "Incidence of drug-induced aggravation in benign epilepsy with centrotemporal spikes," *Epilepsia*, vol. 42, no. 6, pp. 754–759, 2001.

[8] K. Kikumoto, H. Yoshinaga, M. Oka et al., "EEG and seizure exacerbation induced by Carbamazepine in Panayiotopoulos syndrome," *Epileptic Disorders: International Epilepsy Journal with Videotape*, vol. 8, no. 1, pp. 53–56, 2006.

[9] J. Ha¨berle, E. Schmidt, S. Pauli et al., "Gene structure of human carbamylphosphate synthetase 1 and novel mutations in patients with neonatal onset," *Human Mutation*, vol. 21, p. 444, 2003.

[10] J. Häberle, O. A. Shchelochkov, J. Wang et al., "Urea Cycle Disorders Consortium. Molecular defects in human carbamoy phosphate synthetase I: mutational spectrum, diagnostic and protein structure considerations," *Human Mutation*, vol. 32, no. 6, pp. 579–589, 2011.

[11] C. Díez-Fernández, L. Hu, J. Cervera, J. Häberle, and V. Rubio, "Understanding carbamoyl phosphate synthetase (CPS1) deficiency by using the recombinantly purified human enzyme: effects of CPS1 mutations that concentrate in a central domain of unknown function," *Molecular Genetics and Metabolism*, vol. 112, no. 2, pp. 123–132, 2014 1.

[12] H. B. C. Verbiest, J. S. Straver, J. P. Colombo, J. C. M. Vijver, and T. C. A. M. Woerkom, "Carbamyl phosphate synthetase-l deficiency discovered after valproic acid-induced coma," *Acta Neurologica Scandinavica*, vol. 86, no. 3, pp. 275–279, 1992.

[13] P. K. Janicki, D. Bezinover, M. Postula et al., "Increased occurrence of valproic acid-induced hyperammonemia in carriers of T1405N polymorphism in carbamoyl phosphate synthetase 1 gene," *ISRN neurology*, vol. 2013, Article ID 261497, 4 pages, 2013.

[14] S. Sharma and A. Prasad, "Inborn errors of metabolism and epilepsy: current understanding, diagnosis, and treatment approaches," *International Journal of Molecular Sciences*, vol. 18, no. 7, p. 1384, 2017.

9

A Rare Case of Cyclophosphamide-Induced Posterior Reversible Encephalopathy Syndrome in a Patient with Anti-GBM Vasculitis and Review of Current Literature

Taha Nisar, Abdul R. Alchaki, and Erin Feinstein

Rutgers New Jersey Medical School, Newark, USA

Correspondence should be addressed to Taha Nisar; tahanisar@hotmail.com

Academic Editor: Isabella Laura Simone

Posterior reversible encephalopathy syndrome (PRES) is a clinical syndrome of headache, altered mental status, and seizures with reversible mainly posterior leukoencephalopathy on neuroimaging. Precipitating factors for PRES are multifactorial and include autoregulatory failure due to changes in blood pressure, metabolic derangements, and cytotoxic medications. We report the second case of cyclophosphamide-induced PRES in a patient with anti-glomerular basement membrane (Anti-GBM) positive vasculitis. In the acute setting, PRES can be challenging to distinguish from cerebral venous sinus thrombosis or cerebral vasculitis based on clinical presentation. Neuroimaging with magnetic resonance imaging (MRI) of the brain along with a vessel imaging, can help reach the diagnosis.

1. Introduction

Posterior reversible encephalopathy syndrome (PRES) is a clinical syndrome of headache, altered mental status, and seizures with reversible mainly posterior leukoencephalopathy on neuroimaging [1]. Precipitating factors for PRES are multifactorial and include autoregulatory failure due to changes in blood pressure, metabolic derangements, and cytotoxic medications [2]. As the name implies, PRES is generally reversible and resolves by treating the underlying cause [1–3]. The use of immunosuppressants is a known risk factor for the development of PRES [4]. Among cytotoxic medications, cyclosporine is the best reported to cause PRES, but many other medications have also been reported to have PRES as a complication [2, 5]. We report a rare case of a patient who was given cyclophosphamide for the treatment of Anti-glomerular basement membrane (Anti-GBM) positive vasculitis, and developed PRES.

2. Case Report

29-year-old African American woman presented to the emergency department for three weeks of nausea, vomiting, and diarrhea; and five days of anuria. She was found to be uremic with renal failure (Creatinine: 5.5 mg/dl, blood urea nitrogen: 34 mg/dl, creatinine clearance: 6 ml/min). Renal biopsy showed necrotizing glomerulonephritis (Immunoglobulin G, perinuclear anti-neutrophil cytoplasmic antibodies, anti-glomerular basement membrane positive). She was treated with intravenous methylprednisolone started on day 5 of hospitalization (1 g intravenous daily for three days followed by 24 mg twice a day), plasmapheresis on day 8 of hospitalization, and cyclophosphamide (induced at a dose of 510 mg because of renal failure and plasmapheresis) on day 9 of hospitalization. Two days after cyclophosphamide induction, the patient became encephalopathic and developed clinical seizures consisting of left gaze deviation, left neck tonic deviation, left eye blinking, left arm flexion with rhythmic jerking in conjunction with the head. Fosphenytoin (loaded with 20 mg/kg followed by phenytoin maintenance at 100 mg three times a day) was initiated for seizures, and the patient was intubated and sedated on propofol drip. Blood pressure remained normotensive throughout hospitalization (Mean: 122.5/77, Median: 122/78 over a range of ten days of the event). The initial working diagnosis was cerebral vasculitis versus cerebral venous thrombosis. Magnetic

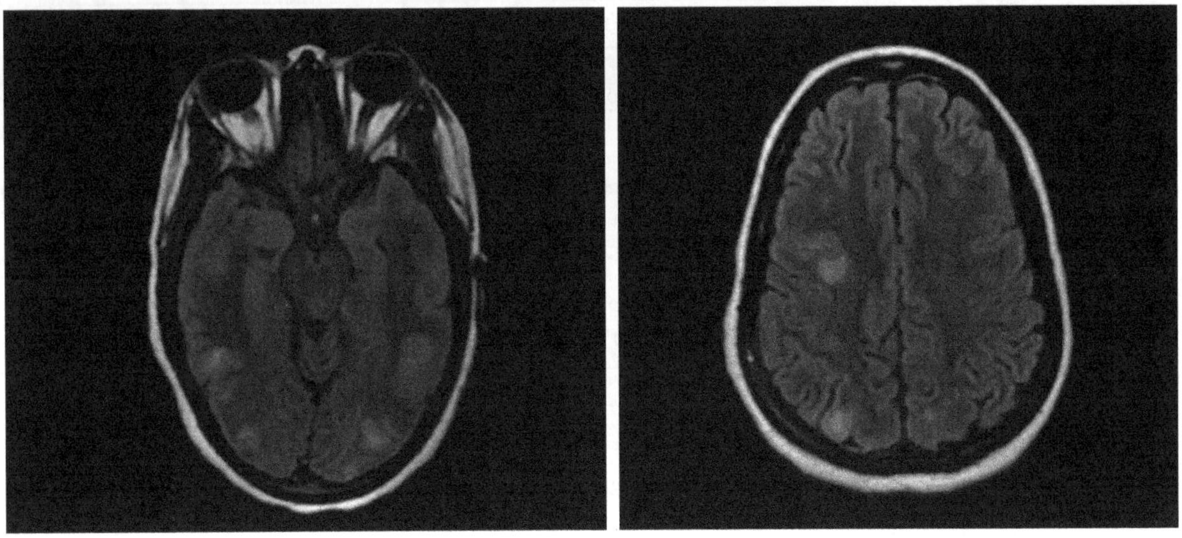

FIGURE 1: MRI brain without contrast showing areas of cortical and subcortical white matter hyperintensities likely secondary to posterior reversal encephalopathy syndrome on the FLAIR sequence. *Abbreviation*: MRI, Magnetic Resonance Imaging; FLAIR, Fluid Attenuation Inversion Recovery.

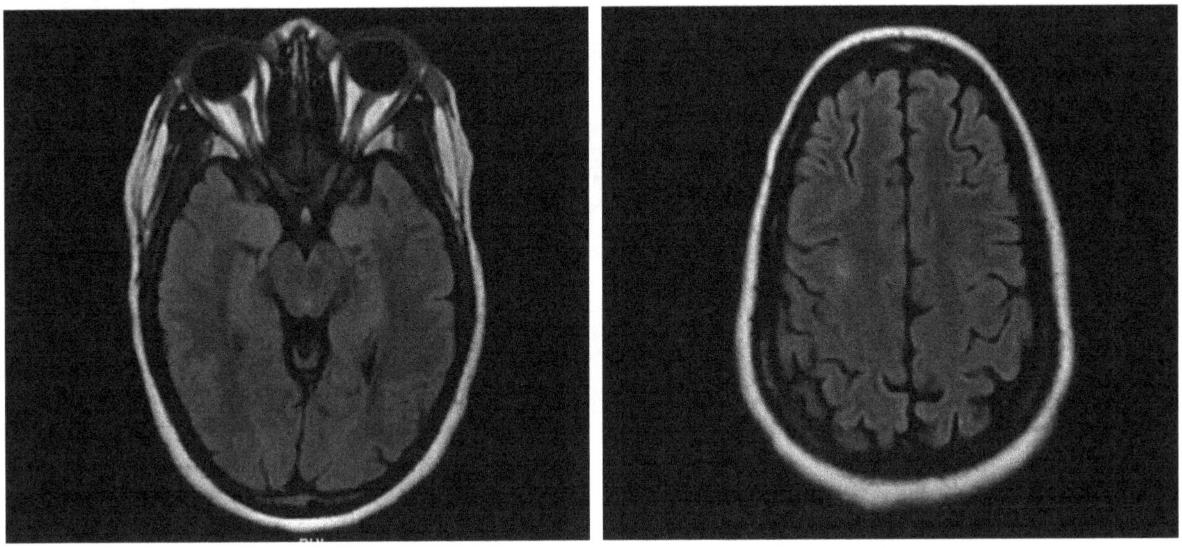

FIGURE 2: MRI brain without contrast five days later showing resolution of previously seen areas of cortical and subcortical white matter hyperintensities on the FLAIR sequence. *Abbreviation*: MRI, Magnetic Resonance Imaging; FLAIR, Fluid Attenuation Inversion Recovery.

resonance angiography (MRA) showed clear patent vessels, with no signs of venous thrombosis. Magnetic resonance imaging (MRI) revealed areas of cortical and subcortical white matter T2 Fluid-attenuated inversion recovery (FLAIR) hyperintensities in bilateral occipital-parietal and the right frontal region, as shown in Figure 1. Continuous electroencephalogram monitoring showed diffuse interictal slowing. Seizures and encephalopathy in the setting of chemotherapy treatment with the radiographic findings were most consistent with PRES. Patient self-extubated three days later and was oriented to person, place, and time with no clear neurologic deficits on examination. Repeat MRI done six days after the initial scan showed resolution of previously seen areas of T2 FLAIR, white matter hyperintensities as shown in Figure 2. She was discharged home on carbamazepine 400 mg BID and taper of phenytoin (100 mg every third day followed by stopping), and a steroid taper (methylprednisolone 16 mg BID for two weeks with a plan to taper by 4 mg BID every two weeks if tolerated).

3. Discussion

First described in 1996, PRES is a clinical syndrome with seizures, headache, altered mental status, and visual disturbances [1]. Data from case series suggest generalized tonic-clonic seizure is the most common presentation, followed by encephalopathy and headache [6, 7]. The exact incidence of PRES is unknown, though it is being increasingly reported [2]. PRES has a female preponderance and usually afflicts middle-aged patients though the range of patient's age can range from 4 years to 90 years [1–4]. Neuroimaging shows symmetrically posterior leukoencephalopathy that improves with time [1, 3]. The classic description is the parietooccipital pattern of vasogenic edema

Table 1: Case reports of posterior reversible encephalopathy syndrome (PRES) in patients given cyclophosphamide.

Case reports	Demographics	Rheumatological condition	Laboratory investigations	Treatments given	MRI findings
Chang-Hoon Lee et al. [30]	42-year-old female	SLE	Cr: 2.68 mg/dl, BUN: 41.7 mg/dl	Cyclophosphamide, steroids, anticonvulsive and antihypertensive medications	T2 hyperintensities involving the bilateral parieto-occipital lobes, frontal lobes, and basal ganglia
Jabrane et al. [28]	16-year-old female	SLE	BUN: 58 mg/dl, CrCl: 5 ml/min, Proteinuria 2.5 g/day	Cyclophosphamide, steroids	T2 hyperintensities on bilateral occipital lobes
Zekić et al. [25]	18-year-old female	SLE	Proteinuria 2.7 g/day	Cyclophosphamide, steroids	T2 hyperintensities involving the bilateral parieto-occipital lobes and right frontal lobe
Jayaweera et al. [27]	33-year-old female	SLE	Cr: 5.79 mg/dl	Cyclophosphamide, steroids, midazolam, phenytoin, valproate, topiramate	T2 hyperintensities on bilateral occipital lobes
Abenza-Abilua et al. [29]	27-year-old male	Anti-GBM disease	Cr: 8.50 mg/dl, BUN: 149 mg/dl, CrCl: 6 ml/min	Cyclophosphamide, steroids	T2 hyperintensities involving the bilateral parieto-occipital lobes
Di Pan et al. [26]	22-year old female	Sjogren's syndrome	Cr: 1.47 mg/dl, BUN: 41.7 mg/dl	Cyclophosphamide, steroids	T2 hyperintensities involving the bilateral parieto-occipital lobes and cerebellum

MRI, Magnetic Resonance Imaging; SLE, Systemic Lupus Erythematosus; Anti-GBM, Anti-Glomerular Basement Membrane; Cr, Creatinine; BUN, Blood Urea Nitrogen; CrCl, Creatinine Clearance.

in predominantly subcortical areas, though cortical involvement is also common [1, 8]. Involvement of parietooccipital lobe (≥98%) is more common than frontal lobe (around 70%), though temporal lobe (around 65%), cerebellar (30–53%), basal ganglia (630%), and midbrain involvement (630%) have also been reported [8]. The findings of PRES are appreciated on MRI on T2 sequences which show punctate or confluent areas of increased signal [8, 9]. The MRI findings usually resolve in 7–14 days [3]. Brain biopsy in PRES reveals edema in white matter with no evidence of vessel wall damage or infarction [10].

Causes of PRES are multifactorial, with a common pathway of autoregulatory failure or endothelial damage, that lead to capillary leakage with vasogenic edema [1, 2, 11]. Uncontrolled hypertension, chemotherapeutic agents, eclampsia, and hypomagnesemia are some factors associated with the development of PRES [1, 4, 12].

The exact mechanism of PRES is unknown; there is evidence to support the notion that autoregulatory failure leading to cerebral hyperperfusion or hypoperfusion is thought to be causative [4]. Schwartz et al. proposed an increase in perfusion using Single Photon Emission Computed Tomography (SPECT) scans, while Bartynski et al. showed a decrease in perfusion on relative cerebral blood volume (rCBV) color maps [13, 14]. Acute and rapid elevation of BP above the limit of autoregulation is a common cause of PRES and is associated with 75% of the cases [1, 11]. Rapid elevation of BP is thought to overwhelm the autoregulatory mechanisms, causing arteriolar dilation and break down of the blood-brain barrier, and leakage of plasma into brain parenchyma [15].

Our patient was normotensive and developed PRES after receiving one dose of cyclophosphamide in addition to three cycles of plasmapheresis and six days of intravenous methylprednisolone. The use of immunosuppressants is a known risk factor for the development of PRES [4]. PRES as a complication of immunosuppression has most often been reported with cyclosporine and tacrolimus, though interferon-alpha, intrathecal methotrexate, bevacizumab, gemcitabine, and sirolimus have also been reported [5, 16–24]. immunosuppressive therapies are thought to have a direct toxic effect on endothelium causing arteriolar and capillary damage with disruption of the blood–brain barrier and subsequent vasogenic edema, causing PRES [1, 22].

There is a paucity of case reports identifying cyclophosphamide as a trigger for PRES in the rheumatologic population. Many of these cases developed PRES in the setting of acute renal failure when treated with cyclophosphamide for a rheumatological condition, similar to our case [25–30]. These cases are summarized in Table 1. Chang-Hoon Lee reported a case of a 42-year-old woman with systemic lupus erythematosus (SLE) who presented with renal failure secondary to glomerulonephritis and developed PRES after two cycles of cyclophosphamide [30]. Jabrane et al. reported a case of a 16-year-old girl with SLE and lupus nephritis who presented with renal failure and developed sudden onset of a headache, blurring of vision, followed by three episodes of generalized seizures after being treated with IV cyclophosphamide pulse therapy at 300 mg/m^2 of the body surface [28]. Zekić et al. reported a case of an 18-year-old girl with of SLE who presented with renal failure due to lupus nephritis and acute arthritis and developed PRES after administration of the second dose of cyclophosphamide [25]. Jayaweera et al. reported a case of a 33-year-old woman who presented with renal failure due to lupus nephritis who developed PRES after the second dose of cyclophosphamide [27].

Abenza-Abildua reported another case of PRES in a 27-year-old man with high blood pressure (HBP) and glomerulonephritis caused by anti-GBM disease treated with cyclophosphamide [29]. Di Pan reported PRES in a 22-year-old woman with a history of Sjogren's syndrome who had an acute respiratory failure from diffuse alveolar hemorrhage concurrent with renal failure from glomerulonephritis, who was treated with cyclophosphamide on day 2, and developed seizures on day 5, with findings concerning for PRES on neuroimaging [26]. All of these case reports are young individuals with an underlying rheumatological condition causing renal failure who developed PRES while receiving cyclophosphamide for their underlying rheumatologic condition. Majority of these cases had SLE with nephritis, however along with Abenza-Abildua et al., our case reports PRES caused by cyclophosphamide use to treat Anti-GBM vasculitis [26]. Our case report provides further insight into the pathophysiology of immunosuppressants causing PRES; specifically in patients with renal failures and Anti-GBM vasculitis undergoing treatment with cyclophosmaphide.

4. Conclusion

To our knowledge, this is only the second reported case in the literature associated with the development of PRES due to cyclophosphamide given for (Anti-GBM) vasculitis. There are several other case reports of young individuals with underlying rheumatological conditions developing renal failure and subsequent PRES after receiving cyclophosphamide. In the acute setting, PRES can be difficult to distinguish from cerebral venous sinus thrombosis, cerebral vasculitis based on clinical findings. Neuroimaging with magnetic resonance imaging (MRI) of the brain along with vascular imaging can help reach the diagnosis.

Disclosure

This case was presented as a poster at the American Academy of Neurology Conference, 2018.

References

[1] J. Hinchey, C. Chaves, B. Appignani et al., "A reversible posterior leukoencephalopathy syndrome," *New England Journal of Medicine*, vol. 334, no. 8, pp. 494–500, 1996.

[2] S. Legriel, F. Pico, and E. Azoulay, "Understanding posterior reversible encephalopathy syndrome," *In Annual Update in Intensive Care and Emergency Medicine*, Berlin Heidelberg J.-L. Vincent, Ed., Springer, pp. 631–653, 2011.

[3] S. O. Casey, Sampaio, R. C. et al., "Posterior reversible encephalopathy syndrome: utility of fluid-attenuated inversion recovery MR imaging in the detection of cortical and subcortical lesions," *American Journal of Neuroradiology*, vol. 21, no. 7, pp. 1199–206, 2000.

[4] G. Leroux, J. Sellam, N. Costedoat-Chalumeau et al., "Posterior reversible encephalopathy syndrome during systemic lupus erythematosus: four new cases and review of the literature," *Lupus*, vol. 17, no. 2, pp. 139–147, 2008.

[5] R. B. Schwartz, S. M. Bravo, R. B. Klufas et al., "Cyclosporine neurotoxicity and its relationship to hypertensive encephalopathy: CT and MR findings in 16 cases," *American Journal of Roentgenology*, vol. 165, no. 3, pp. 627–631, 1995.

[6] E. V. Hobson, I. Craven, and S. C. Blank, "Posterior reversible encephalopathy syndrome: a truly treatable neurologic illness," *Peritoneal Dialysis International*, vol. 32, no. 6, pp. 590–594, 2012.

[7] A. M. McKinney, J. Short, C. L. Truwit et al., "Posterior reversible encephalopathy syndrome: incidence of atypical regions of involvement and imaging findings," *American Journal of Roentgenology*, vol. 189, no. 4, pp. 904–912, 2007.

[8] M. Ollivier, A. Bertrand, F. Clarençon et al., "Neuroimaging features in posterior reversible encephalopathy syndrome: a pictorial review," *Journal of the Neurological Sciences*, vol. 373, pp. 188–200, 2017.

[9] L. Edvinsson, C. Owman, and N. O. Sjoberg, "Autonomic nerves, mast cells, and amine receptors in human brain vessels. a histochemical and pharmacological study," *Brain Research*, vol. 115, no. 3, pp. 377–393, 1976.

[10] D. Schiff and M. B. Lopes, "Neuropathological correlates of reversible posterior leukoencephalopathy," *Neurocritical Care*, vol. 2, no. 3, pp. 303–305, 2005.

[11] W. S. Bartynski, "Posterior reversible encephalopathy syndrome, part 1: fundamental imaging and clinical features," *American Journal of Neuroradiology*, vol. 29, no. 6, pp. 1036–1042, 2008.

[12] M. Almoussa, A. Goertzen, S. Brauckmann, B. Fauser, and C. W. Zimmermann, "Posterior reversible encephalopathy syndrome due to hypomagnesemia: a case report and literature review," *Case Reports in Medicine*, vol. 2018, Article ID 1980638, 6 pages, 2018.

[13] R. B. Schwartz, K. M. Jones, P. Kalina et al., "Hypertensive encephalopathy: findings on CT, MR imaging, and SPECT imaging in 14 cases," *American Journal of Roentgenology*, vol. 159, no. 2, pp. 379–383, 1992.

[14] W. S. Bartynski and J. F. Boardman, "Catheter angiography, MR angiography, and MR perfusion in posterior reversible encephalopathy syndrome," *American Journal of Neuroradiology*, vol. 29, no. 3, pp. 447–455, 2008.

[15] S. Strandgaard and O. B. Paulson, "Cerebral autoregulation," *Stroke*, vol. 15, no. 3, pp. 413–416, 1984.

[16] P. Glusker, L. Recht, and B. Lane, "Reversible posterior leukoencephalopathy syndrome and bevacizumab," *New England Journal of Medicine*, vol. 354, no. 9, pp. 980–982, 2006, discussion 980-210.

[17] R. Kou, D. Greif, and T. Michel, "Dephosphorylation of endothelial nitric-oxide synthase by vascular endothelial growth factor. Implications for the vascular responses to cyclosporin A," *Journal of Biological Chemistry*, vol. 277, no. 33, pp. 29669–29673, 2002.

[18] R. C. S. Seet and A. A. Rabinstein, "Clinical features and outcomes of posterior reversible encephalopathy syndrome following bevacizumab treatment," *QJM*, vol. 105, no. 1, pp. 69–75, 2012.

[19] O. S. Kozak, E. F. M Wijdicks, E. M. Manno, J. T. Miley, and A. A. Rabinstein, "Status epilepticus as initial manifestation of posterior reversible encephalopathy syndrome," *Neurology*, vol. 69, no. 9, pp. 894–897, 2007.

[20] M. R. Junna and A. A. Rabinstein, "Tacrolimus induced leukoencephalopathy presenting with status epilepticus and prolonged coma," *Journal of Neurology, Neurosurgery & Psychiatry*, vol. 78, no. 12, pp. 1410–1411, 2007.

[21] A. Rajasekhar and T. J. George, "Gemcitabine-induced reversible posterior leukoencephalopathy syndrome: a case report and review of the literature," *Oncologist*, vol. 12, no. 11, pp. 1332–1335, 2007.

[22] Y. Ito, Y. Arahata, Y. Goto et al., "Cisplatin neurotoxicity presenting as reversible posterior leukoencephalopathy syndrome," *American Journal of Neuroradiology*, vol. 19, no. 3, pp. 415–417, 1998.

[23] C. L. Bodkin and B. H. Eidelman, "Sirolimus-induced posterior reversible encephalopathy," *Neurology*, vol. 68, no. 23, pp. 2039–2040, 2007.

[24] J. A. Allen, A. Adlakha, and P. R. Bergethon, "Reversible posterior leukoencephalopathy syndrome after bevacizumab/ FOLFIRI regimen for metastatic colon cancer," *Archives of Neurology*, vol. 63, no. 10, pp. 1475–1478, 2006.

[25] T. Zekić, M. S. Benić, R. Antulov, I. Antončić, and S. Novak, "The multifactorial origin of posterior reversible encephalopathy syndrome in cyclophosphamide-treated lupus patients," *Rheumatology International*, vol. 37, no. 12, pp. 2105–2114, 2017.

[26] D. Pan, B. Sabharwal, and F. Vallejo, "Posterior reversible encephalopathy syndrome secondary to cyclophosphamide in the treatment of pulmonary renal syndrome," *Chest*, vol. 152, no. 4, p. A367, 2017.

[27] J. L. Jayaweera, M. R. Withana, C. K. P. Dalpatadu et al., "Cyclophosphamide-induced posterior reversible encephalopathy syndrome (PRES): a case report," *Journal of Medical Case Reports*, vol. 8, no. 1, article no. 442, 2014.

[28] M. Jabrane, Z. A. Lahcen, W. Fadili, and I. Laouad, "A case of PRES in an active lupus nephritis patient after treatment of corticosteroid and cyclophosphamide," *Rheumatology International*, vol. 35, no. 5, pp. 935–938, 2015.

[29] M. J. Abenza-Abildua, B. Fuentes, D. Diaz et al., "Cyclophosphamide-induced reversible posterior leukoencephalopathy syndrome," *BMJ Case Reports*, vol. 2009, pp. bcr0720080467–bcr0720080467, 2009.

[30] C.-H. Lee, Y. M. Lee, S. H. Ahn, D. W. Ryu, J. H. Song, and M.-Su Lee, "Cyclophosphamide-induced posterior reversible encephalopathy syndrome in a patient with lupus nephritis," *Journal of Rheumatic Diseases*, vol. 20, no. 2, pp. 103–107, 2013.

10

Optic Neuropathy with Features Suggestive of Optic Neuritis in Cerebrotendinous Xanthomatosis

Miyuki Miyamoto,[1] Nobuyuki Ishii,[1] Hitoshi Mochizuki,[1] Kazutaka Shiomi,[1] Tomoko Kaida,[2] Hideki Chuman,[3] and Masamitsu Nakazato[1]

[1]*Division of Neurology, Respirology, Endocrinology and Metabolism, Department of Internal Medicine, University of Miyazaki, Miyazaki, Japan*
[2]*Miyata Eye Hospital, Miyakonojo, Miyazaki, Japan*
[3]*Department of Ophthalmology, University of Miyazaki, Miyazaki, Japan*

Correspondence should be addressed to Nobuyuki Ishii; nobuyuki_ishii@med.miyazaki-u.ac.jp

Academic Editor: Peter Berlit

We describe our encounter with a 39-year-old man who exhibited acute painless visual loss and progressive gait disturbance. He had tendinous xanthoma and several neuroophthalmological findings indicative of optic neuropathy in the right eye, including afferent pupillary defect, cecocentral scotoma, and optic disc swelling. Neurological examination showed cerebellar ataxia and pyramidal weakness. Brain magnetic resonance imaging revealed bilateral swelling in the optic nerves with gadolinium-enhancement suggesting optic neuritis, an enlarged fourth ventricle, atrophy of the cerebellum, and hyperintensities in the bilateral dentate nuclei. The patient was diagnosed with cerebrotendinous xanthomatosis (CTX) based on an elevated serum cholestanol level and a homozygous missense mutation in *CYP27A1*. CTX is a genetic lipid storage disease caused by dysfunction of the mitochondrial enzyme sterol 27-hydroxylase. With respect to ophthalmological manifestations, juvenile cataracts and optic neuropathy are common findings in patients with CTX, but there have been no reports of optic neuropathy with features suggestive of optic neuritis. Thus, this case illustrates that clinicians should consider a diagnosis of CTX in patients with cardinal features of CTX even if the patients show signs indicative of optic neuritis.

1. Introduction

Cerebrotendinous xanthomatosis (CTX), an autosomal recessive lipid storage disease, is characterized by various systemic and neurological symptoms, including chronic diarrhea, juvenile cataracts, tendon xanthomas, and developmental delay [1]. With respect to ophthalmological manifestations, apart from cataracts, optic neuropathy with optic disc paleness is a common finding in patients with CTX [2]. However, cases of CTX with optic neuritis have not been previously reported. Here, we present the first case of CTX with optic neuropathy and findings suggestive of optic neuritis, including disc edema and contrast agent enhancement of the peripapillary retina and optic nerve.

2. Case Presentation

A 39-year-old man, born of a consanguineous marriage, had epilepsy since the age of 12 years, as well as dyslipidemia; he was referred to our hospital because of acute painless visual loss and progressive gait disturbance. His visual acuity was 20/16 bilaterally after bilateral cataract surgery at the age of 31 years. His developmental milestones were normal. He denied a history of neonatal jaundice or infantile diarrhea, smoked half a pack of cigarettes per day, and drank socially. His family history was unremarkable. Medications included carbamazepine, phenytoin, clobazam, and bezafibrate.

On physical examination, swelling was observed in the tendons of Achilles, patella, and triceps, which indicated

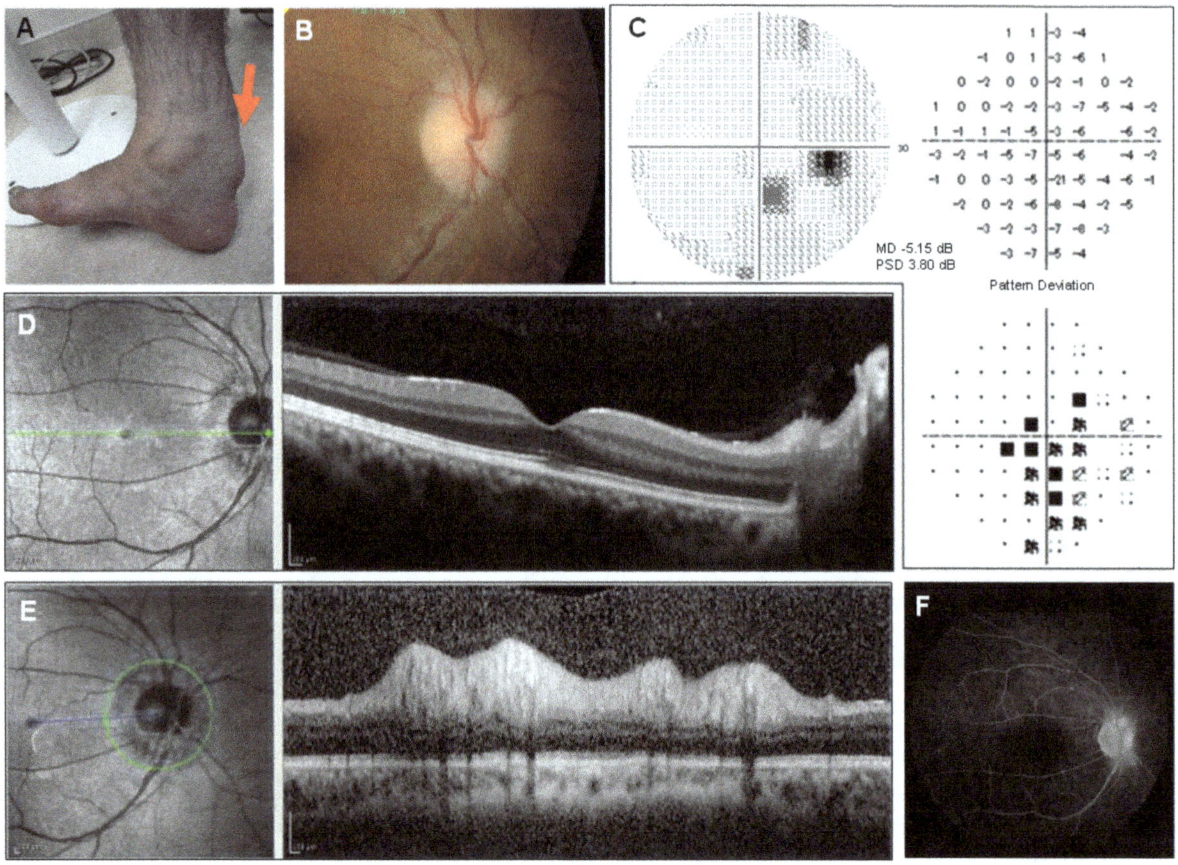

FIGURE 1: The patient's enlarged right Achilles tendon (arrow), which indicated xanthoma (A). Funduscopic examination showed mild swelling in the nasal side of the right optic disc (B). Humphrey 30-2 visual field examination revealed a cecocentral scotoma in the right eye (C). OCT of the right eye demonstrated intact thickness of the retinal nerve fiber layer (RNFL) in the macula (D) and increased thickness of the peripapillary RNFL (E). Fluorescein angiography exhibited profuse dye leakage on the right optic disc (B).

xanthoma (Figure 1(A)). A neuroophthalmological examination showed corrected visual acuities of 20/125 in the right eye and 20/30 in the left eye. The right pupil measured 4 mm with a round shape in dark and 2 mm in light conditions; both pupils constricted briskly in response to light. The right eye exhibited an afferent pupillary defect. A biomicroscopic examination was remarkable for bilateral centrally-fixed intraocular lens. Funduscopic examination showed mild swelling in the nasal side of the right optic disc (Figure 1(B)); the left eye was normal. Humphrey 30-2 visual field examination showed a cecocentral scotoma in the right eye (Figure 1(C)). Optical coherence tomography (OCT) of the right eye showed intact thickness of the retinal nerve fiber layer (RNFL) in the macula (Figure 1(D)), while the peripapillary RNFL thickness had increased. Fundus fluorescein angiography (FAG) showed mild leakage on the nasal side of the right optic disc (Figure 1(F)). Pattern-reversal visual-evoked potentials (VEPs) with check sizes of 7.5', 15', 30', and 60' revealed no clear potentials in both eyes, and the P100 wave could not be identified. All findings indicated optic neuropathy. Neurological examination revealed Minimental State Examination scores of 22/30. The patient exhibited slurred speech, weakness in the lower limbs with spasticity, brisk deep tendon reflexes throughout all extremities, and bilateral positive Babinski sign. His gait was unstable because of truncal ataxia.

Routine laboratory tests revealed the following: normal renal and liver functions, no elevations in inflammatory markers such as erythrocyte sedimentation rate and C-reactive proteins, normal LDL cholesterol, 137 mg/dL, high triglycerides, 331 mg/dL, increased lactic acid levels, 17.3 mg/dL (reference range: 3.0–17.0 mg/dL), and pyruvate levels, 2.02 mg/dL (reference range: 0.3–0.94 mg/dL). Serological analyses of the herpes simplex virus, cytomegalovirus, Epstein-Barr virus, angiotensin-converting enzyme, PR3 and MPO anti-neutrophil cytoplasmic antibodies, anti-nuclear antibody, SS-A and SS-B antibodies, and anti-DNA antibody revealed negative results. Moreover, anti-aquaporin 4 and anti-myelin oligodendrocyte antibodies were not detected. No mitochondrial DNA mutations (i.e., nucleotide positions 3460, 11,778, and 14,484) associated with Leber's hereditary optic neuropathy (LHON) were observed. Cerebrospinal fluid (CSF) analysis revealed no cells but showed an increased protein level (77 mg/dL); isoelectric focusing revealed no oligoclonal bands in the CSF.

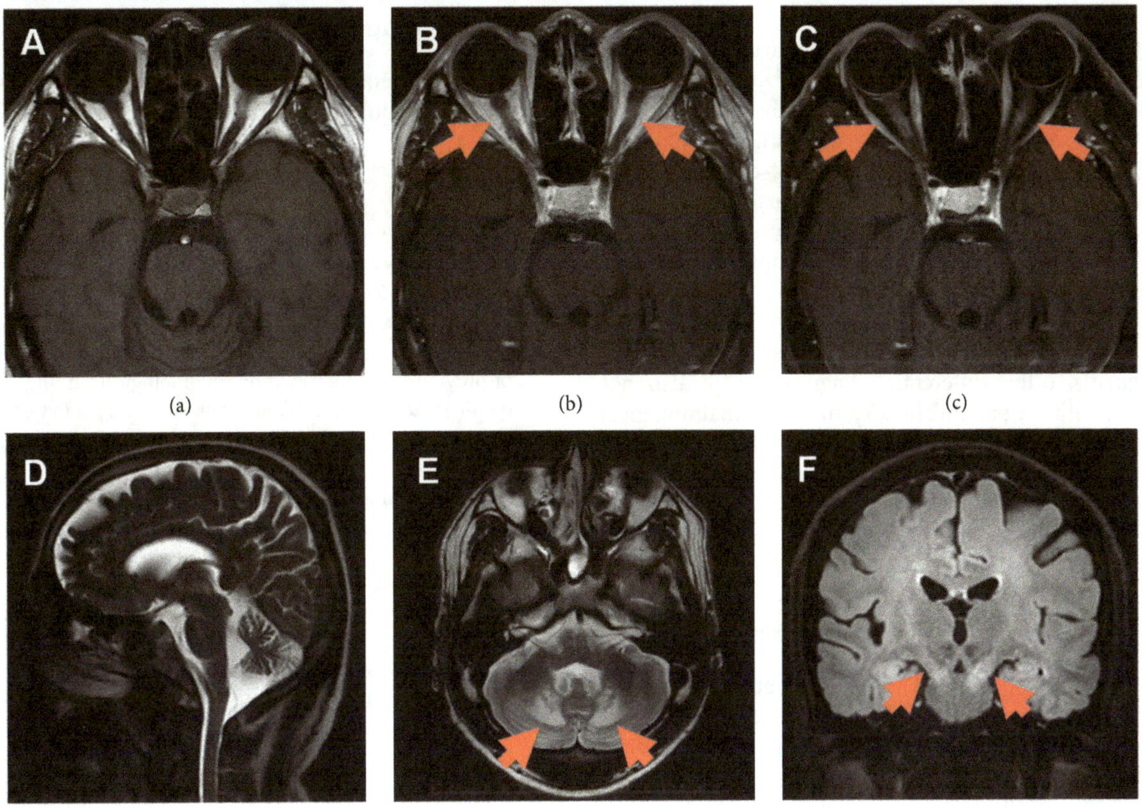

(a) (b) (c) (d) (e) (f)

FIGURE 2: Brain magnetic resonance imaging revealed the following: bilateral swelling of optic nerves on T1-weighted images (a) with enhancement (arrows) on gadolinium-enhanced T1-weighted (b) and T1 weighted fat-suppressed images (c), enlarged fourth ventricle and cerebellar atrophy (d), and hyperintensities in the bilateral dentate nuclei (arrows, (e)) on T2-weighted images; FLAIR images demonstrated hyperintensities in the bilateral dentate nuclei and pyramidal tract (arrows, (f)).

Brain magnetic resonance imaging (MRI) revealed bilateral swelling in the optic nerves on T1-weighted images (Figure 2(a)) and enhancement on gadolinium-enhanced T1-weighted and T1-weighted fat-suppressed images (Figures 2(b) and 2(c)), suggesting optic neuritis. Furthermore, T2-weighted images showed an enlarged fourth ventricle, atrophy of the cerebellum, and hyperintensities in the bilateral dentate nuclei (Figures 2(d) and 2(e)); fluid-attenuated inversion recovery images demonstrated hyperintensities in the bilateral dentate nuclei and the pyramidal tract (Figure 2(f)).

The patient was finally diagnosed with CTX upon observance of an elevated serum cholestanol level of 13.6 μg/mL (reference range: 2.0–3.4 μg/mL) and a homozygous missense mutation (c.1421G>A) in *CYP27A1*.

One month later, before the initiation of oral chenodeoxycholic acid (CDCA) treatment, the patient's visual acuity spontaneously recovered to 20/16 bilaterally, and hyperintensities in the optic nerves were found to be diminished on follow-up MRI. His neurological symptoms, however, were not altered 6 months after administration of CDCA.

3. Discussion

CTX, an autosomal recessive lipid storage disease, is caused by mutations in *CYP27A1*, which encodes the mitochondrial enzyme sterol 27-hydroxylase [1]. A deficiency of this enzyme causes disruption of the formation of bile acid, including cholic acid and chenodeoxycholic acid. Subsequently, cholesterol and cholestanol accumulate in tissues throughout the body, leading to the development of many systemic and neurologic symptoms [1].

Ophthalmological manifestations in CTX include juvenile cataracts, the incidence of which may be up to 90% [1]. In addition, pale optic disc, exophthalmos, xanthelasma, and premature retinal senescence have been reported [1–3]. With respect to optic nerve dysfunction, optic neuropathy may occur in 50% of patients with CTX [2, 3]. Moreover, 50–80% of affected patients exhibit a prolonged or diminished VEP latency in the presence or absence of abnormal fundus [2–4]. Optic neuropathy in CTX is not uncommon; however, optic neuropathy with features suggestive of optic neuritis, including the spontaneous recovery of visual acuity and contrast enhancement of the peripapillary retina and optic nerve, as in our patient, has not been previously reported. Thus, through this case, we discuss whether this patient's optic neuropathy was caused by CTX and whether CTX is accompanied with ophthalmological findings similar to those seen in optic neuritis.

The etiology of optic neuropathy with acute visual loss includes optic neuritis, arteritic and nonarteritic ischemic optic neuropathy, infections, optic nerve compression, LHON, toxic and metabolic optic neuropathy, and traumatic optic neuropathy [5]. Considering the pathophysiology of CTX, which involves the accumulation of cholesterol and cholestanol in virtually all tissues, nonarteritic ischemic optic neuropathy (NAION) is immediately included in the differential diagnosis of a patients with optic neuropathy. However, the presence of contrast-enhanced optic nerves on MRI and spontaneous recovery of visual acuity render NAION a less likely diagnosis [6]. Except for idiopathic optic neuritis, other differential diagnoses were also not compatible with the patient's history, neuroophthalmological examination, and laboratory and imaging findings. Although we could not exclude idiopathic optic neuritis, we speculated that the patient's optic neuropathy was caused by CTX because optic neuropathy is commonly associated with CTX.

We hypothesized that optic neuropathy with findings similar to those seen in optic neuritis in CTX may involve mitochondrial dysfunction, although the exact mechanism remains unclear. Sterol 27-hydroxylase, a mitochondrial enzyme, is impaired in CTX, leading to abnormalities in mitochondrial function as well as lipid metabolism [1]. Indeed, the following findings suggesting mitochondrial dysfunction have been revealed by previous studies: increased lactic acid and pyruvate levels in the blood and CSF [7], a lactate peak on brain MR spectroscopy [8], decreased activities of mitochondrial respiratory chain enzymes [7], and structural abnormalities in the mitochondria [9].

Similarly, LHON is established as a mitochondrial disorder. A typical clinical presentation of LHON includes acute or subacute painless visual loss accompanied by disc swelling, which resembles our patient's clinical course; however, leakage in the fundus FAG and progressive optic nerve atrophy is not typical of LHON [10]. However, several studies have reported fundus edema, dye leakage in FAG, and gadolinium-enhancement of the optic nerve on MRI, masquerading as optic neuritis [11, 12], as well as spontaneous improvement in visual acuity [13] in patients with LHON. The similarities between our case and LHON cases indicate that the ophthalmological findings in our patient may have resulted from mitochondrial dysfunction in CTX. Furthermore, our patient's clinical course might explain the mechanism underlying the optic neuropathy commonly seen in CTX.

To the best of our knowledge, there have been no reports of cases of optic neuropathy with features suggestive of optic neuritis in CTX. The exact underlying mechanisms remain unclear; however, we speculate that mitochondrial dysfunction caused by CTX may be involved. Thus, this case illustrates that clinicians should consider a diagnosis of CTX in patients with cardinal features of CTX, such as xanthomas or hyperintensities of the dentate nuclei on brain MRI, even in the presence of contrast enhancement of the optic discs and optic nerves, indicating optic neuritis.

Consent

Written informed consent was obtained from the patient.

Acknowledgments

This study did not receive any specific grants from funding agencies in the public, commercial, or not-for-profit sectors.

References

[1] G. Salen and R. D. Steiner, "Epidemiology, diagnosis, and treatment of cerebrotendinous xanthomatosis (CTX)," *Journal of Inherited Metabolic Disease*, vol. 40, no. 6, pp. 771–781, 2017.

[2] M. T. Dotti, A. Rufa, and A. Federico, "Cerebrotendinous xanthomatosis: Heterogeneity of clinical phenotype with evidence of previously undescribed ophthalmological findings," *Journal of Inherited Metabolic Disease*, vol. 24, no. 7, pp. 696–706, 2001.

[3] J. R. M. Cruysberg, R. A. Wevers, B. G. M. Van Engelen, A. Pinckers, A. Van Spreeken, and J. J. M. Tolboom, "Ocular and systemic manifestations of cerebrotendinous xanthomatosis," *American Journal of Ophthalmology*, vol. 120, no. 5, pp. 597–604, 1995.

[4] M. Mondelli, A. Rossi, C. Scarpini, M. T. Dotti, and A. Federico, "Evoked potentials in cerebrotendinous xanthomatosis and effect induced by chenodeoxycholic acid," *JAMA Neurology*, vol. 49, no. 5, pp. 469–475, 1992.

[5] A. T. Toosy, D. F. Mason, and D. H. Miller, "Optic neuritis," *The Lancet Neurology*, vol. 13, no. 1, pp. 83–99, 2014.

[6] J. F. Rizzo III, C. M. Andreoli, and J. D. Rabinov, "Use of magnetic resonance imaging to differentiate optic neuritis and nonarteritic anterior ischemic optic neuropathy," *Ophthalmology*, vol. 109, no. 9, pp. 1679–1684, 2002.

[7] M. T. Dotti, L. Manneschi, and A. Federico, "Mitochondrial enzyme deficiency in cerebrotendinous xanthomatosis," *Journal of the Neurological Sciences*, vol. 129, no. 2, pp. 106–108, 1995.

[8] N. De Stefano, M. T. Dotti, M. Mortilla, and A. Federico, "Magnetic resonance imaging and spectroscopic changes in brains of patients with cerebrotendinous xanthomatosis," *Brain*, vol. 124, no. 1, pp. 121–131, 2001.

[9] A. Federico, M. T. Dotti, and N. Volpi, "Muscle mitochondrial changes in cerebrotendinous xanthomatosis," *Annals of Neurology*, vol. 30, no. 5, pp. 734-735, 1991.

[10] C. Meyerson, G. Van Stavern, and C. McClelland, "Leber hereditary optic neuropathy: Current perspectives," *Clinical Ophthalmology*, vol. 9, pp. 1165–1176, 2015.

[11] A. Arianti, H. Chuman, N. Kajihara, N. Sakamoto, and N. Nao-I, "Atypical clinical and neuroimaging findings in leber's hereditary optic neuropathy: A case report," *JOJ Ophthalmology*, vol. 6, no. 5, Article ID 555698, 2018.

[12] C. Lamirel, J. Cassereau, I. Cochereau et al., "Papilloedema and MRI enhancement of the prechiasmal optic nerve at the acute stage of Leber hereditary optic neuropathy," *Journal of Neurology, Neurosurgery & Psychiatry*, vol. 81, no. 5, pp. 578–580, 2010.

[13] T.-K. Hsu, A.-G. Wang, M.-Y. Yen, and J.-H. Liu, "Leber's hereditary optic neuropathy masquerading as optic neuritis with spontaneous visual recovery," *Clinical and Experimental Optometry*, vol. 97, no. 1, pp. 84–86, 2014.

11

Acute Brainstem Dysfunction Caused by Cavernous Sinus Dural Arteriovenous Fistula

Yuwa Oka,[1] Kenichi Komatsu,[1] Soichiro Abe,[1] Naoya Yoshimoto,[2] Junya Taki,[2] and Sadayuki Matsumoto[1]

[1]*Department of Neurology, Kitano Hospital, Tazuke Kofukai Medical Research Institute, Osaka, Japan*
[2]*Department of Neurosurgery, Kitano Hospital, Tazuke Kofukai Medical Research Institute, Osaka, Japan*

Correspondence should be addressed to Kenichi Komatsu; kkomatsu@kuhp.kyoto-u.ac.jp

Academic Editor: Shahid Nimjee

Symptoms of cavernous sinus dural arteriovenous fistula depend on the drainage patterns and are very diverse. Among these, brainstem dysfunction is a rare but serious complication. Here, we describe a case with isolated and rapidly progressive brainstem dysfunction due to cavernous sinus dural arteriovenous fistula. An 80-year-old woman presented with a 2-day history of progressive gait disturbance. Neurological examination revealed mild confusion, dysarthria, and left hemiparesis. Magnetic resonance imaging (MRI) revealed pontine swelling without evidence of infarction. Magnetic resonance angiography suggested a faint abnormality near the cavernous sinus. Dural arteriovenous fistula was suspected, and digital subtraction angiography was planned for the next day. Her condition had progressed to coma by the next morning. Pontine swelling worsened, and hyperintensity appeared on diffusion-weighted imaging. Digital subtraction angiography revealed a right-sided cavernous sinus dural arteriovenous fistula with venous reflux into the posterior fossa. Orbital or ocular symptoms had preceded brainstem symptoms in all nine previously reported cases, but brainstem symptoms were the only presentation in our case, making the diagnosis difficult. Some dural arteriovenous fistulas mimic inflammatory diseases when the clinical course is acute. Prompt diagnosis using enhanced computed tomography or MRI and emergent treatment are needed to avoid permanent sequelae.

1. Introduction

Symptoms of cavernous sinus dural arteriovenous fistula depend on the drainage patterns and are very diverse. Among these, brainstem dysfunction is a rare but serious complication. Here, we describe a case with isolated and rapidly progressive brainstem dysfunction due to cavernous sinus dural arteriovenous fistula.

2. Case Presentation

We report the case of an 80-year-old woman who presented to the neurology department with a 2-day history of progressive gait disturbance. Neurological examination revealed mild confusion, dysarthria, and left hemiparesis. She needed assistance to stand and could not walk unassisted. Magnetic resonance imaging (MRI) revealed fluid-attenuated inversion recovery (FLAIR) hyperintensity, dominant on the right side (Figures 1(a) and 1(b)). Diffusion-weighted imaging (DWI) showed no significant hyperintensity. Magnetic resonance angiography suggested a faint flow signal abnormality posterolateral to the cavernous sinus (CS) (Figure 1(c)). Dural arteriovenous fistula (dAVF) was suspected, and we planned digital subtraction angiography (DSA) for the next day. High-dose methylprednisolone was administered, considering the possibility of inflammatory disease. The next morning, her condition had progressed to coma. Pontine swelling had worsened (Figure 1(d)), and DWI hyperintensity had appeared (Figure 1(e)). T2 star-weighted imaging showed an area of low intensity (Figure 1(f)), suggesting venous congestion and hemorrhage. DSA revealed a right-sided CS dAVF with venous reflux into the brainstem and cerebellar cortical veins *via* the right superior petrosal sinus and petrosal vein (Figures 2(a)–

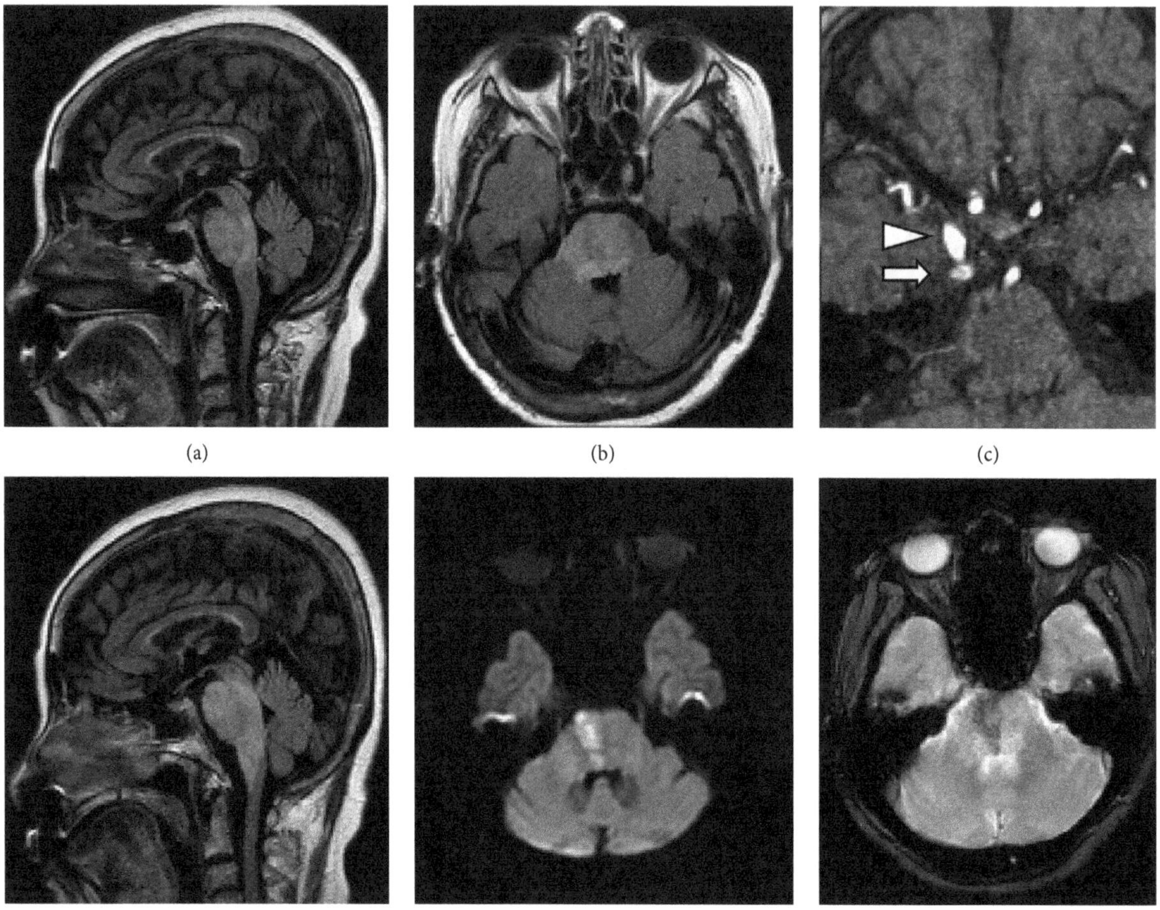

(a) (b) (c)

(d) (e) (f)

Figure 1: Magnetic resonance imaging. (a, b) Fluid-attenuated inversion recovery (FLAIR) imaging showing widespread hyperintensity diffusely involving the right pons on day 1. (c) Magnetic resonance angiography showing an abnormal flow signal (arrow) posterolateral to the cavernous sinus. Arrowhead indicates the right internal carotid artery. (d) FLAIR imaging. Brainstem edema has worsened and expanded rostrocaudally on day 2. (e) Diffusion-weighted showing shows hyperintense lesion within the edematous pons. (f) T2 star-weighted imaging showing an area of low intensity, suggesting venous congestion and hemorrhage.

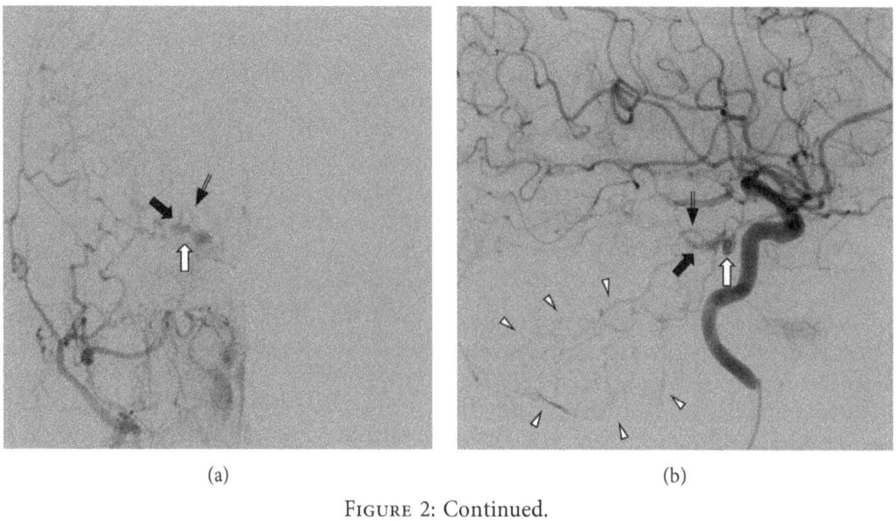

(a) (b)

Figure 2: Continued.

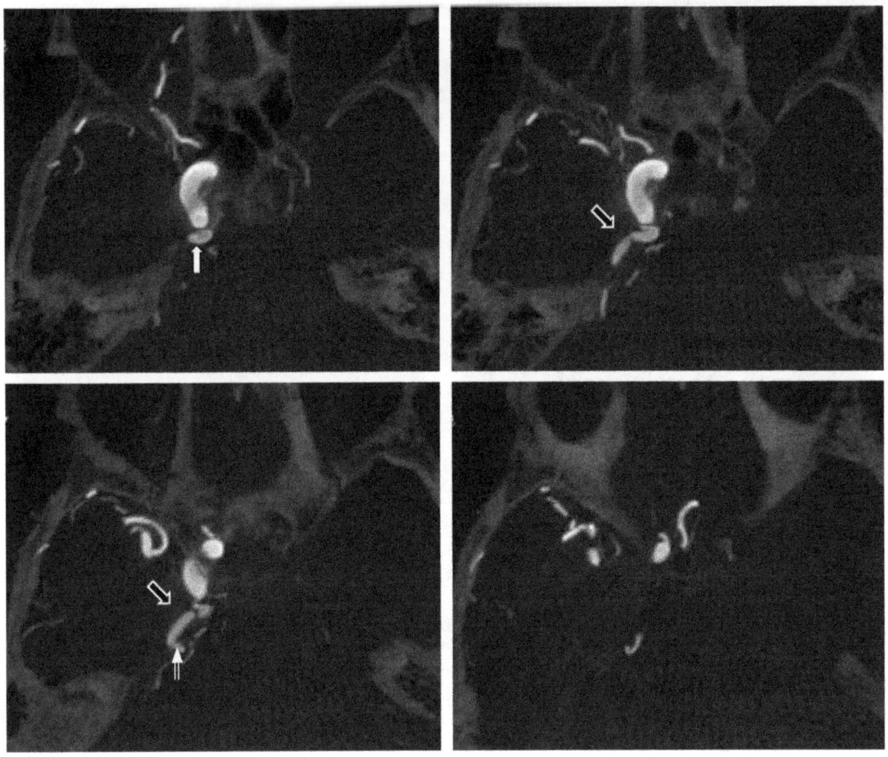

(c)

Figure 2: (a) Anteroposterior view of the right external carotid artery angiogram and (b) lateral view of the right internal carotid artery angiogram demonstrate a right-sided cavernous sinus dural arteriovenous fistula (white arrow) draining into the superior petrosal sinus (black arrow) and petrosal vein (double arrow). Note the retrograde venous drainage into the brainstem and cerebellar cortical veins (arrowheads). (c) Axial maximum intensity projection images of the right internal carotid artery angiogram. White arrow indicates the cavernous sinus dural arteriovenous fistula. No bridging veins other than the superior petrosal sinus (black arrow) and petrosal vein (double arrow) are detected.

2(c)). We attempted transvenous and transarterial embolizations, but could not approach close to the shunt pouch. Another approach was to surgically close the petrosal vein with a craniotomy. However, respiratory failure developed, and the patient was intubated during the transcatheter procedure. As a poor prognosis was predicted by severe neurological deficit and high age, we refrained from further intervention. Strict antihypertensive and antiedema therapies were initiated. MRI after 5 days showed spontaneous occlusion of the fistula. T2 star hypointensity at the pons persisted, and the hemorrhagic infarction was confirmed. Her level of consciousness gradually improved, and she was transferred for rehabilitation 3 months later, with severe weakness of the left extremities.

3. Discussion

Symptoms of CS dAVF depend on the drainage patterns and are very diverse, including orbital, ocular, cranial nerve, and cerebral symptoms. Cerebral symptoms occur in 3–5% of cases [1, 2]. Among these, brainstem dysfunction is a rare but serious complication. In our case, major drainage routes had been obliterated, and the right CS was isolated. Previous reports have pointed that increased venous pressure causes the thickening of the intima of the affected sinus and other draining vessels and can obliterate the drainage routes [3, 4]. We could not find direct evidence of a thrombus in the cavernous sinus or superior ophthalmic vein, but probably obliteration occurred as a natural history of dAVFs. Compartmentalizaion of the CS may have played a role. Single drainage route *via* the right petrosal vein caused venous reflux into posterior fossa, and subsequent focal venous congestion caused acute brainstem dysfunction and hemorrhagic infarction. Orbital or ocular symptoms had preceded brainstem symptoms in all nine cases previously reported in the English literature [5–10], but brainstem symptoms were the only presentation in our case, making the diagnosis difficult.

Some dAVFs lack orbital or ocular symptoms and mimic inflammatory diseases when the clinical course is acute. Prompt diagnosis using enhanced CT or MRI and emergent treatment are needed to avoid permanent sequelae.

References

[1] D. C. Suh, J. H. Lee, S. J. Kim et al., "New concept in cavernous sinus dural arteriovenous fistula," *Stroke*, vol. 36, no. 6, pp. 1134–1139, 2005.

[2] H. Kiyosue, Y. Hori, M. Okahara et al., "Treatment of intracranial dural arteriovenous fistulas: current strategies based on location and hemodynamics, and alternative techniques of

transcatheter embolization," *Radiographics*, vol. 24, no. 6, pp. 1637–1653, 2004.
[3] K. Misaki, N. Uchiyama, M. Mohri et al., "Unique venous drainage of a sphenoid wing dural arteriovenous fistula with ocular symptoms," *Neuroradiology*, vol. 51, pp. 175–181, 2009.
[4] M. Nishijima, A. Takaku, S. Endo et al., "Etiological evaluation of dural arteriovenous malformations of the lateral and sigmoid sinuses based on histopathological examinations," *Journal of Neurosurgery*, vol. 76, no. 4, pp. 600–606, 1992.
[5] T. Miyagishima, M. Inoue, H. Ohno et al., "Pontine venous congestion due to dural arteriovenous fistula of the cavernous sinus: case report and review of the literature," *Surgical Neurology International*, vol. 3, no. 1, p. 53, 2012.
[6] A. Uchino, A. Kato, Y. Kuroda, S. Shimokawa, and S. Kudo, "Pontine venous congestion caused by dural carotid-cavernous fistula: report of two cases," *European Radiology*, vol. 7, no. 3, pp. 405–408, 1997.
[7] S. Takahashi, N. Tomura, J. Watarai, K Mizoi, and H Manabe, "Dural arteriovenous fistula of the cavernous sinus with venous congestion of the brain stem: report of two cases," *AJNR. American Journal of Neuroradiology*, vol. 20, no. 5, pp. 886–888, 1999.
[8] S. Shintani, S. Tsuruoka, and T. Shiigai, "Carotid-cavernous fistula with brainstem congestion mimicking tumor on MRI," *Neurology*, vol. 55, no. 12, pp. 1929–1931, 2000.
[9] Y. Kai, J.-I. Hamada, M. Morioka, S. Yano, and Y. Ushio, "Brain stem venous congestion due to dural arteriovenous fistulas of the cavernous sinus," *Acta Neurochirurgica*, vol. 146, no. 10, pp. 1107–1112, 2004.
[10] M. Iwasaki, K. Murakami, T. Tomita, Y. Numagami, and M. Nishijima, "Cavernous sinus dural arteriovenous fistula complicated by pontine venous congestion. A case report," *Surgical Neurology*, vol. 65, no. 5, pp. 516–518, 2006.

12

Long-Lasting Unruptured Large Intracranial Aneurysm in Bilateral Moyamoya Disease: Case Report

Eunyoung Chae,[1] **Soomin Jeong**,[1] **and Chan-Hyuk Lee**[2]

[1]*Medical School, Jeonbuk National University, Jeonju, Republic of Korea*
[2]*Department of Neurology, Asan Medical Center, Seoul, Republic of Korea*

Correspondence should be addressed to Chan-Hyuk Lee; bluewave0210@gmail.com

Academic Editor: Peter Berlit

Introduction. The rupture risk of intracranial aneurysms in patients with moyamoya disease is higher than that in the general population. We report a confirmed case of moyamoya disease with bilateral middle cerebral artery (MCA) occlusion with a large and long-lasting aneurysm. *Case.* A 71-year-old woman visited the clinic with a large intracranial aneurysm. The patient was diagnosed with an ischemic stroke 2 months ago. She exhibited weakness in the left upper and lower extremities and dysarthria and was taking aspirin. The brain magnetic resonance imaging showed complete occlusion in the bilateral MCA proximal (M1) and a large 11 × 11 mm nonruptured cerebral aneurysm in the A3 segment of the left anterior cerebral artery. On transfemoral cerebral angiography, the patient was diagnosed with Suzuki grade VI moyamoya disease with bilateral MCA occlusion. After 7 years, the cerebral aneurysm size further increased, but it remained unruptured. *Conclusions.* Here, the patient had moyamoya disease with a large aneurysm, but aneurysmal rupture did not occur even after 7 years. Our case report might help in understanding the mechanisms of cerebral aneurysm occurrence and rupture in moyamoya patients.

1. Introduction

Moyamoya disease is a chronic cerebrovascular disease involving slowly progressing cerebral artery stenosis, including the Willis' circle, without clear pathophysiology. Although its incidence is high in Asian countries, it has been reported worldwide. The incidence of intracranial aneurysms in moyamoya patients (3.4–14.8%) is higher than that in the general population (1–3%). Additionally, the rupture risk of intracranial aneurysms is high in moyamoya patients [1]. Here, we report a patient diagnosed with moyamoya disease with bilateral middle cerebral artery (MCA) occlusion and a large aneurysm in the left A3 segment, which has not ruptured for >7 years.

2. Case Presentation

A 71-year-old woman presented with an intracranial aneurysm. The patient was earlier diagnosed with acute ischemic stroke in the right periventricular white matter and centrum semiovale at another hospital 2 months ago after exhibiting weakness in the left upper and lower extremities and was prescribed aspirin. On admission, mild dysarthria and left upper and lower extremity muscle weakness (Medical Research Council Grade IV) were observed. The brain magnetic resonance imaging (MRI) showed complete occlusion in the bilateral proximal MCA (M1) and a large 11 × 11 mm nonruptured cerebral aneurysm in the A3 segment of the left anterior cerebral artery (ACA) (Figure 1). Perfusion delay was observed in both MCA regions on the brain perfusion MRI. On transfemoral cerebral angiography, the patient was diagnosed with Suzuki grade VI moyamoya disease with bilateral MCA occlusion. After 7 years, a brain MRI was performed for the observation of the cerebral aneurysm. The aneurysm increased to 17 × 13 mm in size, but it remained unruptured. The patient provided informed consent, and the study conforms to the provisions of the Declaration of Helsinki (as revised in Tokyo 2004).

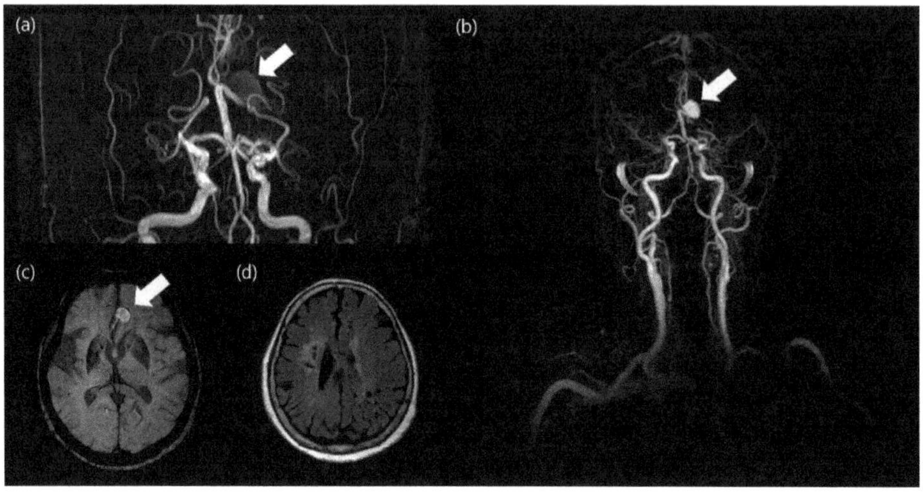

FIGURE 1: The brain MR images in moyamoya disease patients with a large intracranial aneurysm. (a) Brain TOF-MRA presenting a bilateral middle cerebral artery occlusion with a large aneurysm (arrow). (b) Brain MRA with gadolinium enhancement in the same patient with a large aneurysm (arrow). (c) SWI image presenting with large intracranial aneurysms (arrow). (d) FLAIR image showing multiple old ischemic lesions in the parenchyma.

3. Discussion

Long-term hemodynamic changes due to major cerebrovascular occlusion may lead to a high frequency of intracranial aneurysms in moyamoya patients. High shear stress not only affects the early development of aneurysms in moyamoya patients, but it also increases the levels of nitric oxide synthase, matrix metalloproteinase-2, and -9 in the aneurysmal tissue, impairing endothelial cell homeostasis. [2].

The high incidence of intracranial aneurysm in moyamoya patients may be associated with the pathological similarities between the two diseases (intracranial aneurysm and moyamoya disease). Decreased mesothelial thickness and structural defects are pathological findings in the intracranial aneurysm. In moyamoya disease, hyperproliferative vascular smooth muscle cells invade the endothelium, destroying the vascular endothelium and narrowing the lumen. The vascular mesothelium becomes fibrous and weak. Therefore, both aneurysms and moyamoya disease cause destruction of the internal elastic lamina and weaken the vascular mesothelium. Recently, derangement of the peri-endothelial matrix in moyamoya disease also increased the fragility by wall shear stress. [3].

Researchers at Nara University conducted a retrospective analysis of 111 moyamoya patients with cerebral aneurysms to study the location of the accompanying cerebral aneurysms. Of the 131 aneurysms identified in the patients, 56% were located in the circle of Willis, 18% in the basal ganglia, and 26% in the collateral vessel. In the circle of Willis, the posterior part was most common (33%), followed by the anterior part (23%). In a similar study on 2,230 moyamoya patients at Zhengzhou University Hospital, 209 cerebral aneurysms were found in 182 (8.2%) patients. Among them, 53 cases were present in the internal carotid artery, 47 cases in the anterior communicating artery or ACA, and 41 cases in the vertebrobasilar or posterior cerebral artery. Furthermore, aneurysm size >5 mm, irregular shape, and occurrence at the basilar tip or moyamoya vessels were risk factors for rupture in moyamoya patients with cerebral aneurysms.

According to the PHASES score for estimating the rupture risk of cerebral aneurysms, our patient was classified in the high-risk group for rupture (PHASES score of 14) [4]. However, the aneurysm in our patient has not ruptured for many years. We suggest two explanations for this condition. The first explanation is the aneurysmal location. Generally, arterial bifurcation aneurysms have a higher rupture risk due to hemodynamic effects [5]. However, our patient had an aneurysm slightly distal to the single A2 bifurcation. Therefore, the shear stress might have been reduced to some extent due to the turbulent flow in the branching area. In the second explanation, a fairly wide preaneurysmal artery diameter (4.3 mm) might have contributed to lowering the shear stress. A large diameter leads to an increase in the cross-sectional area, which contributes to lowering the shear stress. [6].

Aneurysms of a small diameter could be regressed by surgical procedures. Researchers in Germany investigated the microaneurysms of moyamoya vessels by using MRI. They found that one case of a microaneurysm naturally improved after bypass surgery [7]. Reduced hemodynamic stress might have contributed to the alleviation of the aneurysm.

Here, the patient with moyamoya disease did not experience an aneurysm rupture for a long period despite having a large aneurysm. Previous case studies suggest that various factors are involved in aneurysm rupture in moyamoya patients. This study will help in understanding the mechanisms of cerebral aneurysm occurrence and rupture in moyamoya patients.

Abbreviations

MR: Magnetic resonance
TOF: Time of flight

SWI: Susceptibility weighted imaging
FLAIR: Fluid-attenuated inversion recovery.

References

[1] H. Yang, L. Zhang, M. Wang, J. Wang, L. Chen, and H. Lu, "Clinical features of and risk factors for intracranial aneurysms associated with moyamoya disease," *International Journal of Stroke*, vol. 16, no. 5, pp. 542–550, 2021.

[2] Z. Wang, J. Kolega, Y. Hoi et al., "Molecular alterations associated with aneurysmal remodeling are localized in the high hemodynamic stress region of a created carotid bifurcation," *Neurosurgery*, vol. 65, no. 1, pp. 169–178, 2009.

[3] M. Matsuo, S. Nadanaka, M. Soga et al., "Vulnerability to shear stress caused by altered peri-endothelial matrix is a key feature of Moyamoya disease," *Scientific Reports*, vol. 11, no. 1, 2021.

[4] S. Huang, Z. N. Guo, M. Shi, Y. Yang, and M. Rao, "Etiology and pathogenesis of Moyamoya Disease: an update on disease prevalence," *International Journal of Stroke*, vol. 12, no. 3, pp. 246–253, 2017.

[5] S. Gholampour and S. Mehrjoo, "Effect of bifurcation in the hemodynamic changes and rupture risk of small intracranial aneurysm," *Neurosurgical Review*, vol. 44, no. 3, pp. 1703–1712, 2021.

[6] X. Zhang, T. Karuna, Z. Q. Yao et al., "High wall shear stress beyond a certain range in the parent artery could predict the risk of anterior communicating artery aneurysm rupture at follow-up," *Journal of Neurosurgery*, vol. 131, no. 3, pp. 868–875, 2019.

[7] T. Matsushige, M. Kraemer, M. Schlamann et al., "Ventricular microaneurysms in moyamoya angiopathy visualized with 7T MR angiography," *American Journal of Neuroradiology*, vol. 37, no. 9, pp. 1669–1672, 2016.

13

Tumoral Calcinosis of the Cervical Spine Associated with a Pathologic Odontoid Fracture

Andy Y. Wang,[1] **Joseph N. Tingen**,[1] **Eric J. Mahoney**,[2] **and Ron I. Riesenburger**[1]

[1]*Department of Neurosurgery, Tufts Medical Center, Boston, MA, USA*
[2]*Department of Surgery, Tufts Medical Center, Boston, MA, USA*

Correspondence should be addressed to Andy Y. Wang; andy.wang@tufts.edu

Academic Editor: Peter Berlit

Tumoral calcinosis involves focal calcium deposits in the soft tissues surrounding a joint and most commonly occurs in the hips and elbows, rarely in the cervical spine. Furthermore, it has not been known to be associated with pathologic fractures. To the best of our knowledge, our case report highlights the first case of a pathologic type II odontoid fracture associated with adjacent tumoral calcinosis, resulting in pain, dysphagia, and severe spinal stenosis. The patient underwent a posterior occipitocervical fusion and C1 laminectomy, along with planned tracheostomy and gastrostomy to avoid expected difficulty with postoperative extubation and dysphagia. Additionally, we present a review of existing literature on tumoral calcinosis in the upper cervical spine.

1. Introduction

Tumoral calcinosis is a rare clinical disease typified by focal and/or multifocal calcium masses in the soft tissue surrounding a joint in the body, typically in the juxta-articular regions [1, 2]. The first cases of calcifying masses were presented by Giard in 1898 and Duret in 1899, where they found deposition in the connective tissue surrounding a joint [3, 4]. Subsequently, the term "tumoral calcinosis" was first used by Inclan et al. in 1943, characterizing large juxta-articular lobular calcified masses showing multiple calcium-filled cysts [5]. There are several similar differentials to consider such as calcific tendonitis and calcific myonecrosis, for which imaging can aid in distinguishing [2]. Tumoral calcinosis has been found to mostly affect patients in the first two decades of life, especially in populations of African descent and without sex predominance [6]. Most of the depositions occur surrounding larger joints, including, in descending order, the hip, elbow, shoulder, foot, and wrist [6]. Tumoral calcinosis in the cervical spine is especially rare, with only a handful of reported cases.

In this case presentation, we report the first known instance of tumoral calcinosis in the cervical spine associated with a pathologic type II odontoid fracture. Typically, tumoral calcinosis patients have shown a lack of osseous destruction. However, this case demonstrates the possible association of tumoral calcinosis in the cervical spine with pathologic fracture, highlighting the need for increased awareness of tumoral calcinosis involvement in the cervical spine and the possibly increased risk of cervical instability in such patients predisposed to the disease.

2. Case Presentation

A 73-year-old female presented to our neurosurgery clinic with cervical pain. The patient uses a walker but did not remember any obvious fall or injury mechanism and presented 3 weeks prior to an outside clinic with moderate aching pain at her midposterior neck. The pain was relieved with ibuprofen, with no radiation, numbness, tingling, burning, or paresthesias. The patient did have dysphagia supported by swallow studies from an outside institution, but no decreased appetite nor dyspnea. Imaging completed at that time showed a type II odontoid fracture, and she was placed in a hard cervical collar. Past medical history is notable for tumoral calcinosis in the shoulder, hyperparathyroidism, Parkinson's disease, difficult intubation, essential hypertension, and osteoarthritis. Past surgical history is notable for multiple elbow surgeries for tumoral calcinosis. Physical exam was limited in the upper extremities with her history of shoulder surgeries, though patellar reflexes were 2+ bilaterally and negative for Babinski sign and ankle clonus.

Noncontrast computed tomography (CT) of the head and neck revealed an unstable type II odontoid fracture with significant anterolisthesis of the odontoid over C2 (Figure 1(a)). The left and right parasagittal CT images confirmed a large amount of abnormal bone ventral to C2 consistent with tumoral calcinosis which displaces the pharynx (Figure 1(b)). Magnetic resonance imaging (MRI) of the cervical spine showed C1-2 subluxation with the anteriorly displaced posterior arch of C1 resulting in severe stenosis (Figure 1(c)).

Based on the abovementioned findings along with the patient's history of tumoral calcinosis in the shoulder, we determined the diagnosis of pathological type II odontoid fracture secondary to tumoral calcinosis with C1 stenosis and cervical instability resulting in pain and dysphagia. The patient opted for surgical intervention and underwent a posterior occipitocervical fusion (occiput to C3) with posterior C1 laminectomy. She also underwent planned tracheostomy and G-tube placement under the same anesthetic to avoid likely difficulties with postoperative extubation and dysphagia.

The patient was brought to the operating room and intubated under general anesthesia with placement of a Foley catheter and neuromonitoring leads to monitor for intact motor and somatosensory evoked potentials. Upon exposure, the C1-C2 area appeared very unstable. The occipital keel plate was placed, and three midline keel screws were placed with bilateral purchase. Bilateral C2 pars screws and bilateral C3 lateral mass screws were placed, and rods were placed to stabilize the occipitocervical junction (Figure 2). For the decompression, a wide C1 laminectomy was performed. The thecal sac appeared well decompressed. Locally harvested autograft was denuded of soft tissue and combined with osteomatrix bone graft extender and laid along the posterior decorticated posterolateral elements to complete the arthrodesis. Final somatosensory evoked potentials, and motor evoked potentials were stable and intact.

Subsequently, general surgery performed the tracheostomy and Stamm gastrostomy under the same anesthetic. During the tracheostomy, it was noticed that her tracheal rings were calcified. Attempt at percutaneous G-tube placement failed, as the mass effect from the tumoral calcinosis posterior to the pharynx prevented the passage of the endoscope. Therefore, an open G-tube was placed. The patient tolerated the procedure well and was discharged to rehab. Postoperative visits showed well-positioned hardware, and the tracheostomy was discontinued without event after 2 weeks. Her swallowing also improved slowly, and the G-tube was removed three months after surgery. She reports doing well 6 months following surgery with improvement in her neck pain.

3. Discussion

Tumoral calcinosis is characterized by calcium deposition in the juxta-articular regions and is known to occur mostly in regions outside of the spine such as the hip and elbow. Calcification in the spine is much less common since it consists of much smaller joints, and tumoral calcinosis in the cervical spine is rarer. The patient described in this case report was found to have a pathological type II odontoid fracture secondary to tumoral calcinosis with C1 stenosis and cervical instability. Smack et al.'s classification of tumoral calcinosis separated the disease into three subtypes—normophosphatemic primary, hyperphosphatemic primary, and secondary tumoral calcinosis [7]. Due to our patient's previous history with hyperparathyroidism, her ultimate diagnosis was secondary tumoral calcinosis. However, unlike any other reported cases of tumoral calcinosis in the cervical spine, our patient's cervical instability is associated with a pathological fracture. This case report raises the concern for pathologic fractures to be considered when determining the diagnosis and management of tumoral calcinosis.

We considered several differential diagnoses (Table 1). In terms of the other calcifying disorders, calcific tendinitis shows increased calcium levels centered within a tendon but does not involve deposition of calcium into a mass. Synovial osteochondromatosis involves calcification in the sheath between joints and tendons but occurs in an intra-articular location rather than periarticular like in tumoral calcinosis. Other differential diagnoses such as myositis ossificans, heterotopic ossification, and tophaceous gout are characterized by nonlobular masses [2, 6]. Imaging is particularly helpful to help differentiate findings specific to tumoral calcinosis. On radiographs, tumoral calcinosis has distinguishable features in the periarticular region, including amorphous, cystic, and multilobulated calcifications [6]. These masses can be better distinguished by CT scans, particularly showing fluid-fluid levels due to calcium layering in a process termed the sedimentation sign. The CT scans in Figure 1 include findings of cystic loculi and calcium layering, aiding in our diagnosis of tumoral calcinosis. The primary treatment for tumoral calcinosis in all joint regions is surgical excision of the calcified mass [6]. Since recurrence is common, some have attempted to use low phosphate diets or phosphate binders.

Compared to other case reports of tumoral calcinosis in the cervical spine, this patient's associated pathologic fracture with tumoral calcinosis is singly unique. Only 22 reported cases involve tumoral calcinosis around C1 or C2, and none of these cases have been associated with a pathological fracture (Table 2). Many of the cases in the upper cervical spine were also presented with spinal stenosis and dysphagia [8–19]; however, tumoral calcinosis and anterolisthesis resulting in a fracture of the cervical joint are essentially absent from the literature. This case report provides a valuable addition to the currently limited available literature. The current literature tends to focus on the pathological etiology and how tumoral calcinosis has been associated with chronic renal failure, systemic sclerosis,

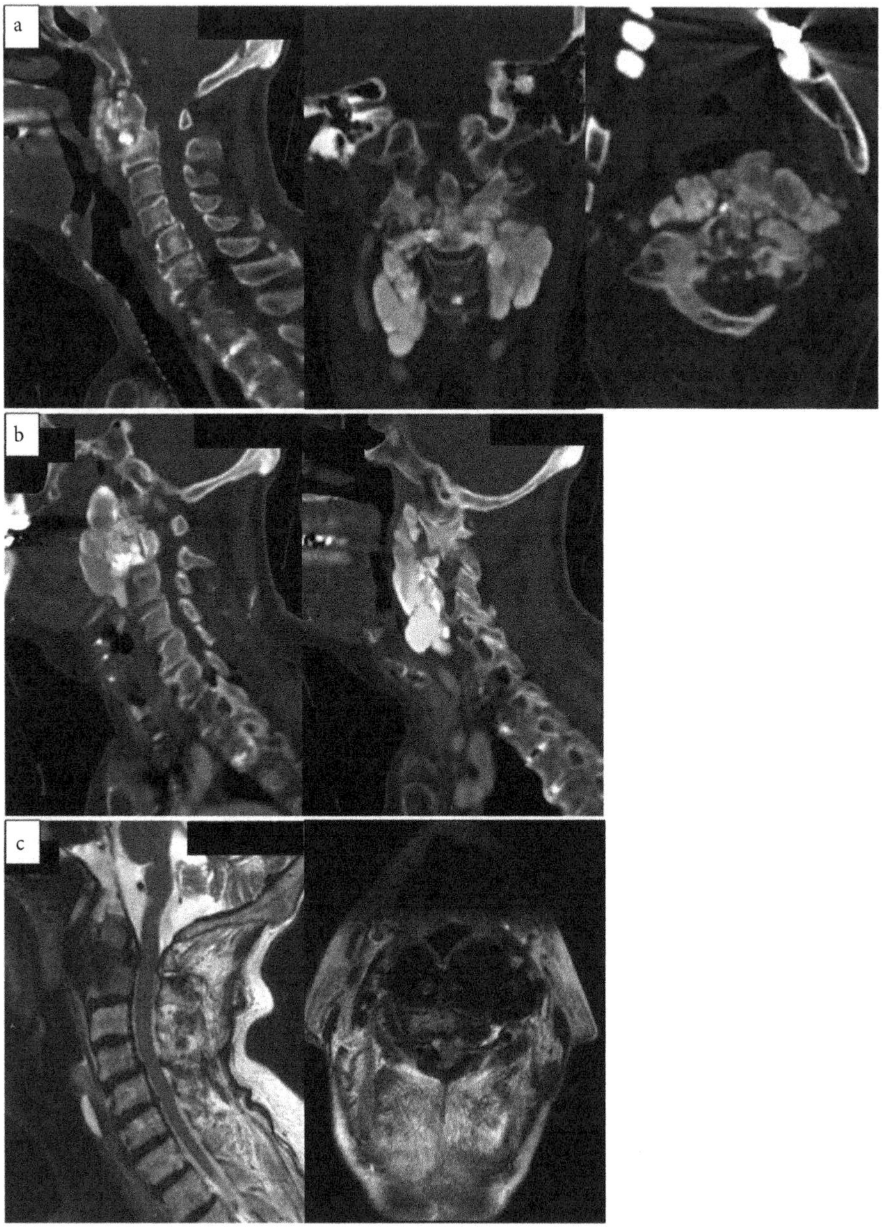

FIGURE 1: Noncontrast CT scans and T2-weighted MRI of preoperative odontoid fracture with associated tumoral calcinosis. (a) Sagittal, coronal, and axial CT images, respectively from left to right, show pathological type II odontoid fracture, (b) left: left parasagittal CT image shows extensive tumoral calcinosis; right: right parasagittal CT image shows extensive tumoral calcinosis, and (c) left: T2-weighted sagittal MRI shows spinal cord compression at C1-C2; right: T2-weighted axial MRI at C1-C2.

and collagen and vascular disorders. We present a new perspective, emphasizing a new risk that may emerge from tumoral calcinosis. Although a pathological fracture secondary to tumoral calcinosis in the cervical spine does not appear in the literature, Miura et al. presented a case of tumoral calcinosis in the thoracic spine with an associated fracture that parallels our patient's condition [20]. It is imperative that these factors are considered in the possible association of fracture risk with tumoral calcinosis. Our current patient also presents with Parkinson's disease, not described as a comorbidity with the other case reports. Patients with compromised motor control may be at further risk of spinal cord instability and injury, which may necessitate further precautions in preventing a joint fracture.

To our knowledge, this is the first report of tumoral calcinosis in the cervical spine with an associated pathological type II odontoid fracture. This case raises the possibility of tumoral calcinosis involving surrounding regions, which may apply to tumoral calcinosis outside of the spine as well. Further research is needed to better understand the biochemical underpinnings of this process, such as the role of inflammatory markers [20]. Physicians and clinicians should be wary of the possibility of pathologic fracture in patients with tumoral calcinosis.

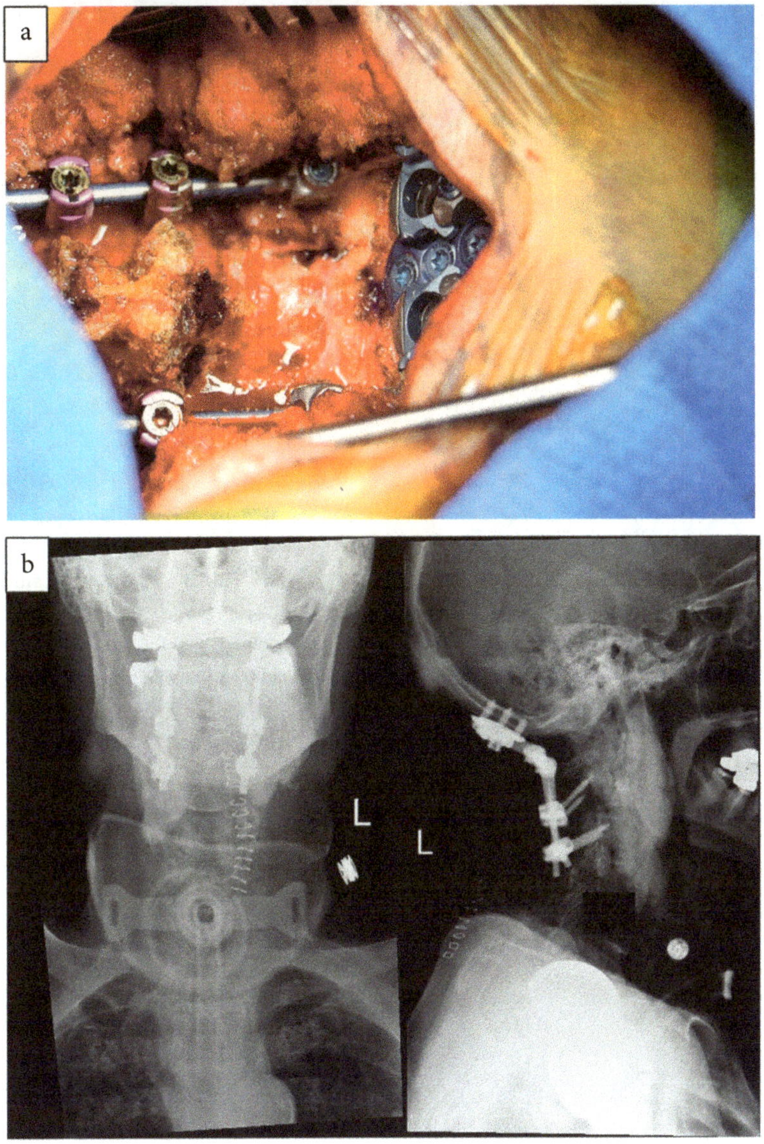

FIGURE 2: (a) Intraoperative photo of the posterior occipitocervical (occiput to C3) fusion with a posterior C1 laminectomy. (b) Postoperative AP and lateral x-rays of the cervical spine showing the construct.

TABLE 1: Differential diagnoses considered.

Differential diagnosis	Rationale
Infection	No local (redness, swelling, and other skin findings) nor systemic signs (fever) and no disc space involvement
Type I odontoid fracture secondary to trauma	Type I involves avulsion of the rostral tip of the odontoid process; in this case, the fracture is at the base
Type III odontoid fracture secondary to trauma	Type III involves fracture through the body of C2; in this case, the fracture is at the base
Type II odontoid fracture secondary to trauma alone	Type II involves fracture through the base of the odontoid process, which matches this case, but there is no identifiable fall or injury mechanism
Pathologic type II odontoid fracture secondary to primary bone tumor or bone metastases	No evidence of primary bone tumor or metastases on imaging, no clinical symptoms such as weight loss, and no personal or family history
Pathologic type II odontoid fracture secondary to tumoral calcinosis	This differential matches the type of odontoid fracture and explains why there is a fracture despite no obvious injury mechanism. The patient has a history of tumoral calcinosis and along with the radiological findings, differentiates tumoral calcinosis from other calcifying conditions

Table 2: Existing case reports of tumoral calcinosis involving the upper cervical spine at C1 or C2.

Authors, year	Sex	Age	Location	Associated conditions	Clinical presentation	Treatment
Kokubun et al., 1996	F	68	C1-C2	NP	Neck pain below the occiput	Resection, laminectomy
Arginteanu et al., 1997 [9]	F	65	C1–C5	SS	Neck pain	Decompression, resection, fusion
Mooney et al., 1997	M	17 mo.	C1-C2	NP	Torticollis	Resection, limited laminectomy
Ward et al., 1997	F	62	C1-C2	SS	Left-side neck pain, limited range of motion, tenderness	CT-guided aspiration
Durant et al., 2001 [8]	M	78	C1-C2	OA, HTN	Pannus from RA	Posterior fusion, excision
Matsukado et al., 2001 [1]	F	54	C2–C4	RF, RM	Cervical pain, weakness	C-2 laminectomy, C3-4 laminoplasty
Van de Perre et al., 2003	F	74	C2–C7	SS	Increasing joint/neck pain	NS
Olsen et al., 2004	F	75	C2–C4	SS	Torticollis, swelling	CT-guided biopsy and excision
Smucker et al., 2006 [11]	M	60	C1-C2	SS	Severe upper neck pain, myelopathy	Decompression, resection, fusion
Smucker et al., 2006 [11]	F	59	C2–C5	SS	Neck pain	Laminectomy, resection, fusion
Tuy et al., 2008	F	50	C2-C3	RF, previous scleroderma	Neck pain	Resection
Shoji et al., 2012	F	34	C1-C2	SS	Severe headache, narrowed face	NS
Bisson-Vaivre et al., 2013	F	72	C1-C2	SS	Severe upper neck pain	Colchicine treatment
Chang et al., 2013	F	44	C1-C2	RF, HTN	Severe neck soreness, headache	C1 laminectomy, fixation, fusion
Daumas et al., 2013	F	60	C2–C5	SS	NS	NS
Lebl et al., 2013	F	63	C1-C2	SS	Severe neck pain, limited range of motion	Physical therapy, steroid injections
Al-Khudairi et al., 2015 [16]	F	62	C2–C6	SS	Weakness, altered sensation, inability to mobilize	Decompression, fusion
Ashraf et al., 2015	M	5 mo.	C2-C3	Familial RA	Torticollis	CT-guided biopsy, excision
Fatehi et al., 2016	F	73	C2-C3	HTN, RF	Growing painful mass	Only hemodialysis
Mooney et al., 2017 [18]	F	60	C1-C2	HTN	Dysphagia, neck pain	Transoral decompression
Ebot et al., 2019	F	71	C1-C2	NS	Neck pain	C1-C2 laminectomy
Steward et al., 2019	F	4 mo.	C1-C2	NS	Loss of head control, neck hypotonia	Surgical excision
Current case report	F	73	C1-C2	HTN, Parkinson's, HP	Achy neck pain, dysphagia, pathological fracture	Occ-cervical fusion, C1 laminectomy, tracheostomy

M: male, F: female, HP: hyperparathyroidism, OA: osteoarthritis, NP: no particular cause, NS: not specified, HTN: hypertension, RA; rheumatoid arthritis, RF: renal failure, RM: radiculomyelopathy, SS: systemic sclerosis/scleroderma, RI: renal insufficiency.

References

[1] K. Matsukato, T. Amano, O. Itou, F. Yuhi, and S. Nagata, "Tumoral calcinosis in the upper cervical spine causing progressive radiculomyelopathy," *Neurologia Medico-Chirurgica*, vol. 41, pp. 411–414, 2001.

[2] I. Fathi and M. Sakr, "Review of tumoral calcinosis: a rare clinico-pathological entity," *World Journal of Clinical Cases*, vol. 2, no. 9, pp. 409–414, 2014.

[3] A. Giard, "Sur la calcification hibernale," *Comptes Rendus des Séances de la Société de Biologie et de ses Filiales*, vol. 10, pp. 1013–1015, 1898.

[4] M. H. Duret, "Tumours multiples et singulieres des bourses sereuses," *Bull Mem Soc Anat Paris*, vol. 74, pp. 725–733, 1899.

[5] A. Inclan, P. P. Leon, and M. Camejo, "Tumoral calcinosis," *Journal of the American Medical Association*, vol. 121, no. 7, pp. 490–495, 1943.

[6] K. M. Olsen and F. S. Chew, "Tumoral calcinosis: pearls, polemics, and alternative possibilities," *Radio Graphics*, vol. 26, no. 3, pp. 871–885, 2006.

[7] D. P. Smack, S. A. Norton, and J. E. Fitzpatrick, "Proposal for a pathogenesis-based classification of tumoral calcinosis," *International Journal of Dermatology*, vol. 35, no. 4, pp. 265–271, 1996.

[8] D. M. Durant, L. H. Riley 3rd, P. C. Burger, and E. F. McCarthy, "Tumoral calcinosis of the spine a study of 21 cases," *Spine*, vol. 26, no. 15, pp. 1673–1679, 2001.

[9] M. S. Arginteanu and N. I. Perin, "Paraspinal calcinosis associated with progressive systemic sclerosis," *Journal of Neurosurgery*, vol. 87, no. 5, pp. 761–763, 1997.

[10] J. G. Ojemann, R. L. Grubb, M. Kyriakos, and K. B. Baker, "Calcium carbonate apatite deposition in the cervical spine with associated vertebral destruction," *Journal of Neurosurgery*, vol. 86, no. 6, pp. 1022–1026, 1997.

[11] J. D. Smucker, J. G. Heller, H. H. Bohlman, and T. E. Whitesides, "Surgical treatment of destructive calcific

lesions of the cervical spine in scleroderma: case series and review of the literature," *Spine*, vol. 31, no. 17, pp. 2002–2008, 2006.

[12] A. P. Carlson, H. M. Yonas, and P. T. Turner, "Disorders of tumoral calcification of the spine," *Journal of Spinal Disorders & Techniques*, vol. 20, no. 1, pp. 97–103, 2007.

[13] W. Jackson, A. Sethi, J. Carp, G. Talpos, and R. Vaidya, "Unusual spinal manifestation in secondary hyperparathyroidism: a case report," *Spine*, vol. 32, no. 19, pp. E557–E560, 2007.

[14] N. Miyakoshi, Y. Shimada, Y. Kasukawa, and S. Ando, "Progressive myelopathy due to idiopathic intraspinal tumoral calcinosis of the cervical spine," *Journal of Neurosurgery: Spine*, vol. 7, no. 3, pp. 362–365, 2007.

[15] R. H. Wong, A. P. Bhansali, and E. M. Doppenberg, "Cervical spine instability from tumoral calcinosis," *Acta Neurochirurgica*, vol. 155, no. 7, pp. 1245-1246, 2013.

[16] N. Al-Khudairi, S. Kobayashi, and A. Meir, "A case of symptomatic cervical spine calcinosis in systemic sclerosis," *The Spine Journal*, vol. 15, no. 9, pp. 2099-2100, 2015.

[17] A. Al-Sukaini, N. R. Paulino Pereira, E. W. Yu, I. Chebib, M. A. Bredella, and J. Schwab, "Idiopathic tumoral calcinosis-like lesion in the lower cervical spine causing acute central cord syndrome: case report," *Journal of Neurosurgery: Spine*, vol. 26, no. 1, pp. 97–102, 2017.

[18] M. A. Mooney, M. E. Oppenlander, U. K. Kakarla, and N. Theodore, "Tumoral calcinosis of the craniovertebral junction as a cause of dysphagia with treatment by transoral decompression: case report," *Journal of Neurosurgery: Spine*, vol. 26, no. 5, pp. 567–571, 2017.

[19] S.-I. Motegi, A. Sekiguchi, S. Toki, H. Amano, and O. Ishikawa, "Progressive myelopathy in systemic sclerosis patient with cervical intraspinal calcinosis," *The Journal of Dermatology*, vol. 44, no. 2, pp. 209-210, 2017.

[20] I. Miura, M. Kubota, K. Takebayashi et al., "Tumoral calcinosis of thoracic spine associated with vertebral fracture and inflammatory reactions," *Case Reports in Orthopedics*, vol. 2020, Article ID 8881698, 5 pages, 2020.

14

Something Got Your Tongue? A Unique Cause of Hypoglossal Nerve Palsy

Alan Tesson,[1] **Peter Kranz**,[2] **Ali Zomorodi**,[3] **and Joel Morgenlander**[4]

[1]*Inova Neuroscience Service Line, Inova Health System, 8081 Innovation Park Dr, Fairfax, VA 22031, USA*
[2]*Department of Radiology, Duke University Medical Center, 2301 Erwin Rd, Durham, NC 27710, USA*
[3]*Department of Neurosurgery, Duke University Medical Center, 2301 Erwin Rd, Durham, NC 27710, USA*
[4]*Department of Neurology, Duke University Medical Center, 2301 Erwin Rd, Durham, NC 27710, USA*

Correspondence should be addressed to Alan Tesson; alan.tesson@duke.edu

Academic Editor: Dominic B. Fee

Introduction. The authors report a rare cause of isolated hypoglossal nerve palsy caused by a high cervical osteophyte. This case increases clinical knowledge of an underreported condition and teaches the clinician radiologic pearls in making the diagnosis. To their knowledge, this is the first case report showing surgical remediation of this condition. *Symptoms and Clinical Findings.* A 73-year-old female presented with several months of occipital headache, progressive dysarthria, dysphagia, and tongue deviation to the right. Her neurologic exam was significant for atrophy of the right hemitongue with tongue fasciculations. On protrusion, her tongue deviated rightward. *Diagnosis and Therapeutic Intervention.* Careful review of her initial head computed tomography (CT) imaging revealed that a high cervical osteophyte caused unilateral, isolated hypoglossal nerve palsy. Neurosurgery performed a right, far lateral approach for decompression of this osteophyte and over the ensuing months her symptoms improved. *Conclusion.* High cervical osteophyte is an underrecognized cause of isolated hypoglossal nerve palsy. The imaging investigation should be systematic and focus on the skull base with magnetic resonance imaging (MRI) or CT. This is a rare occasion when high resolution CT of the skull base can actually be the more helpful imaging modality. As shown in this case, an osteoarthritic cause can be surgically ameliorated.

1. Case

A 73-year-old woman with a history of osteoarthritis and hypertension complained of a chronic but progressive right occipital headache and was developing problems with her tongue. Six weeks prior to presentation, she noticed uncoordinated tongue movements, tongue deviating right on protrusion, and dysarthria. She had difficulty manipulating a food bolus in her mouth and continually bit her right cheek and tongue. Subsequently she had lost ten pounds. She denied facial weakness, ptosis, diplopia, facial sensory changes, or taste perversion.

Her neurologic exam was significant for atrophy of the right hemitongue with tongue fasciculations. On protrusion, her tongue deviated rightward. Taste was preserved. The remainder of her cranial nerve, facial motor, and peripheral motor exam, including muscle bulk and tone were normal. There were no peripheral fasciculations. Sensory exam and reflexes were normal.

Without detailed history of tongue weakness, an initial noncontrast head CT was read as normal. MRI brain with and without contrast showed atrophy of the right tongue associated with subtle fatty infiltration and T2 hyperintensity suggestive of denervation atrophy. Lumbar puncture and erythrocyte sedimentation rate were normal. Electromyography (EMG) with nerve conduction study was performed to evaluate for more diffuse neuromuscular disease. The only abnormal finding on EMG was a subacute right hypoglossal neuropathy.

After reviewing the head CT and MRI with neuroradiology and including clear clinical information, degenerative osteophytes were seen projecting from the right atlanto-

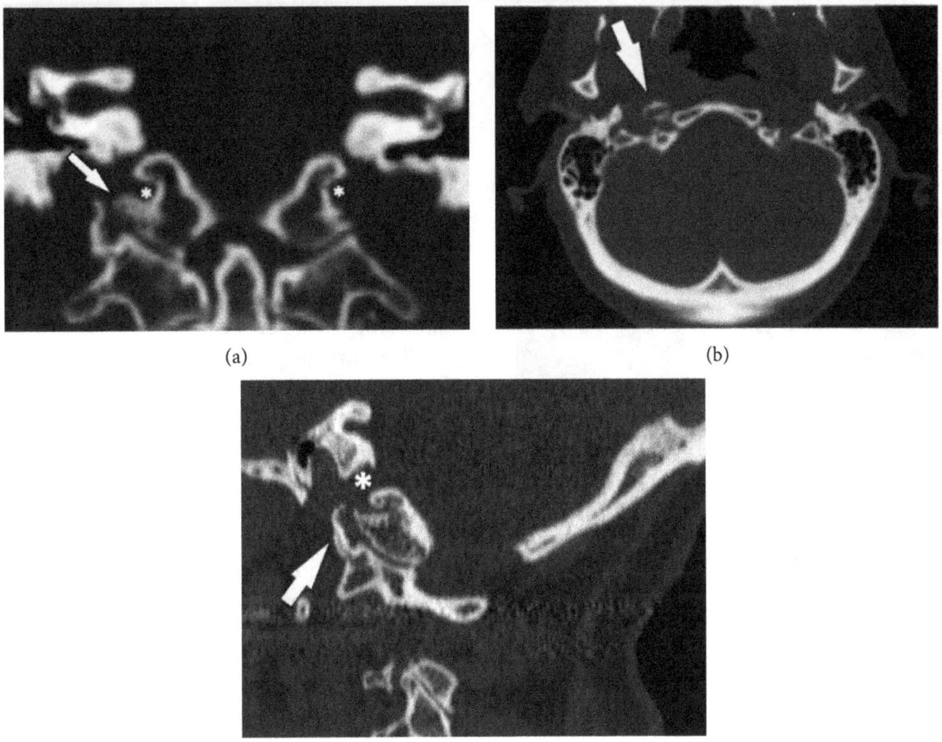

(a) (b) (c)

Figure 1: (a) Coronal reformatted CT image shows osteophytosis (arrow) of the atlanto-occipital articulation on the right. The osteophyte arising from the occipital condyle narrows the hypoglossal canal (asterisks). (b) Axial CT showing osteophyte in the right hypoglossal canal. (c) Sagittal CT showing osteophyte in the right hypoglossal canal.

occipital joint laterally to the adjacent right carotid space, best seen on the CT (Figures 1(a)–1(c)). The osteophyte could be seen at the exit of the right hypoglossal canal on axial MRI images but it was much more difficult to visualize (Figure 2).

Based on our patient's workup, we concluded that she had an isolated hypoglossal nerve palsy from an atlanto-occipital osteophyte compressing the nerve as it exited the hypoglossal canal. Neurosurgery was consulted. To decompress the nerve and stabilize her condition, surgery was indicated.

The patient was taken to the operating room for a right, far lateral approach for decompression of this osteophyte. Subperiosteal dissection was used to expose the suboccipital bone and the mastoid bone. The high-speed drill was used to turn a suboccipital craniotomy and perform a partial mastoidectomy to decompress the sigmoid sinus and the jugular bulb. The high cervical region was then dissected. The occipital and C1 condyles were exposed and the drill was used to resect the condyle down to the level of the hypoglossal canal. This decompressed the hypoglossal nerve adequately without having to remove the osteophyte. The dura was then closed in a water tight fashion. The bone was replaced using the plating system. The muscles were reapproximated. The scalp was then closed in layers. Postoperative CT is shown in Figure 3.

She noticed improvement within months that has persisted over 3 years. Her tongue function including eating and swallowing was much improved. The right half of her tongue was less atrophic. The tongue now protruded midline. Her right occipital headache had resolved. Only some mild numbness around her surgical scar remained. From her

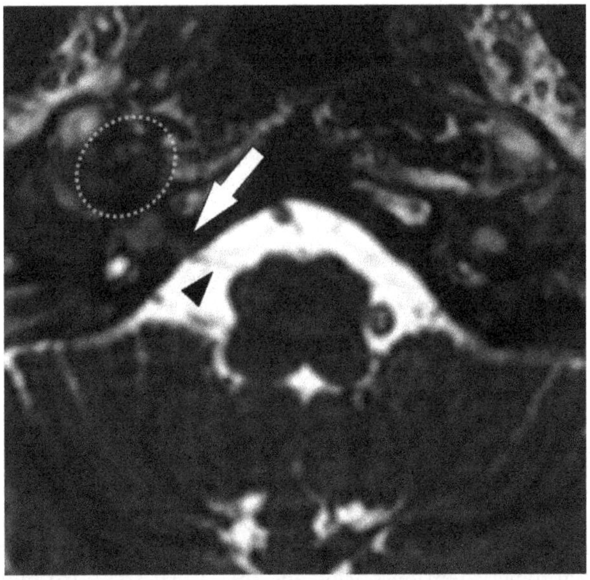

Figure 2: Axial steady-state free procession MR image through the skull base shows the hypoglossal nerve (arrowhead) passing through the hypoglossal canal (arrow). The osteophyte (dashed oval) lies just anterior to the hypoglossal canal, along the expected path of the hypoglossal nerve.

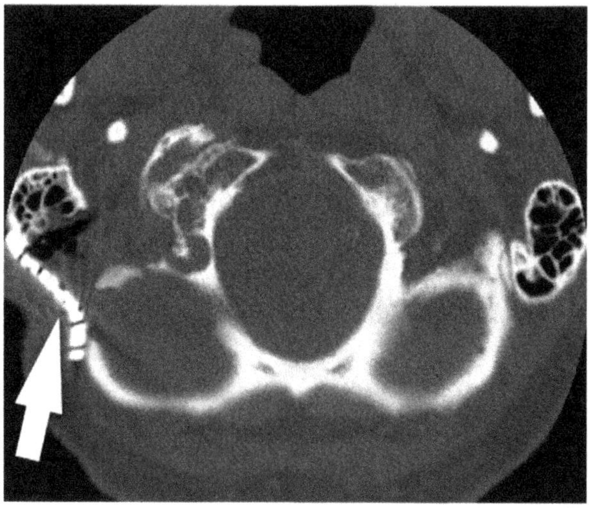

Figure 3: Axial CT image showing postoperative appearance. The hypoglossal canal was decompressed laterally via partial mastoidectomy, high cervical dissection, and partial resection of the occipital condyle. Metallic plating (arrow) covers the postoperative site.

perspective, she was pleased with the surgical outcome. To the best of our knowledge, this is the first described surgically ameliorated case of hypoglossal nerve palsy caused by high cervical osteophyte.

2. Discussion

Hypoglossal nerve injury is not uncommon when it occurs with other lower cranial nerve palsies [1], but isolated hypoglossal nerve palsy is rare. Isolated hypoglossal nerve palsy has been previously reviewed [2, 3]. The best way to ascertain the cause of hypoglossal nerve injury is to use an anatomical segmental approach. By subdividing the course of the hypoglossal nerve into five sections (brain stem, premedullary cistern, skull base/hypoglossal canal, nasopharyngeal/carotid area, and sublingual area), the number of differential causes in each area becomes more manageable and easier for the clinician to remember [3].

The most common cause of isolated hypoglossal nerve palsy is skull base tumor (either metastasis or primitive malignant or benign tumor), accounting for up to 50% of cases [2, 3]. Cranial trauma producing occipital condyle fracture is the second most common cause. This cranial trauma tends to occur in two ways—deceleration trauma from road accidents [4] or surgical trauma. The most common surgical injury is neck surgery or prolonged cervical hyperextension during anesthesia [3]. The third most common cause of isolated hypoglossal injury is internal carotid artery dissection. Cervical rheumatoid arthritis and cervical osteophytes from osteoarthritis have been more rarely implicated [5–7]. In children and adolescents, infectious mononucleosis should be investigated [2].

More modern case series are questioning if hypoglossal nerve palsy caused by craniocervical junction (CCJ) degenerative disease is an under-recognized entity because of provider unawareness compounded by difficulty in identifying the offending lesions on initial CT or MRI standard formats [7]. This was highlighted by our case. Alerting the radiologist to one's suspicion of this diagnosis is critical so they can dedicate attention to the skull base and perform CT reconstructions if necessary. A retrospective series from the Mayo Clinic of 18 patients with hypoglossal nerve palsy from CCJ degenerative disease concluded that a small field of view; thin-section (≤2 mm) axial, coronal, and sagittal soft tissue; and bone reconstructions centered at the hypoglossal canal are more effective at identifying the offending CCJ degenerative disease [7].

The imaging investigation should be systematic and focus on the skull base with MRI or CT [1]. This is one of those rare occasions when high resolution CT of the skull base can actually be the more helpful imaging modality. This was the case with our patient. As shown in our case, an osteoarthritic cause can be surgically ameliorated. The patient was pleased at the improvement in most neurologic symptoms and resolution of her right occipital headache. Since the osteophyte was left in place postoperatively, the headache was likely due to associated CCJ degenerative disease and improved after the surgery. Retrospective case series of 18 patients with hypoglossal nerve palsy from CCJ degenerative disease identified major associated complaint of new or worsening headache or suboccipital pain in 13 of 18 patients [7]. Her timely presentation and surgery within two months of symptom onset likely contributed to the favorable outcome.

Acknowledgments

This research did not receive specific funding. It was performed as part of the routine employment of the authors at Duke University Health System.

References

[1] A. M. Stino, B. E. Smith, M. Temkit, and S. N. Reddy, "Hypoglossal nerve palsy: 245 cases," *Muscle & Nerve*, vol. 54, no. 6, pp. 1050–1054, 2016.

[2] J. R. Keane, "Twelfth-nerve palsy. Analysis of 100 cases," *Archives of Neurology*, vol. 53, no. 6, pp. 561–566, 1996.

[3] A. Guarnizo, R. Glikstein, and C. Torres, "Imaging features of isolated hypoglossal nerve palsy," *Journal of Neuroradiology*, vol. 47, no. 2, pp. 136–150, 2020.

[4] B. Castling and K. Hicks, "Traumatic isolated unilateral hypoglossal nerve palsy - case report and review of the literature," *British Journal of Oral and Maxillofacial Surgery*, vol. 33, no. 3, pp. 171–173, 1995.

[5] V. Patron, P. Y. Roudaut, J. Lerat, M. Vivent, J. P. Bessede, and K. Aubry, "Isolated hypoglossal palsy due to cervical osteophyte," *European Annals of Otorhinolaryngology, Head and Neck diseases*, vol. 129, no. 1, pp. e44–e46, 2012.

[6] S. N. Patro, C. Torres, and R. Riascos, "An unusual case of isolated hypoglossal nerve palsy secondary to osteophytic projection from the atlanto-occipital joint," *The Neuroradiology Journal*, vol. 27, no. 3, pp. 361–364, 2014.

[7] S. M. Weindling, R. D. Goff, C. P. Wood, D. DeLone, and J. Hoxworth, "Is hypoglossal nerve palsy caused by craniocervical junction degenerative disease an underrecognized entity?" *AJNR Am J Neuroradiol*, vol. 37, no. 11, pp. 2138–2143, 2016.

15

Transient Dyschromatopsia, Static Form Agnosia and Prosopagnosia Observed in a Patient with Anti-NMDA Receptor Encephalitis

Ritsuo Hashimoto,[1] **Asako Tagawa,**[2] **Noriyo Komori,**[3]
Tomoko Ogawa,[1] **and Hiroyuki Kato**[1]

[1]*Department of Neurology, International University of Health and Welfare Hospital, Japan*
[2]*Department of Neurology, Hiratsuka City Hospital, Japan*
[3]*Department of Language and Hearing Sciences, International University of Health and Welfare, Japan*

Correspondence should be addressed to Ritsuo Hashimoto; ritsuo@iuhw.ac.jp

Academic Editor: Norman S. Litofsky

We presented a case of a 19-year-old woman who suffered from anti-*N*-methyl-D-aspartate (NMDA) receptor encephalitis associated with ovarian teratoma. The patient showed a variety of higher visual symptoms which changed over the recovery phase of the disease. In chronological order, she experienced cortical blindness, amblyopia, dyschromatopsia, static form agnosia, and prosopagnosia. Among these symptoms, the most intriguing was the static form agnosia. Although she could recognize the forms of moving objects, she could not make out those of stationary ones. All of these visual symptoms were transient, implying that she might have incidentally regained the function of the distinct cortical visual areas in the time course of follow-up. This case further suggests that visual functions concerned with the perceptions of static form and form-from-motion could be dissociable and may rely on distinct brain regions.

1. Introduction

Anti-*N*-methyl-D-aspartate (NMDA) receptor encephalitis is an autoimmune disease first reported over a decade ago among women who were diagnosed with ovarian teratoma and who presented with a variety of neurological symptoms, including behavioral changes, hallucinations, memory deficits, seizures, decreased level of consciousness, and central hypoventilation [1]. A definitive association between anti-NMDA autoantibodies and encephalitis was established by Josep Dalmau and colleagues in 2007 [2]. Here, we report a case of a young woman with anti-NMDA receptor encephalitis associated with ovarian teratoma who showed a variety of cortical visual symptoms including dyschromatopsia, static form agnosia, and prosopagnosia during the recovery phase of the disease. Among these symptoms, the most intriguing was the static form agnosia, wherein she could recognize the forms of moving objects but not of stationary objects. We discuss a possible underlying mechanism of the symptom.

2. Case Report

A 19-year-old right handed woman was referred to our hospital with complaints of persistent fever and headache from 3 days before. At the time of initial symptoms, her family members reported strange behavior as the patient had repeatedly asked the same questions. On admission, she still retained consciousness and could recognize her family members, but was disorientated to time and place. Magnetic resonance imaging (MRI) on admission demonstrated no signal abnormalities in the brain, including the medial temporal areas. Cerebrospinal fluid (CSF) examination on admission revealed lymphocyte dominant pleocytosis (lymphocytes 168/mm^3, polymorphonuclear cells 13/mm^3) with a

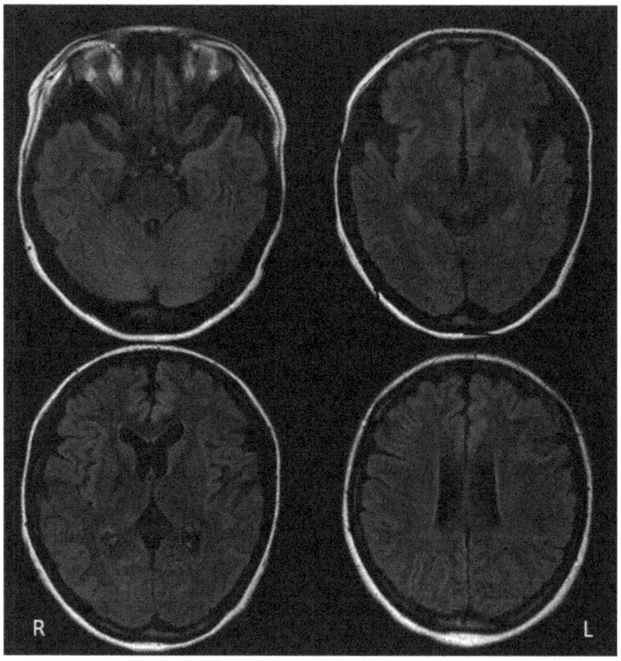

Figure 1: Axial fluid-attenuated inversion recovery (FLAIR) images of the brain two months after admission. Note the slight high intensities in the bilateral occipital cortices and subcortical white matter, which were somewhat prominent on the right side, as well as small subcortical high intensities in the right frontal lobe. However, there were no signal abnormalities in the medial temporal areas.

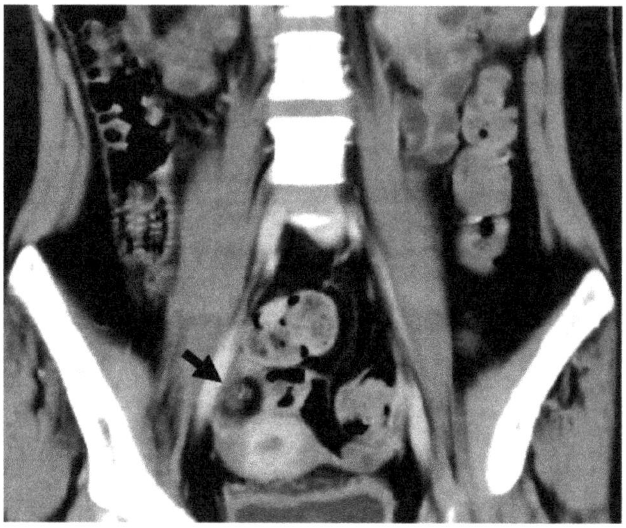

Figure 2: Abdominal CT after 8 months of admission demonstrating a small ovarian calcified cystic mass on the right side (arrow).

protein level of 46 mg/dL (normal 15–40 mg/dL) and a sugar level of 61 mg/dL (normal 50–70 mg/dL). A clinical diagnosis of encephalitis was made and an intravenous administration of acyclovir, fosphenytoin sodium hydrate, and glycerol was initiated. On the second day of admission, she developed repeated generalized tonic-clonic convulsions leading to a convulsive status. She required supportive therapy involving intubation, mechanical ventilation, and sedation. A test for herpes simplex virus (HSV)-PCR of the CSF was negative. Antibodies against GluN1/GluN2 heteromers of the NMDA receptor were detected in serum at two different times (Table 1). From this evidence, a diagnosis of anti-NMDA receptor encephalitis was made. Two months after admission, fluid-attenuated inversion recovery (FLAIR) images of brain MRI showed areas of slightly high intensity in the bilateral occipital cortices and subcortical white matter, which were somewhat prominent on the right side, as well as small subcortical high intensities in the right frontal lobe (Figure 1). Over the following several months, orofacial dyskinesia and bibrachial spasm occurred frequently despite immunotherapy with high-dose methylprednisolone (1000 mg/day for 3 days) twice and intravenous immunoglobulin (400 mg/kg/day for 5 days) once. She was weaned off the ventilator 6 months after admission, though she was still unconscious.

Abdominal computed tomography (CT) and MRI for the purpose of detecting ovarian tumor were both negative on initial examinations. However, a repeated abdominal CT after 8 months of admission revealed a small ovarian calcified cystic mass on the right side (Figure 2). The patient had the tumor removed, which was diagnosed as a mature cystic ovarian tumor on pathological examination. After the removal of the tumor, she received high-dose methylprednisolone and intravenous immunoglobulin therapy again. Three months after these treatments (12 months after admission), the patient's consciousness improved gradually and she was slowly able to respond to verbal commands.

At this time, she stated that she could not see anything. Ophthalmological examination revealed that pupillary reaction and extraocular movements were normal. In addition, there were no abnormalities in the anterior and posterior components of the eyes, including the lens, retina, and optic fundi. The patient's exact visual acuity was difficult to estimate because she complained of fatigue and often refused to continue the test. Regarding color perception, she could differentiate a red cup from a blue cup; however, she could not distinguish a blue cup from a green cup. On behavioral observations, she behaved like a blind person; although she could walk while holding hands with a caregiver, she frequently collided with doors. When she attempted to pick up her comb or toothbrush from a table, she explored these objects by palpating with her hand across the table. She could not recognize stationary objects by visual inspection alone, but she could identify them by tactility or hearing the sounds that they made. Around this time, it was incidentally noticed that she could successfully respond to the examiner's motions. For example, when the examiner waved their hand, she waved back. On a different occasion, when the examiner swayed their body, the patient immediately imitated the movements. These observations suggested the patient was able to see moving objects better than stationary objects, despite her serious visual impairment.

Subsequently, we further examined her visual abilities in detail. First, the patient was asked to detect stationary visual stimuli presented on a computer screen placed 30 cm

Table 1: Laboratory data.

WBC	16700/μL	(3500–9700)	Influenza A	-	
RBC	$490 \times 10^4/\mu$L	($376–516 \times 10^4$)	Influenza B	-	
Plt	$28.7 \times 10^4/\mu$L	($14.0–37.9 \times 10^4$)	ANA	<40	(<79)
AST	12 IU/L	(8–38)	CEA/CLIA	1.1	(0.0–5.0)
ALT	10 IU/L	(4–44)	CA19-9	<=1.0	(0.0–37.0)
BUN	4.2 mg/dL	(8.0–20.0)	CA125	13.4	(0.0–35.0)
Cr	0.55 mg/dL	(0.47–0.79)	NSE/RIA	14.8	(0.1–16.3)
CPK	109 IU/L	(43–165)	CA602	10	(0–63)
UA	2.2 mg/dL	(2.7–7.0)	CSF		
Na	142 mEq/L	(135–145)	cell count	185/mm^3	(0–15/mm^3)
K	4.3 mEq/L	(3.5–5.0)	mono	168/mm^3	
Cl	105 mEq/L	(98–108)	poly	13/mm^3	
Glucose	105 mg/dL	(70–109)	protein	46 mg/dL	(15–45)
CRP	0.48	(0.00–0.30)	glucose	61 mg/dL	(50–75)
TSH	0.39μIU/ml	(0.40–4.00)	HSV-PCR	-	
FT3	2.33 pg/ml	(1.71–3.71)			
FT4	1.19 ng/ml	(0.70–1.48)			
			Serum Anti-NMDAR antibodies	1:800	2 months after admission
				1:3200	4 months after admission

(), Normal range; Anti-NMDAR antibodies, Anti-*N*-methyl-D-aspartate receptor antibodies.

Table 2: Results of dot detection and figure recognition tasks.

	Stationary condition	Moving condition	Statistical values[a]
Dot detection	1/10 (correct/total)	8/10 (correct/total)	$p < 0.001$
Figure recognition	3/18 (correct/total)	7/18 (correct/total)	$p = 0.06$

[a] Calculated by χ^2 test using a 2 × 2 contingency table.

from her eyes. We prepared two different stimuli, a black dot with 1 cm in diameter (approximately 2 degrees in visual angle) and another with 0.4 cm in diameter. They were presented randomly for three seconds on each of the five points, comprised of four corners and the center of the screen. She was able to identify the larger stimuli perfectly (10/10: correct/total) indicating that she had no obvious hemianopsia or quadrantanopsia of the cortical type, although she often missed the smaller ones (2/10: correct/total). Second, the patient was tested for her ability to detect the motion of a visual stimulus. A small black dot 0.4 cm in diameter was presented in the center of the screen for 3 seconds with no motion (stationary condition), or with rightward lateral motion with a velocity of 2 cm/sec (moving condition) (Figure 3(a)). She was able to detect the moving stimuli better (8/10: correct/total) than stationary ones (1/10: correct/total). Third, the patient was tested to see if the motion of a figure influenced her ability to identify the shape of the figure. Four different figures in black: a circle, a star, a triangle, and a square, were inscribed in a circle with a diameter of 1 cm. Each figure was presented in the center of the screen with no motion for 4 seconds (stationary condition) or with a clockwise rotational movement from the center tracing on a circle of a 4 cm diameter with a velocity of 2 cm/sec for 4 seconds (moving condition) (Figure 3(b)). She showed a tendency to recognize the shape of moving figures better (7/18: correct/total) than stationary ones (3/18: correct/total) (Table 2). The test results suggested that the patient retained some capacity of form-from-motion perception: i.e., an ability to recognize the shape of an object under motion.

The patient's visual symptoms and general cognitive function gradually improved. Fifteen months after admission, she was able to recognize stationary objects as well as moving ones in everyday life. She also was able to pick up an object with appropriate preshaping of her fingers. At this time, the patient scored 28/30 on the revised Hasegawa dementia scale (normal >21/30). Further, we administered Visual Perception Test for Agnosia (VPTA) to her. On VPTA, a mistake or failure in performance is each scored 1 or 2 points according to the criteria. Thus, greater score indicates more severe visual disability. The patient showed a partial impairment in her basic visual perception (VPTA score 6/24), yet she was able to read kana and kanji characters. Notably, we observed severe impairment in perceiving famous faces (VPTA score 10/10). She could not tell if a photograph of a person was young or old, or man or a woman, but was able to identify if two faces presented were identical or not. The patient also demonstrated difficulties in identifying family members by visual inspection alone, stating "I can recognize my family members when I hear their voice but cannot by sight alone because their faces look dark and ambiguous." On the other

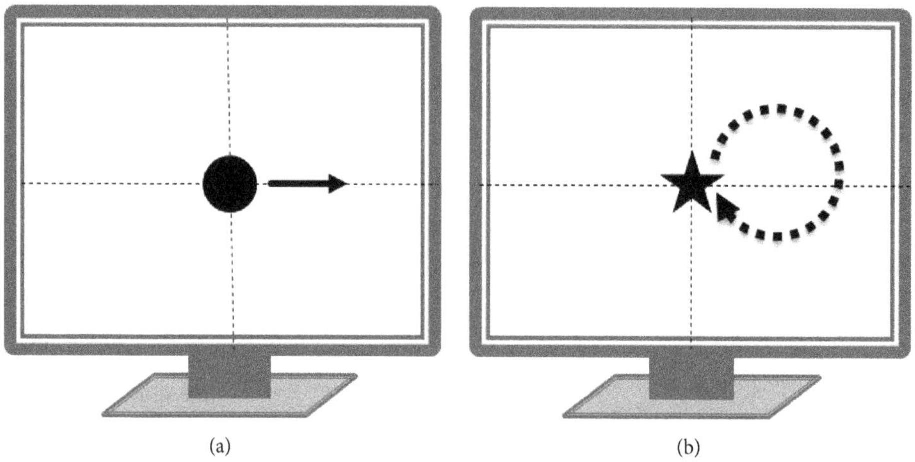

Figure 3: (a) Dot detection task. The patient was tested to see if motion of a visual stimulus affected her visual ability. A small black dot 0.4 cm in diameter was presented in the center of the screen for 3 seconds with no motion (stationary condition) or with right side lateral motion with a velocity of 2 cm/sec (moving condition). (b) Figure recognition task. The patient was tested to see if motion of a figure could influence her ability to identify it. Four different figures black in color were prepared; a circle, a star, a triangle, and a square, each of which was inscribed in a circle with a diameter of 1 cm. Each figure was presented in the center of the screen with no motion for 4 seconds (stationary condition) or with clockwise rotatory movement from the center tracing on a circle of 4 cm diameter with a velocity of 2 cm/sec for 4 seconds (moving condition).

hand, her color perception had recovered to near normal levels (VPTA score 2/30).

She was discharged 18 months after admission, and had become able to identify family members and medical staff on sight, with no complaints of any visual symptoms. Brain MRI performed on discharge showed no signal abnormalities except for subcortical small high intensities in the occipital lobes.

3. Discussion

NMDA receptor encephalitis involves antibodies against the GluN1 subunit of the NMDA receptor. These antibodies probably cause the binding, capping, and cross-linking of NMDA receptors leading to internalization of the receptors from the neuronal membrane surface, resulting in dysfunction of signal transmission mediated by glutaminergic synapses [3, 4]. A previous study of brain metabolism patterns using fluorodeoxyglucose (FDG)-PET/CT revealed that decreased occipital lobe metabolism was more prominent in patients with anti-NMDA receptor encephalitis compared to other definite autoimmune encephalitis [5]. Furthermore, the study reported that among patients with anti-NMDA receptor encephalitis, patients with the greatest neurologic disability were more hypometabolic compared with less severe disability in the visual cortical and occipital brain regions [5]. Thus, it is not surprising that patients with anti-NMDA receptor encephalitis, especially those with serious neurologic disability, would exhibit notable cortical visual symptoms. However, there has been only one case report describing visual symptoms in detail in an encephalitis patient [6]. The present case took the severe disease course, and we inferred that it could relate to her characteristic visual symptoms.

There are many disorders of higher visual processing that result from damage to specific areas of the cerebral cortex which have a specific role in processing certain aspects (modalities) of vision. These can be grouped into those that affect the ventral, or "what?" pathway (e.g., object agnosia, cerebral achromatopsia, prosopagnosia, topographagnosia, and pure alexia), and those that affect the dorsal, or "where?" pathway (e.g., akinetopsia, simultagnosia, and optic ataxia) [7, 8]. The dorsal pathway may be subdivided further into two pathways: (1) the dorso-dorsal stream that extends from the primary visual cortex (V1) to the superior parietal lobule, which is supposed to be involved in implicit perception of an object's spatial position, motion, and form, and (2) the dorso-ventral stream that directs to the inferior parietal lobule being engaged in the conscious perception of an object's motion or spatial location [9].

Our patient showed a variety of higher visual symptoms which changed over recovery phase of the disease. In chronological order, she experienced cortical blindness, amblyopia, dyschromatopsia, relative difficulty in identifying stationary objects more than moving objects (static form agnosia), and prosopagnosia. On discharge, these visual symptoms recovered to the point where she had no complaints of disability in perceiving any visual stimuli. This implies that the patient may have unequally regained function of the aforementioned distinct visual areas in the time course of recovery. The areas involved in the dorsal pathway were likely improved initially, and those areas engaged in the ventral pathway were successively convalesced.

An intriguing observation in the present case was that, during the initial phase of her recovery, she demonstrated static form agnosia. Vania [10] previously reported a visually agnostic patient who suffered from bilateral occipital lesions, extending ventrally into the medial temporal areas. Similar to the present case, Vania's case showed impaired static form perception with preserved motion perception, including low-level motion perception (i.e., an ability to detect coherent motion when proportion of dots move coherently against a background of random dots), form-from-motion (i.e., an ability to detect kinetic boundaries defining shape), and biological motion perception (i.e., an ability to identify a point-light walker in the dark). Conversely, Blanke et al. [11] reported a case of impaired form-from-motion perception with preserved static form and low-level motion perception after damage to the ventral temporal lobe. These cases demonstrate a double dissociation suggesting that visual areas engaged in processing static form perception and form-from-motion perception rely upon functionally distinct regions. Consistent with this, functional MRI studies showed that the lateral occipital cortex and other ventral occipitotemporal cortices are activated when subjects were involved in detecting form-from-motion [12, 13], and there seemed to be little overlap in activation to static form stimuli and form-from motion stimuli within this region [14].

Because the patient suffered from encephalitis and the MRI revealed lesions with vague boundaries, detailed lesion localization in the present case was difficult to determine. However, it seems that two distinct visual areas (an area engaged in processing form-from-motion perception and an area involved in static form perception) recovered at different rates, with the former regaining function earlier.

Of note, the form-from motion task undertaken in our case is different from previous studies. In previous studies, form-from-motion tasks are performed as follows: a proportion of background dots in a random dot display move in one direction (or at a set velocity) comprising the background, and the remainder of dots comprising the foreground object (such as a letter) moving in another direction (or at a different velocity) [10–14]. The difference in the tasks performed in the present case and previous studies may prove difficult to directly compare results. However, the tasks in previous studies (and ours) both evaluated the subject's ability to detect kinetic boundaries. Moreover, the peculiar visual symptom demonstrated in the present case, i.e., "can see moving figures better than stationary ones," suggests that these two visual perceptual abilities can be dissociable.

In conclusion, we presented a case of a variety of cortical visual symptoms in the recovery phase of anti-NMDA receptor encephalitis. The case further provides clinical evidence for functional segregation of static form and form-from-motion processing in the visual cortex.

Acknowledgments

The authors thank Professor Josep Dalmau (Service of Neurology, Hospital Clinic-IDIBAPS, University of Barcelona; Catalan Institution of Research and Advanced Studies, Barcelona, Spain; and Department of Neurology, University of Pennsylvania) for analysis of the antibodies against NMDA receptor.

References

[1] R. Vitaliani, W. Mason, B. Ances, T. Zwerdling, Z. Jiang, and J. Dalmau, "Paraneoplastic encephalitis, psychiatric symptoms, and hypoventilation in ovarian teratoma," *Annals of Neurology*, vol. 58, no. 4, pp. 594–604, 2005.

[2] J. Dalmau, E. Tüzün, H.-Y. Wu et al., "Paraneoplastic anti-N-methyl-D-aspartate receptor encephalitis associated with ovarian teratoma," *Annals of Neurology*, vol. 61, no. 1, pp. 25–36, 2007.

[3] E. G. Hughes, X. Peng, A. J. Gleichman et al., "Cellular and synaptic mechanisms of anti-NMDA receptor encephalitis," *The Journal of Neuroscience*, vol. 30, no. 17, pp. 5866–5875, 2010.

[4] J. Dalmau, "NMDA receptor encephalitis and other antibody-mediated disorders of the synapse," *Neurology*, vol. 87, no. 23, pp. 2471–2482, 2016.

[5] JC. Probasco, L. Solnes, and A. Nalluri, "Decreased occipital lobe metabolism by FDG-PET/CTAn anti-NMDA receptor encephalitis biomarker," *Neurology: Neuroimmunology Neuroinflammation*, vol. 5, pp. e413-10–e413-20, 2018.

[6] H. Sawamura, T. Yamamoto, R. Ohtomo, T. Bannnai, M. Wakakura, and S. Tsuji, "Anti-NMDA receptor encephalitis associated with transient cerebral dyschromatopsia, prosopagnosia and lack of stereopsis," *Journal of Neuro-Ophthalmology*, vol. 34, no. 3, pp. 144–148, 2014.

[7] A. D. Milner and M. A. Goodale, "Two visual systems re-viewed," *Neuropsychologia*, vol. 46, no. 3, pp. 774–785, 2008.

[8] S. Haque, MS. Vaphiades, and CJ. Lueck, "The visual agnosias and related disorders," *Journal of Neuro-Ophthalmology*, vol. 0, pp. 1–14, 2017.

[9] G. Rizzolatti and M. Matelli, "Two different streams form the dorsal visual system: anatomy and functions," *Experimental Brain Research*, vol. 153, no. 2, pp. 146–157, 2003.

[10] LM. Vaina, "Functional segregation of colour and motion processing in the human visual cortex: Clinical evidence," *Cerebral Cortex*, vol. 5, pp. 555–572, 1994.

[11] O. Blanke, A. Brooks, M. Mercier et al., "Distinct mechanisms of form-from-motion perception in human extrastriate cortex," *Neuropsychologia*, vol. 45, no. 4, pp. 644–653, 2007.

[12] P. Dupont, B. de Bruyn, R. Vangenberghe et al., "The kinectic occipital region in human visual cortex," *Cerebral Cortex*, vol. 7, pp. 283–297, 1997.

[13] J. Grèzes, P. Fonlupt, B. Bertenthal, C. Delon-Martin, C. Segebarth, and J. Decety, "Does perception of biological motion rely on specific brain regions?" *NeuroImage*, vol. 13, no. 5, pp. 775–785, 2001.

[14] B. Gulyas, C. A. Heywood, D. A. Popplewell, P. E. Roland, and A. Cowey, "Visual form discrimination from color or motion cues: functional anatomy by positron emission tomography.," *Proceedings of the National Acadamy of Sciences of the United States of America*, vol. 91, no. 21, pp. 9965–9969, 1994.

16

New Onset British Accent, Acute Behavioral Changes and Seizures: A Unique Presentation of NMDAR Encephalitis

Mohankumar Kurukumbi,[1] Tulsi S. Shah,[2] Jose A. Castillo,[2] Rahul U. Nayak,[2] and Jahnnavi Madiraju[2]

[1]*Department of Neurology, Inova Fairfax Hospital, Falls Church VA, USA*
[2]*Virginia Commonwealth University School of Medicine, Inova Campus, Falls Church VA, USA*

Correspondence should be addressed to Mohankumar Kurukumbi; mohan311@gmail.com

Academic Editor: Peter Berlit

The leading cause of autoimmune encephalitis is N-methyl-D-aspartate receptor (NMDAR) encephalitis. Symptoms can present as prominent behavioral abnormalities prompting inaccurate psychiatric diagnoses. Psychiatric features such as bizarre behavior, agitation, anxiety, delusions, and hallucinations are well noted in the current literature, but a manifestation of foreign accent syndrome has, to our knowledge, never been reported in cases of encephalitis. Once diagnosed, initiation of therapy can result in effective treatment. Here, we present a case of a 32-year-old female with new onset seizures and marked behavioral changes, such as speaking in a foreign accent, who was empirically treated for NMDAR encephalitis due to strong clinical suspicion, showed no improvement with first line therapy with IVIG and IV steroids, and finally had rapid resolution of symptoms with the early initiation of second line therapy of rituximab. In a young female presenting with nonspecific behavioral changes, NMDAR encephalitis should be on the differential and, although CSF antibodies are definitively diagnostic, there should be a low threshold to start empiric therapy and escalate to second line treatment.

1. Introduction

NMDAR encephalitis is one of the most common autoimmune encephalitis syndromes; however symptoms can often be difficult to distinguish from psychiatric etiologies. In addition, it often takes time for definitive diagnostic lab results, which can be detrimental given that research has shown that early intervention can lead to a better prognosis and decreased risk of relapse. Once the treatment has been initiated, the ideal timeline of escalation to second line therapies has not been completely elucidated. Here we present an interesting case of a 32-year-old female with new onset seizure activity and multiple acute behavioral changes, including a rare finding of foreign accent syndrome, found to have NMDAR encephalitis which was resolved with empiric treatment and early escalation to second line therapy.

2. Case Presentation

A 32-year-old female with a history of hyperthyroidism status after radiation resulting in hypothyroidism and no history of seizures presented with an acute onset of behavioral changes and witnessed seizure activity. Family history is remarkable for thyroid disease in multiple relatives, but negative for seizure or psychiatric disorders. Behavioral changes included uncontrolled laughter, screaming, signs of agitation, spitting on the floor, complete lack of appetite, and speaking in a British accent. A further history revealed that the patient is of Caucasian descent, was born in Germany, moved to the United States when she was a baby, and has no ties to Britain.

She had two seizures both involving tongue biting and postictal confusion with combative behavior. Her workups for seizures, including but not limited to head CT, urine drug screen, and electrolyte levels, were all within normal limits.

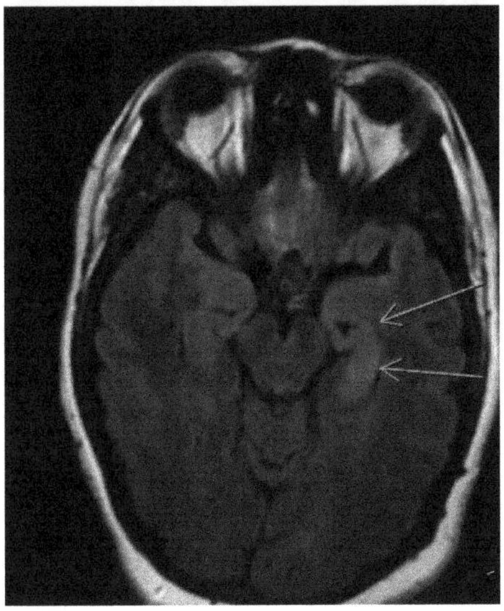

FIGURE 1: Asymmetric increased flair signal over the left hippocampus.

She, as well as her family, refused MRI and subsequently was discharged on levetiracetam for new onset seizures. On the fourth day of illness (DOI), the patient was admitted to a local community hospital with continued behavioral changes, where an MRI and lumbar puncture (LP) were found to be unremarkable, with a WBC count of 1 cell per mm^3. Other CSF parameters include a RBC count of 10 cells per mm^3, glucose of 53 mg per dL, and protein of 26 mg per dL. She was subsequently transferred to our hospital care on the fourteenth day of illness because of persisting and worsening behavioral changes. Upon revisiting the initially unremarkable impression of the MRI, abnormal T2 flair hyperintensity in the mesial temporal lobes was noted, with left lobe hyperintensity greater than that of the right lobe (Figure 1). These features raised suspicion for limbic encephalitis.

Titers for serum anti-NMDAR and paraneoplastic antibody panel were sent on clinical suspicion. Video EEG (Figure 2) showed frequent focal onset electrographic seizures from the left frontocentral and left frontotemporal region. Some of these electroclinical seizures showed delta brushes (Figure 3). With strong clinical suspicion for an anti-NMDAR or paraneoplastic antibody related encephalitis, before even receiving antibody titer results, the patient was started on five-day IV steroids on the fourteenth DOI, and IVIG course started on the fifteenth DOI.

At this point, multiple differential diagnoses were being considered including autoimmune encephalitides. During hospital admission, the patient continued to remain afebrile. Repeat LP showed lymphocytic pleocytosis, with a quantitative value of 54 cells per mm^3 with 98% lymphocytes, after which she was started on empiric acyclovir until HSV PCR was later confirmed to be negative. All other CSF findings were insignificant, with a normal protein level of 16.8 mg per dL, no RBCs, and an elevated glucose level of 95 mg per dL. She continued to have seizures requiring Lacosamide followed by an addition of Lamotrigine. On the fifth day of IVIG course and twentieth DOI, NMDAR antibody was found to be positive in the serum. CT of the chest, abdomen, and pelvis showed no evidence for neoplasms and a transvaginal ultrasound was negative for ovarian teratoma. CSF was positive for NMDAR antibody with a titer of 1:64. After completion of IV steroids and IVIG, there was no significant clinical improvement. She was started on rituximab on DOI 27 for a total of 4 weeks given weekly, with subsequent clinical improvement in addition to no clinical seizures on EEG and resolution of her new onset British accent.

The patient continued to have subclinical focal seizures, catatonia, and orofacial dyskinesias with subsequent gradual improvement in her behavior at discharge. When seen for follow-up as an outpatient, she still was found to have some residual memory and cognitive processing deficits. The patient continues to follow up in the hospital for rituximab infusions which is controlling her anti-NMDAR encephalitis and she has now returned back to baseline health.

3. Discussion

According to epidemiologic studies, NMDAR encephalitis is not only the best characterized of autoimmune encephalitis syndromes, but also the most common. The California Encephalitis Project, established in 1998 to better understand the epidemiology of encephalitis and its etiologies, found that, of the 761 cases of uncertain etiologies of encephalitis, the leading cause was by far anti-NMDAR encephalitis, present in 32 of 79 identified etiologies. Anti-NMDAR encephalitis was identified more than 4 times more frequently than HSV-1, West Nile virus, or Varicella Zoster virus [1].

Interestingly, anti-NMDAR receptor encephalitis was initially thought to be solely a paraneoplastic disorder associated with young females with immature ovarian teratomas [1]. However, further studies revealed that approximately 80% of patients with anti-NMDAR encephalitis are women, and, in women above the age of 18, only about 50% have an ovarian teratoma. Other studies also confirmed that it can occur in both males and females, children and adults, and is not in fact always associated with a neoplastic cause [2], as in our case. In our patient, CT abdomen/pelvis and transvaginal ultrasound were both negative, likely excluding the presence of a teratoma. Though retrospectively, we recognize that a pelvic MRI is most sensitive for teratoma screening; this imaging modality was not done in our patient.

In NMDAR encephalitis, it has been shown that the NMDAR antibodies cause increased internalization of the receptor leading to effective loss of NMDAR signaling via disruption of the GluN1/N2b interaction with Ephrin-B2. [1, 3]

Many patients initially present with headache, fever, or a viral-like condition, which in a few days usually progress to include prominent psychiatric features such as bizarre behavior, agitation, anxiety, delusions, and hallucinations. In addition, other characteristic clinical symptoms of anti-NMDAR encephalitis include seizures, stupor, autonomic

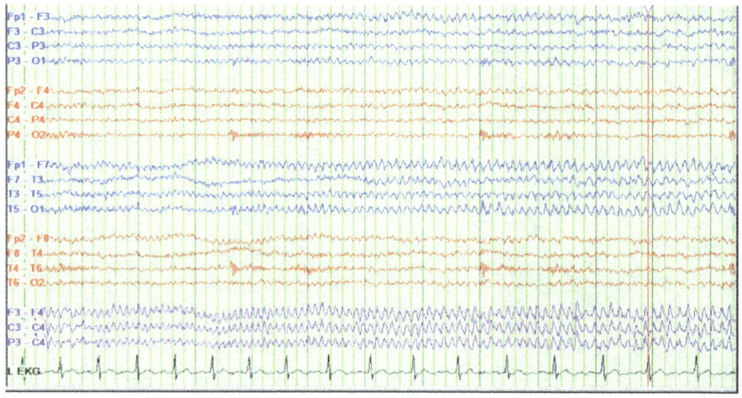

Figure 2: Electroclinical seizure: rhythmic theta discharges originating from left frontocentral/ frontotemporal region.

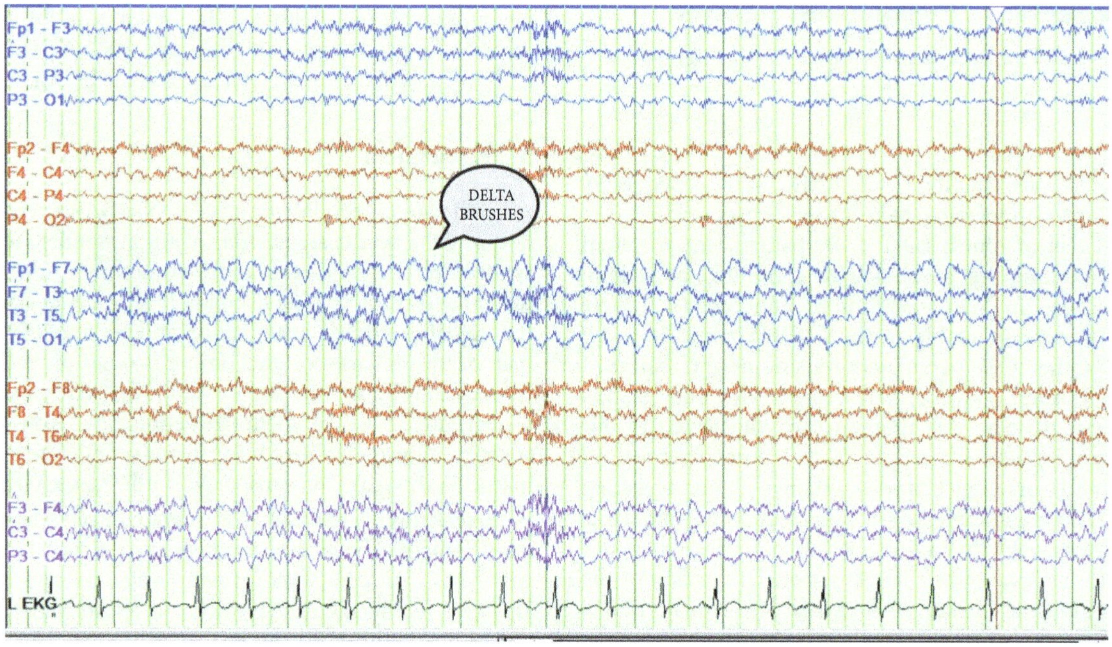

Figure 3: Electroclinical seizure: rhythmic delta activity originating from left frontotemporal region.

instability, dyskinesias, memory deficits, and language dysfunction [4]. A manifestation of foreign accent syndrome, as seen in our patient, has to our investigation never been reported.

Interestingly, Dalmau et al. reported in a case study of 100 participants that 77 were initially evaluated by psychiatry [4]. This can make properly identifying anti-NMDAR encephalitis symptoms difficult. NMDAR encephalitis is a differential that must always be kept in mind when a young female acutely presents with psychiatric symptoms.

From all of the possible manifestations of anti-NMDAR encephalitis, our patient presented with seizures, bizarre behavior, agitation, and a change in language function. Interestingly our patient was using a British accent upon presentation.

This phenomenon, known as foreign accent syndrome (FAS), is well appreciated with functional or structural neurologic disorders like conversion disorders and strokes, but not as a manifestation of encephalitis.

FAS is a rare disorder where the affected person speaks in an accent that the listener perceives as foreign. Although most cases have left hemisphere lesions, some may be functional. It was first described by French neurologist Pierre Marie in 1907 with a patient who was recovering from a left hemisphere subcortical stroke. Since then there have been over 60 reported cases with etiology consistent with stroke or traumatic brain injury and a few associated with underlying psychological disorder. Interestingly, neither was the case in our patient as the diagnosis was that of an inflammatory process and not a structural or psychological one.

Currently the cause behind this syndrome is unknown. It has been proposed that it results from lesions of the dominant language cortex (usually the left hemisphere). Our patient had only mesial temporal lobe involvement found via MRI.

There are many types of speech disorders, including stuttering disfluencies, speech substitutions, and defects in the rhythm and sound of speech, which could present in the form of a foreign accent [5, 6]. The current literature shows reports of various foreign accents including Welsh and French, and, now in our case, a patient with a British accent.

This syndrome is diagnosed clinically. MRI findings can be used in support of a structural cause for the syndrome, like a stroke or traumatic brain injury [5].

Currently no proven treatment options exist for this phenomenon, besides attempting to correct the underlying structural or functional pathology and pursuing supportive measures like speech therapy or insight-oriented counseling [6]. Most reported cases endorse resolution of the foreign accent with time but some also mention continued periods of foreign accent speech. Though our patient initially presented with a British accent, these findings completely resolved by the end of her clinical course.

MRI is helpful in the clinical setting but findings are neither unique nor diagnostic for this disorder. A MRI of the brain is abnormal in only 30-50% of patients with NMDAR encephalitis [3]. Whether or not an MRI is more likely to indicate a pathologic process if done at a certain time of the disease course has not been definitively studied. However, one study found that, with initially normal MRI findings, further findings tend to remain normal or show minimal changes, despite the severity and duration of symptoms [2].

If it is indicative of an underlying pathology, a T2-weighted fluid-attenuated inversion recovery (flair) brain MRI frequently shows hyperintense signals in the grey and/or white matter, and commonly present in the medial temporal lobes [4].

A continuous video EEG mainly excludes a nonconvulsive seizure. Anti-NMDAR encephalitis shows some common nonspecific EEG patterns which include epileptiform activity, focal and/or generalized slowing, and periodic lateralized epileptiform discharges [7]. A unique finding in approximately one-third of people affected by anti-NMDAR encephalitis is a pattern in the EEG tracing called extreme delta brush, that is now becoming recognized as characteristic for anti-NMDAR encephalitis [8]. Our patient had EEG findings indicative of anti-NMDAR encephalitis, including focal slowing and delta brush, as seen in one of the figures.

The sensitivity of anti-NMDAR antibody testing was found to be higher in the CSF when compared to serum [9]. The diagnosis of anti-NMDAR encephalitis is therefore confirmed by the presence of antibodies, specifically immunoglobulin G (IgG), to the NMDAR's GluN1 subunit in the CSF.

The mainstay treatment option for anti-NMDA receptor encephalitis is immunosuppression [10]. Most patients have a favorable prognosis when treatment is started early [11]. Particularly, improvement of the prognosis probability was higher with administration of immunotherapy at <40 days of illness when compared to >40 days; however, comparison for earlier dates has yet to be studied [11]. Evidently in our case, treatment was started on the fourteenth DOI.

One study found that patients with delays in diagnosis and treatment are more likely to have persistent impairments, such as deficits in executive function and memory, when compared to those with early intervention [12]. Our patient on follow-up as an outpatient initially had some residual deficits but showed gradual improvement in her behavior and with continuous follow-up with rituximab infusions showed complete resolution.

The literature for treatment is in support of an escalation approach with promise being evident when the first line agents being used are steroids and IVIG or plasma exchange [10].

The regimen most frequently used is a combination of steroids and IVIG. The literature regarding whether the efficacy of IVIG or plasma exchange is equivalent to treating anti-NMDAR encephalitis has yet to be further explored. If there is no evidence of improvement with first line agents, second line therapies should be administered including rituximab, cyclophosphamide, or a combination of both. One series confirmed this by showing that 75-80 percent of patients showed improvement by 24 months when this was the case [10].

In this case the patient's symptoms were refractory to IVIG and steroids. Second line therapy of rituximab was started and showed significant clinical improvement, and therefore the patient was continued on rituxan infusions.

Management and treatment of anti-NMDAR encephalitis still hold a lot of uncertainties, as timeline, duration, combination, and efficacy of treatment options are still unclear. However, it is clear that management should not be limited to first line agents and if the patient is not showing improvement of symptoms, second line therapies should always be taken into consideration and can completely change the clinical picture.

4. Conclusion

This case is reported due to the unique presentation of anti-NMDAR encephalitis, which included a never before seen symptom of FAS that resolved with correction of the underlying pathology. FAS may apparently also be of autoimmune or inflammatory etiology.

For any patient who presents with psychiatric manifestations with no underlying psychiatric history and seizures, it is vital to consider anti-NMDAR encephalitis as well as CSF studies in the workup. Additionally, it is important to note that management should not be limited to IVIG and steroid therapy; rituximab infusions should be a secondary treatment if deemed necessary.

Abbreviations

CT:	Computed tomography
EEG:	Electroencephalogram
MRI:	Magnetic Resonance Imaging
LP:	Lumbar puncture
NMDA:	N-methyl-D-aspartate
NMDAR:	N-methyl-D-aspartate receptor
IV:	Intravenous
IVIG:	Intravenous immunoglobulin

HSV-1: Herpes Simplex Virus-1
FLAIR: Fluid-attenuated inversion recovery
VGKC: Voltage gated potassium channel
WBC: White blood cell
AED: Antiepileptic drug
CSF: Cerebrospinal fluid
IgG: Immunoglobulin G
DOI: Day of illness.

References

[1] M. S. Gable, H. Sheriff, J. Dalmau, D. H. Tilley, and C. A. Glaser, "The frequency of autoimmune N-methyl-D-aspartate receptor encephalitis surpasses that of individual viral etiologies in young individuals enrolled in the california encephalitis project," *Clinical Infectious Diseases*, vol. 54, no. 7, pp. 899–904, 2012.

[2] C. Liu, J. Zhu, X. Zheng, C. Ma, and X. Wang, "Anti-N-methyl-D-aspartate receptor encephalitis: a severe, potentially reversible autoimmune encephalitis," *Mediators of Inflammation*, vol. 2017, Article ID 6361479, 14 pages, 2017.

[3] J. Dalmau, E. Lancaster, E. Martinez-Hernandez, M. R. Rosenfeld, and R. Balice-Gordon, "Clinical experience and laboratory investigations in patients with anti-NMDAR encephalitis," *The Lancet Neurology*, vol. 10, no. 1, pp. 63–74, 2011.

[4] J. Dalmau, A. J. Gleichman, E. G. Hughes et al., "Anti-NMDA-receptor encephalitis: case series and analysis of the effects of antibodies," *The Lancet Neurology*, vol. 7, no. 12, pp. 1091–1098, 2008.

[5] O. Lee, L. Ludwig, R. Davenport, and J. Stone, "Functional foreign accent syndrome," *Practical Neurology*, vol. 16, no. 5, pp. 409–411, 2016.

[6] J. F. Baizabal-Carvallo and J. Jankovic, "Speech and voice disorders in patients with psychogenic movement disorders," *Journal of Neurology*, vol. 262, no. 11, pp. 2420–2424, 2015.

[7] N. D. Lawn, B. F. Westmoreland, M. J. Kiely, V. A. Lennon, and S. Vernino, "Clinical, magnetic resonance imaging, and electroencephalographic findings in paraneoplastic limbic encephalitis," *Mayo Clinic Proceedings*, vol. 78, no. 11, pp. 1363–1368, 2003.

[8] S. E. Schmitt, K. Pargeon, E. S. Frechette, L. J. Hirsch, J. Dalmau, and D. Friedman, "Extreme delta brush; a unique EEG pattern in adults with anti-NMDA receptor encephalitis," *Neurology*, vol. 79, no. 11, pp. 1094–1100, 2012.

[9] N. Gresa-Arribas, M. J. Titulaer, A. Torrents et al., "Antibody titres at diagnosis and during follow-up of anti-NMDA receptor encephalitis: a retrospective study," *The Lancet Neurology*, vol. 13, no. 2, pp. 167–177, 2014.

[10] M. J. Titulaer, L. McCracken, I. Gabilondo et al., "Treatment and prognostic factors for long-term outcome in patients with anti-NMDA receptor encephalitis: an observational cohort study," *The Lancet Neurology*, vol. 12, no. 2, pp. 157–165, 2013.

[11] M. Nosadini, S. S. Mohammad, S. Ramanathan, F. Brilot, and R. C. Dale, "Immune therapy in autoimmune encephalitis: a systematic review," *Expert Review of Neurotherapeutics*, vol. 15, no. 12, pp. 1391–1419, 2015.

[12] C. Finke, U. A. Kopp, H. Prüss, J. Dalmau, K.-P. Wandinger, and C. J. Ploner, "Cognitive deficits following anti-NMDA receptor encephalitis," *Journal of Neurology, Neurosurgery & Psychiatry*, vol. 83, no. 2, pp. 195–198, 2012.

17

On Neuropsychiatric Manifestations of Basal Ganglia Injury: A Report of Three Cases and Literature Review

Heela Azizi,[1] Alexander Kilpatrick,[1] Olaniyi Olayinka,[2] Olusegun Poopola,[2] Maleeha Ahmad,[1] Alexa Kahn,[1] Tasmia Khan,[3] Dina Rimawi,[1] Shantale Williams,[1] Sinthuja Jayaraj,[1] Ivan Leung,[4] Sherina Langdon,[1] Mirna Iskander,[1] Ali Chohan,[1] Deepa Nuthalapati,[1] Ulunma Umesi,[3] Geetha Vyas,[1] Ayotomide Oyelakin,[2] Kodjovi Kodjo,[2] Chiedozie Ojimba,[2] Oluwole Jegede,[2] Carolina Nisenoff,[2] and Ayodeji Jolayemi[2]

[1]*American University of Antigua College of Medicine, Department of Psychiatry, Interfaith Medical Center, Brooklyn, New York, USA*
[2]*Department of Psychiatry, Interfaith Medical Center, Brooklyn, New York, USA*
[3]*Medical University of the Americas, Department of Psychiatry, Interfaith Medical Center, Brooklyn, New York, USA*
[4]*Saba University School of Medicine, Department of Psychiatry, Interfaith Medical Center, Brooklyn, New York, USA*

Correspondence should be addressed to Heela Azizi; heelaa@auamed.net

Academic Editor: Peter Berlit

The basal ganglia have been considered to primarily play a role in motor processing. A growing body of theoretical and clinical evidence shows that in addition to the motor functions the basal ganglia play a key role in perceptual and visual disturbances. This role may be evident in patients with basal ganglia pathology and subsequent manifestation of symptoms that include cognitive, perceptual, and affective disturbances. We present three cases with basal ganglia pathology that demonstrate affective and psychotic symptoms. Two of the cases presented with late onset psychotic disturbances suggesting likely neurological etiologies. The third case presented with treatment refractory psychosis and symptoms that are rare for a diagnosis of schizophrenia. The role of incidental bilateral basal ganglia calcifications in all the cases is discussed. A review of current literature highlighting various neuropsychiatric manifestations of basal ganglia pathologies in various patients with psychiatric symptoms is presented.

1. Introduction

The basal ganglia neural circuits are utilized in movement selection, planning, and learning. A much less researched feature of the basal ganglia is its function in cognition and perceptual function [1–3]. A few cases in literature have suggested the possible link between basal ganglia damage and visual hallucinations and psychosis [4, 5]. The symptoms exhibited by patients are consistent with varying degrees of hallucinations, delusions and flashbacks [6, 7]. The utilization of advanced imaging techniques such as Magnetic Resonance Imaging (MRI) might provide the means to identify organic causes of new onset psychoses and further knowledge of the functions of the basal ganglia. These lesions and associated symptoms give us insight into the complex pathways within the basal ganglia that have not been fully explored. A comprehensive investigation exploring damaged basal ganglia will allow us to elucidate potential causes of psychosis and hallucinations and open up new avenues of pharmacotherapy targeting the neural networks involved in hallucinations and psychosis. We present three patients with affective and psychotic symptoms who share brain imaging findings of incidental basal ganglia pathology. We also review relevant literature of symptoms reported for patients with bilateral basal ganglia calcifications (BGC).

2. Case Presentations

2.1. Case One. The first case was a 59-year-old African American male with a past medical history notable for

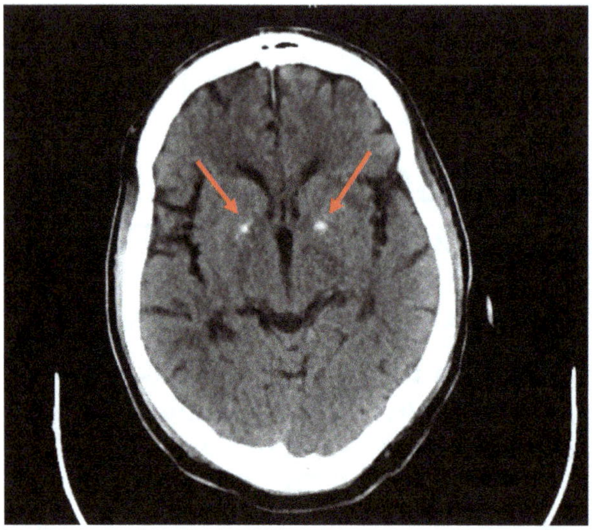

FIGURE 1: CT scan without contrast showing bilateral basal ganglia calcification.

schizoaffective disorder, depression, and substance abuse who was brought in to the emergency room for disorganized behavior and agitation in the community. At the time of admission the patient demonstrated disorientation, repetitive motor behavior, and an alternation between agitation and psychomotor retardation. He had poor response to communication and tactile stimuli. A suspicion of altered mental status due to organic causes was suspected with the possibility of catatonic excitement and retardation. He was admitted to the medical floor, with a work-up revealing a positive toxicology screen for cocaine and opioids. The patients CBC and BMP were within normal limits except for his ammonia level which was 80 mg/dl. The patient was initially treated with Chlorpromazine Hcl 50 mg orally daily for his agitated behavior as well as Naltrexone 50 mg orally daily for his opiate intoxication.

The patient exhibited incoherent thought process in addition to mumbled speech that made a significant portion of his assessment evaluation difficult. During evaluation, he displayed abnormal movements of his arms and face, with tremors and restlessness. His affect was flat. He did not display any perceptual disturbances or delusions. An assessment for cognitive impairment was noncontributory during his most recent admission. The patient received Mirtazapine 45 mg orally at bedtime and Olanzapine 10 mg orally daily in his treatment and by day three of admission had shown improvement in his disorganized behavior with supportive care. The patient demonstrated more effort to directly communicate with house staff after treatment began.

The patient reported a past history of psychiatric illness that was late in onset. His first presentation at the age of 51 years was significant for depressed mood, paranoid delusions, and auditory hallucinations for which he was diagnosed with a major mood disorder. His symptoms responded poorly to medications including antidepressants. His disease course involved increasing periods of impulsive behavior and agitation. He became noncompliant with his prescribed medications. He was later admitted to the medical floors at the age of 54 years for "repetitive behavior" during which he was found moving from his bed to the bathroom repeatedly as if he wanted to use the bathroom all the time. He also showed some abnormal rocking movements during this time period. A medical work-up for seizure was negative. He was discharged with a presumptive diagnosis of a psychotic disorder. Thereafter, at the age of 56 years he had an episode of property destruction in the community and it was noted that he had "abnormal body movements" in addition to lability of mood. His diagnosis was revised to schizoaffective disorder and he was treated for mood lability at the time with risperidone.

Given the late onset of his neuropsychiatric symptoms, a computed tomography scan (CT) of his brain was done during his presentation, as seen in Figure 1. Reviewing his chart, it was noted that the calcifications were apparent in his first head CT taken in January of 2012 with no changes to the current CT in January of 2019.

2.2. Case Two. The second case is of a 71-year-old African American man, who presented following an episode of agitation and combativeness in the community. The patient had a late onset psychiatric history starting at the age of 57 with a diagnosis of schizophrenia. He was found to demonstrate symptoms of pressured speech, loose association, paranoid delusions, grandiose delusions, and lability of mood. He was very restless during the interview and paced around multiple times as he could not sit still. He also demonstrated constant oral movements initially thought to be responding to internal stimuli. However, he denied auditory hallucinations and stated he could not control his mouth movements. A mental status examination (Montreal Cognitive Assessment) revealed a score of 22/30 with significant deficits in memory and executive control. This was consistent with his psychiatric evaluation which revealed significant confabulation in his history. The patient was started on haloperidol 2 mg orally twice daily and risperidone

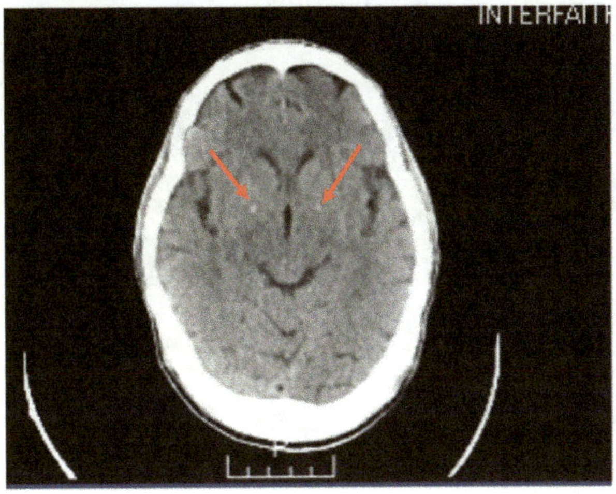

FIGURE 2: CT scan without contrast showing bilateral basal ganglia calcification.

0.5mg orally twice daily for his psychotic symptoms. The patient reports he has been noncompliant with medications previously. On systemic review, the patients CBC was within normal limits and he had a negative toxicology screen. The patients BMP had abnormal glucose values of 172 mg/dl and vitamin D level of 6.4ng/dl. An initial CT scan at the time of first diagnosis noted basal ganglia calcifications. A repeat CT scan of the brain was done (shown in Figure 2) and showed small bilateral basal ganglia calcifications, consistent with the image findings during his first episode of psychotic disturbance.

The patient showed some improvement in lability with medication compliance but his cognitive impairment, paranoid delusions, and grandiose delusions did not significantly improve. His extrapyramidal symptoms were not amenable to pharmacological interventions of anticholinergic benztropine.

2.3. Case Three. The third case reported is a 69-year-old English/Creole speaking Haitian female. Her initial admission was for an acute episode of mixed mood symptoms and psychotic symptoms at the age of 61. The patient reported constant restlessness with inner anxiety and preoccupation with delusions of control. She had a past history of treatment for chronic progressive paranoid delusions, cognitive dysfunction, and disorganized thought believed to be due to schizophrenia that responded poorly to treatment. At the time of her initial admission to our clinic, the diagnosis was revised to schizoaffective disorder considering the mood disturbances. A change in medications from risperidone 3 mg orally twice daily to fluphenazine 5 mg orally twice daily was also done. She showed no improvement in her psychosis and affective symptoms. At the time of her second admission, the patient was brought in by husband on account of bizarre behavior and disorganized thought in the context of medication noncompliance. Her symptoms had evolved to include visual hallucinations of Buddha, visual hallucinations of demons, and perceptual distortions of the floor. She endorses bizarre delusions stating there is a demon inside of her and that an "agent" took the place of her husband. She also exhibited depressive symptoms with worsening restlessness and cognitive functioning. Urine toxicology was negative on admission, with full blood count and metabolic panel within normal limits. Risperdal 2 mg orally twice daily was continued for psychosis. Paliperidone 156 mg intramuscularly one-time depot shot was added, with a second dose five days later of 117 mg intramuscularly one time. She continued to endorse visual hallucinations of "the head of the devil" that "moves like a shadow". Other notable findings were a Montreal Cognitive Assessment score of 22/30 with deficits in memory and executive functioning. Given the refractory nature of her disease and onset of new symptoms specifically of a visual nature, a head CT without contrast was ordered to rule out organic pathology. The images showed small bilateral basal ganglia calcifications, in addition to mild to moderate bilateral periventricular and deep white matter low attenuation suggestive for chronic small vessel ischemic disease (Figure 3).

On day 9 of admission, patient remained internally preoccupied with a disorganized thought process. Throughout the following week, she continued to hear voices of "the devil" with beliefs that the "evil spirits attack me and my husband". Haloperidol 5 mg orally twice daily was added for treatment of psychosis, and no side effects of the medications were reported by the patient. Her antipsychotic regimen of fluphenazine 5 mg orally twice daily that was eventually increased to 7.5 mg orally twice daily, as delusions of persecution with auditory and visual hallucinations, continued to be present.

A differential diagnosis of psychosis due to a neurological condition was added, with possible role of basal ganglia injury considered in light of the visual hallucinations, akathisia symptoms, and cognitive dysfunction. The patient was treated symptomatically with fluphenazine Hcl (Prolixin) 5 mg orally twice daily, hydroxyzine Hcl 10 mg orally twice daily, and benztropine 1 mg twice daily. Although her visual hallucinations and delusions did not resolve significantly with medications, an augmentation with psychoeducation, supportive therapy, and cognitive behavior therapy helped the patient cope with her symptoms.

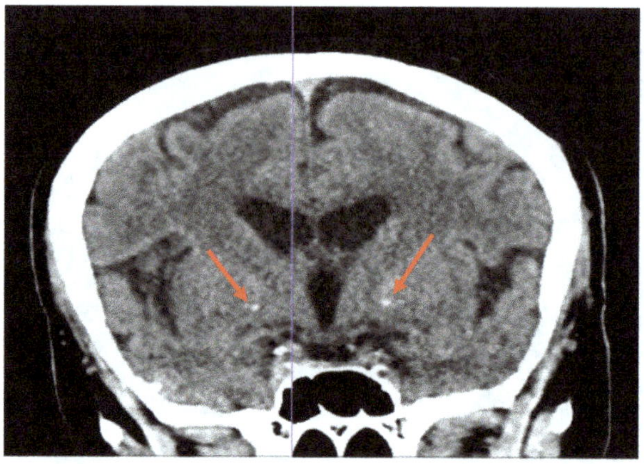

FIGURE 3: CT scan without contrast showing mild to moderate bilateral periventricular and deep white matter low attenuation along with trace bilateral basal ganglia calcification.

3. Discussion

The basal ganglia have been postulated to play a role in motor control, emotional processing, perception, and cognitive function [8]. Consequently, an insult to any part of this circuit should reveal abnormal symptoms of perception, emotional processing, and cognition. Our cases demonstrated progressive disturbances in mood and perception (particularly auditory and visual) in the context of basal ganglia pathology. The possibility of attributing these symptoms to basal ganglia pathology is informed by the evolving understanding of the role of the basal ganglia and brain imaging [8].

In the first and second cases, the late onset of the symptoms raises the index of suspicion for an underlying neurological cause. Mufaddel et al. reported that patients with BGC tend to develop psychiatric symptoms later in life than other psychiatric patients and have higher rates of medical comorbidities [9]. In the third case, the patient had a chronic diagnosis of schizophrenia. The presence of refractory symptoms and visual hallucinations usually motivate a medical work-up for underlying organic etiology which in her case revealed bilateral basal ganglia calcification like the other two cases. Cummings et al. [10] reported a case of basal ganglia calcification that presented with schizophrenia like symptoms as early as age of 17 years; similar observations have been noted in the literature [11]. The image findings reflected a pathology of the basal ganglia bilaterally along with peripheral calcifications of the posterior occipital lobe and central tentorium like those reported in prior literature [8, 10, 12, 13].

The similar natures of the three cases led the team to conduct a literature review on the varying symptoms reported in patients with basal ganglia pathology. Consequently, PubMed was searched for peer-reviewed articles that reported psychiatric symptoms and also had evidence of basal ganglia calcification(s). The search was not restricted by timeframe or language. The search was conducted using the keywords and MeSH terms: "basal ganglia" "calcification" and "function." We also searched the reference list of eligible articles to identify additional papers relevant to this study. Screening for eligible articles was conducted independently by five authors. Eligible studies were those that focused on symptomatology of basal ganglia injury and respective behavior in human subjects.

Given the paucity of articles on this topic, all types of studies were considered for analysis including experimental, cohort, meta-analysis, case-control, case series, and case reports. Any disagreement regarding the eligibility of an article was resolved by discussion among the authors. Relevant data from eligible articles were extracted and entered onto a data abstraction form designed by the authors using Microsoft Excel. Data extracted from eligible articles include title of the article, gender and age of the patient, signs and symptoms elicited, and lab findings/imaging recorded. The literature review table is shown in Table 1.

Bilateral basal ganglia calcification was confirmed by CT scan in a total of 316 patients, ranging from 7 to 96 years old. 125 patients were male and 191 were female. Sixteen percent were ages 7-30 years old, 31% were ages between 20 and 50 years old, about 32% were ages 50 to 70 years old, and 21% were 70 years and older. In terms of location, 33% had no specification of the basal ganglia calcification, while 51% were in the globus pallidum and 18% in the putamen. Twenty-two percent of the cases had other areas of calcification outside the basal ganglia including the thalamus, cerebral white matter, the cerebellar dentate nuclei, and the putamen.

About 53% of cases reported no psychiatric symptoms. Of the 47% that reported symptoms, the symptoms included both affective symptoms (19% of cases) and psychotic symptoms (26% of cases). The most commonly reported symptoms included delusions (12%), extrapyramidal symptoms (9%), mood lability (9%), visual hallucinations (3%), and agitation (1%). Cognitive dysfunctions were reported in less than 1% of cases. Five percent of cases presented with symptoms that met the criteria for schizophrenia, and 2% presented with symptoms that met criteria for mania. No cross correlation was reported between the different symptoms. There was also no report of correlation between the size of the calcification, location of the calcifications in the basal ganglia, the duration of the calcifications, and the symptoms presented. In

TABLE 1: A review of selected literature on basal ganglia injury resulting in neuropsychiatric manifestations.

Researchers	Article Title	Number & Gender of Participants	Age	Signs & Symptoms	Lab Findings/Imaging Studies
Shirahama, M., Akiyoshi, J., Ishitobi, Y., et al.	A young woman with visual hallucinations, delusions of persecution and a history of performing arson with possible three-generation Fahr disease [14]	1 F	23	Visual hallucinations, delusion of injury, irritability, mood lability	CT: bilateral calcifications of the basal ganglia (globus pallidus)
Ber, I. L., Marié, R., Chabot, B., et al.	Neuropsychological and 18FDG-PET studies in a family with idiopathic basal ganglia calcifications [2]	5 M Pts. 3 F Pts.	7-73	Schizophrenia like psychosis with late EPS	CT & MRI: basal ganglia calcification
Pan, B., Liu, W., Chen, Q., et al.	Idiopathic basal ganglia calcification presenting as schizophrenia-like psychosis and obsessive-compulsive symptoms: A case report [15]	1 M	41	Schizophrenia-like psychosis and obsessive-compulsive symptoms	CT: symmetrical calcifications in the basal ganglia
Kasuga, K., Konno, T., Saito, K., et al.	A Japanese family with idiopathic basal ganglia calcification with novel SLC20A2 mutation presenting with late-onset hallucination and delusion [16]	1 F	73	Auditory Hallucinations, heard swear words of neighboring children, and delusions she has been eavesdropped on	CT: symmetric calcification in the basal ganglia, thalamus, white matter, occipital cortex, and cerebellar dentate nuclei
Chabot, B., Roulland, C., & Dollfus, S.	Schizophrenia and familial idiopathic basal ganglia calcification: a case report [12]	3 M 2 F	36 - 68 (36, 38, 39, 46, 68)	Schizophrenia relapse	CT: bilateral and symmetrical basal ganglia calcifications

Table 1: Continued.

Researchers	Article Title	Number & Gender of Participants	Age	Signs & Symptoms	Lab Findings/Imaging Studies
Nicolas, G., Guillin, O., Borden, A., et al.	Psychosis revealing familial idiopathic basal ganglia calcification [17]	F	39	Auditory hallucinations and delusions	CT: basal ganglia calcifications in the proband and in her two asymptomatic parents.
Lauterbach, E. C., Spears, T., Prewett, M. J., et al.	Neuropsychiatric disorders, myoclonus, and dystonia in calcification of basal ganglia pathways [18]	2 M	Patient 1: 44 Patient 2: 40	Both patients had cognitive dysfunction, temporal lobe-like symptoms (including amnestic state, perceptual distortions, or complex visual hallucinations), and myoclonus	Patient 1: CT with contrast: Bilateral medial and lateral pallidal calcification anteromedially. Thyroid T3, I"4, T, and thyroid-stimulating hormone were all normal. Patient 2: MRI: bilateral holo-anterior globus pallidus calcification measuring 1 cm on the right and 1/2 cm on the left at the time of examination.
Flint, J., & Goldstein, L. H.	Familial calcification of the basal ganglia: a case report and review of the literature [19]	Pt 1: M Pt 2: F	Patient 1: 31 Patient 2: 67	Delusions that celebrities were jealous of his song-writing talent and were threatening him, third person auditory hallucinations, thought broadcasting and the belief that people knew what he was thinking. Slight choreiform movements of the arms; repetitive movements were slow and poor coordination.	Serum calcium, phosphate, alkaline phosphatase and PTH were all normal. Radiologic evaluation: bilateral calcification of the globus pallidus.
Forstl, H., Krumm, B., Eden, S., et al.	Neurological disorders in 166 patients with basal ganglia calcification: a statistical evaluation [20]	59 M 107 F	16-86	No evidence of a significantly increased risk of dementia, cerebral infarction, epilepsy, vertigo, headache, or alcoholism	CTs: 97% of BGC group had calcification in the globus pallidus and 46% had calcification in the putamen. 25 BGC patients showed a circumscribed unilateral calcification of the globus pallidus, and 143 patients showed bilateral mineralization

Table 1: Continued.

Researchers	Article Title	Number & Gender of Participants	Age	Signs & Symptoms	Lab Findings/Imaging Studies
Francis, A.	Familial Basal Ganglia Calcification and Schizophreniform Psychosis [21]	5 M 3 F	9-53 (9, 13, 27,32, 35,42,44,53)	Persecutory delusions, aggressive behavior and auditory and visual hallucinosis, coarse involuntary movements of the head and trunk, Parkinsonian facies and gait, flattened affect, elevation of mood, pressured speech, paranoia, EPS.	Skull X-ray: bilateral calcifications of the basal ganglia
Vakaet, A., Rubens, R., Reuck, J. D., et al.	Intracranial bilateral symmetrical calcification on CT-scanning [22]	1 F	57	Tonic fit, LOC, tongue biting, urinary incontinence (hx of epilepsy), global dementia, dysarthria, EPS (rigidity) in all four limbs, positive Chvostek's sign.	CT: extensive bilateral symmetrical calcification in the region of the basal ganglia, nuclei of the cerebellum and the cerebral and cerebellar white matter.
Geschwind, D. H., Loginov, M., & Stern, J. M.	Identification of a Locus on Chromosome 14q for Idiopathic Basal Ganglia Calcification (Fahr Disease) [23]	3 M 9 F	9-73 (9,10,38,40, 41,46,43,58, 52,50,70,76)	Psychosis and schizophreniform psychosis	Whole-genome scan using polymorphic microsatellite markers: Genomic study establishes the first chromosomal locus (IGBC1) and linkage analysis regarding age of onset of familial IBGC produced results consistent with genetic anticipation. CT scan: IBGC
Roiter, B., Pigato, G., & Perugi, G.	Late-onset Mania in a Patient with Movement Disorder and Basal Ganglia Calcifications: A Challenge for Diagnosis and Treatment [24]	1 M	58	Severe delirious-manic episode consisting of irritability, dysphoria, talkativeness, racing thoughts, hyperactivity, distractibility, grandiosity, persecutory delusions, psychomotor agitation, aggressiveness, insomnia, and mental confusion	CT: mild diffuse cortical atrophy and small basal ganglia calcifications but these findings were considered not clinically relevant. CT and brain MRI (for the second episode): moderate diffuse cortical atrophy, especially in frontal and occipital regions, posterior white matter lesions due to chronic vascular ischemia, and small bilateral pallidal calcifications

Table 1: Continued.

Researchers	Article Title	Number & Gender of Participants	Age	Signs & Symptoms	Lab Findings/Imaging Studies
Johnson, J. M., Legesse, B., Camprodon, J. A., et al.	The clinical significance of bilateral basal ganglia calcification presenting with mania and delusions [25]	1 M	37	New-onset psychotic mania presented with increase in guilt, elated and expansive mood, pressured speech, grandiose delusions (i.e. claiming he was Christ), increased energy, erratic thoughts and activity, impulsive and risk-taking. Presence of delusions of reference.	Complete blood count, basic metabolic panel, liver function tests, TSH, CRP, ESR, were unremarkable, with negative RPR. Serum calcium and intact PTH were within normal limits. Urine drug screen was negative. He did have a positive ANA, at 1:30, in a nonspecific speckled pattern. A heavy-metal screen was negative for arsenic, lead, mercury, and cadmium. CT: small bilateral basal ganglia calcifications.
Philpot, M. P., & Lewis, S. W.	The Psychopathology of basal ganglia calcification [26]	12 M 24 F	Mean affected M- 60 Mean affected F- 71	No psychiatric diagnosis was specifically associated with BGC although calcification of the putamen and the caudate was only found in patients with functional disorders.	No abnormalities of calcium or phosphate metabolism were found.
Trautner, R. J., Cummings, J. L., Read, S. L., et al.	Idiopathic basal ganglia calcification and organic mood disorder [27]	5 M	Pt 1: 55 Pt 2: 47 Pt 3: 56 Pt 4: 56 Pt 5: 49	Organic mood changes, including one patient with secondary mania. Symptoms resemble those of other disorders affecting subcortical structures and support an association between mood, affect, cognition, and the extra-pyramidal nuclear system.	Lab studies were normal amongst all cases. CT of Case 1: dense basal ganglia calcification and periventricular gray matter structures. CT of Case 2: calcification of putamen in basal ganglia. CT of Case 3: calcification in the putamen, caudate, pulvinar, deep sulci of frontal cortex and dentate nuclei. Skull X-ray of Case 3: dense basal ganglia calcification. CT of Case 4: extensive basal ganglia calcification in caudate nuclei, thalami, and dentate nuclei of cerebellum. CT of Case 5: massive intracranial calcifications of basal ganglia, cerebellum, and areas of cerebral white matter.

Table 1: Continued.

Researchers	Article Title	Number & Gender of Participants	Age	Signs & Symptoms	Lab Findings/Imaging Studies
Cummings, J. L., Gosenfeld, L. F., Houlihan, J. P., et al.	Neuropsychiatric disturbances associated with idiopathic calcification of the basal ganglia [10]	1 M	56	Schizophrenia like psychosis: auditory hallucinations, ideas of reference and influence, psychomotor retardation, and circumstantial speech. Depressed mood.	CT: calcifications symmetrically deposited in the putamen, the pulvinar, a few sulci of the frontal cortex and the dentate nuclei. Skull X-rays: dense calcifications of the basal ganglia and the dentate nuclei of the cerebellum. CSF protein was elevated
Shakibai, S. V., Johnson, J. P., & Bourgeois, J. A.	Fahr's Disease: An Incidental Finding in a Case Presenting with Psychosis [28]	1 M	24	Aggressive behavior, abusive language, smiling to self, talking to self and ghosts, fear of others, irregular sleep patterns, delusions of persecution, auditory hallucinations.	MRI: symmetrical large areas and foci of calcification in bilateral basal ganglia, thalami, cerebellar parenchyma and subcortical regions of bilateral cerebral hemispheres
König, P.	Psychopathological alterations in cases of symmetrical basal ganglia sclerosis [29]	25 M 37 F	Varies	31 cases initially presented neurological symptoms, 25 psychiatric, and 6 cases had no symptoms. Initial Symptoms in Bilateral Symmetrical Basal Ganglia Sclerosis (n = 62; 6 Cases Incidental Discovers) Primary Neurological 50%, Seizures 6%, TIA 6% syncopes 5% Paresis/apoplexia 10% Cephalea/vertigo 13%, EPS-movement disorders 10%, Primary Psychiatric 40%, Organic affective 21% Organic paranoid/hallucinatory 1.6% Compulsions 1.6% Alcoholism 8%. Oligophrenia 1.6% Dementia 8%.	For both psychiatric and neurological symptoms, no correlations between either localization or volume of intracerebral calcification were noted, excepting cases of dementia, which showed larger hyperdensities. As basal ganglia calcification inflicts morphological damage to the CNS, a deterioration of brain function should occur and, in fact, was identified in terms of either neurological and/or psychiatric symptoms.
Shakibai, S. V., Johnson, J. P., & Bourgeois, J. A.	Paranoid Delusions and Cognitive Impairment Suggesting Fahr's Disease [7]	1 F	62	Multiple paranoid delusions; beliefs that people were controlling her by manipulating electrical dials, unknown other people were "listening through the walls" of her home, fears that her bed was "magnetized".	CT: bilateral symmetric basal ganglia calcifications

"M", males; "F", females; "Pt", patient; "MRI", Magnetic Resonance Imaging; "CT", computed tomography.

addition, there were no reports on the course and evolution of the symptoms reported in the literature. Further studies may be needed to explore these factors in understanding the neuropsychiatry of basal ganglia pathology.

Limitations. (1) To explore functional image studies that may also reveal dysfunction in other areas of the brain causing the pathology (2). Being a report of three individual cases, the need for a larger number of cases may provide a clearer picture of correlation.

4. Conclusion

A growing body of theoretical and clinical evidence shows that the basal ganglia play a key role in perceptual disturbances in addition to motor function. Our three cases demonstrate affective and psychotic symptoms concurrent with basal ganglia pathology. It is consistent with a literature review of the symptoms reported in patients with basal ganglia pathology. More appreciation of neuropsychiatric presentation of basal ganglia injury is needed with studies characterizing the correlation between basal ganglia pathology including onset and subnuclei location with symptoms. In doing so, we may improve the diagnosis, management and treatment following injury.

Consent

The patient's consent was obtained orally.

Authors' Contributions

All authors have participated in the procurement of this document and agree with the submitted case report.

References

[1] F. A. Middleton and P. L. Strick, "Basal ganglia and cerebellar loops: motor and cognitive circuits," *Brain Research Reviews*, vol. 31, no. 2-3, pp. 236–250, 2000.

[2] I. Le Ber, R.-M. Marié, B. Chabot, C. Lalevée, and G.-L. Defer, "Neuropsychological and 18FDG-PET studies in a family with idiopathic basal ganglia calcifications," *Journal of the Neurological Sciences*, vol. 258, no. 1-2, pp. 115–122, 2007.

[3] S. A. Kotz, M. Schwartze, and M. Schmidt-Kassow, "Non-motor basal ganglia functions: A review and proposal for a model of sensory predictability in auditory language perception," *Cortex*, vol. 45, no. 8, pp. 982–990, 2009.

[4] N. Adachi, T. Watanabe, H. Matsuda, and T. Onuma, "Hyperperfusion in the lateral temporal cortex, the striatum and the thalamus during complex visual hallucinations: single photon emission computed tomography findings in patients with charles bonnet syndrome," *Psychiatry and Clinical Neurosciences*, vol. 54, no. 2, pp. 157–162, 2000.

[5] F. A. Middleton and P. L. Strick, "Basal ganglia output and cognition: Evidence from anatomical, behavioral, and clinical studies," *Brain and Cognition*, vol. 42, no. 2, pp. 183–200, 2000.

[6] A. Rosenblatt and I. Leroi, "Neuropsychiatry of Huntington's disease and other basal ganglia disorders," *Psychosomatics*, vol. 41, no. 1, pp. 24–30, 2000.

[7] S. V. Shakibai, J. P. Johnson, and J. A. Bourgeois, "Paranoid delusions and cognitive impairment suggesting Fahr's disease," *Psychosomatics*, vol. 46, no. 6, pp. 569–572, 2005.

[8] L. L. Brown, J. S. Schneider, and T. I. Lidsky, "Sensory and cognitive functions of the basal ganglia," *Current Opinion in Neurobiology*, vol. 7, no. 2, pp. 157–163, 1997.

[9] A. A. Mufaddel, O. T. Osman, G. Al-Hassani, S. Al-Bedwawi, and M. J. Hashim, "Basal ganglia calcification in psychiatric inpatients: a case-control study," *Cognitive and Behavioral Neurology*, vol. 29, no. 3, pp. 139–143, 2016.

[10] J. L. Cummings, L. F. Gosenfeld, J. P. Houlihan, and T. McCaffrey, "Neuropsychiatric disturbances associated with idiopathic calcification of the basal ganglia," *Biological Psychiatry*, vol. 18, no. 5, pp. 591–601, 1983.

[11] E. D. Caine and I. Shoulson, "Psychiatric syndromes in Huntington's disease," *The American Journal of Psychiatry*, vol. 140, no. 6, pp. 728–733, 1983.

[12] B. Chabot, C. Roulland, and S. Dollfus, "Schizophrenia and familial idiopathic basal ganglia calcification: a case report," *Psychological Medicine*, vol. 31, no. 4, pp. 741–747, 2001.

[13] P. Entezami, M. Raff, and S. Bonner, "Visual hallucinations secondary to infarction of the caudate," *Journal of Neurology Neurophysiology*, vol. 6, no. 3, p. 298, 2015.

[14] M. Shirahama, J. Akiyoshi, Y. Ishitobi et al., "A young woman with visual hallucinations, delusions of persecution and a history of performing arson with possible three-generation Fahr disease," *Acta Psychiatrica Scandinavica*, vol. 121, no. 1, pp. 75–77, 2010.

[15] B. Pan, W. Liu, Q. Chen et al., "Idiopathic basal ganglia calcification presenting as schizophrenia-like psychosis and obsessive-compulsive symptoms: a case report," *Experimental and Therapeutic Medicine*, vol. 10, no. 2, pp. 608–610, 2015.

[16] K. Kasuga, T. Konno, K. Saito, A. Ishihara, M. Nishizawa, and T. Ikeuchi, "A Japanese family with idiopathic basal ganglia calcification with novel SLC20A2 mutation presenting with late-onset hallucination and delusion," *Journal of Neurology*, vol. 261, no. 1, pp. 242–244, 2014.

[17] G. Nicolas, O. Guillin, A. Borden, S. Bioux, R. Lefaucheur, and D. Hannequin, "Psychosis revealing familial idiopathic basal ganglia calcification," *General Hospital Psychiatry*, vol. 35, no. 5, 2013.

[18] E. C. Lauterbach, T. E. Spears, M. J. Prewett, S. T. Price, J. G. Jackson, and A. D. Kirsh, "Neuropsychiatric disorders, myoclonus, and dystonia in calcification of basal ganglia pathways," *Biological Psychiatry*, vol. 35, no. 5, pp. 345–351, 1994.

[19] J. Flint and L. H. Goldstein, "Familial calcification of the basal ganglia: A case report and review of the literature," *Psychological Medicine*, vol. 22, no. 3, pp. 581–595, 1992.

[20] H. Förstl, B. Krumm, S. Eden, and K. Kohlmeyer, "Neurological disorders in 166 patients with basal ganglia calcification: a statistical evaluation," *Journal of Neurology*, vol. 239, no. 1, pp. 36–38, 1992.

[21] A. F. Francis, "Familial basal ganglia calcification and schizophreniform psychosis," *The British Journal of Psychiatry*, vol. 135, no. 4, pp. 360–362, 1979.

[22] A. Vakaet, R. Rubens, J. de Reuck, and H. vander Eecken, "Intracranial bilateral symmetrical calcification on CT-scanning. A case report and a review of the literature," *Clinical Neurology and Neurosurgery*, vol. 87, no. 2, pp. 103–111, 1985.

[23] D. H. Geschwind, M. Loginov, and J. M. Stern, "Identification of a locus on chromosome 14q for idiopathic basal ganglia calcification (Fahr disease)," *American Journal of Human Genetics*, vol. 65, no. 3, pp. 764–772, 1999.

[24] B. Roiter, G. Pigato, and G. Perugi, "Late-Onset mania in a patient with movement disorder and basal ganglia calcifications: a challenge for diagnosis and treatment," *Case Reports in Psychiatry*, vol. 2016, Article ID 1393982, 5 pages, 2016.

[25] J. M. Johnson, B. Legesse, J. A. Camprodon, E. Murray, and B. H. Price, "The clinical significance of bilateral basal ganglia calcification presenting with mania and delusions," *The Journal of Neuropsychiatry and Clinical Neurosciences*, vol. 25, no. 1, pp. 68–71, 2013.

[26] M. P. Philpot and S. W. Lewis, "The psychopathology of basal ganglia calcification," *Behavioural Neurology*, vol. 2, no. 4, Article ID 643807, pp. 227–233, 1989.

[27] R. J. Trautner, J. L. Cummings, S. L. Read, and D. F. Benson, "Idiopathic basal ganglia calcification and organic mood disorder," *The American Journal of Psychiatry*, vol. 145, no. 3, pp. 350–353, 1988.

[28] S. Srivastava, M. S. Bhatia, V. Sharma, S. Mahajan, and G. Rajender, "Fahr's disease: An incidental finding in a case presenting with psychosis," *German Journal of Psychiatry*, vol. 13, no. 2, pp. 86–90, 2010.

[29] P. König, "Psychopathological alterations in cases of symmetrical basal ganglia sclerosis," *Biological Psychiatry*, vol. 25, no. 4, pp. 459–468, 1989.

18

A Case of Poisoning with *Abrus precatarius* Complicated with Bilateral Basal Ganglia Haemorrhage

Arun Rajaratnam, Kishan Dissanayake, Kiertie Kularatne, and Sunil Bowattage

Teaching Hospital Kandy, Kandy, Sri Lanka

Correspondence should be addressed to Arun Rajaratnam; nura321@hotmail.com

Academic Editor: Dominic B. Fee

Abrus precatarius is a tropical climber, whose seeds contain abrin, which is known to cause toxicity in humans. We report a case of a young girl, who presented with haemorrhagic enterocolitis, bilateral septal vein thrombosis, and basal ganglia haemorrhage leading to seizures and coma, following ingestion of toxic *A. precatarius* seeds. To the best of our knowledge, this is the first ever case to describe such an intracranial complication of abrin poisoning.

1. Introduction

Abrus precatarius, also referred to as rosary pea or jequirity pea, is a woody, Leguminosae climber found in many parts of Asia and Australia. The plant is widely distributed in Sri Lanka and its seeds are used in local board games and are used in Ayurvedic medical practice. The seeds are small, ovoid, glossy, and scarlet coloured with a black eye at the hilum, making those attractive for accidental consumption by children. Despite this, cases of abrin poisoning are rarely encountered and reported from the country. The seeds, roots, and leaves are considered poisonous, but toxicity occurs commonly from accidental or deliberate consumption of seeds. The hard protective outer covering needs to be breeched for the toxic contents to be released into the alimentary tract. Seeds of *A. precatarius* are toxic primarily due to a potent haemagglutinin called *Abrus agglutinin* and four other water-soluble toxic abrin (named "*a*" to "*d*") that are eliminated via the renal route [1]. Abrin (lectins) contains two subunits (A and B chains) involved in toxic pathogenesis. The B chain facilitates the intracellular entry of the A chain by binding to galactosyl terminated cell surface receptors, whereas the A chain inactivates 60 S ribosomal activity of Elongation Factors (1 and 2) leading to impaired protein translation and eventual cell death [2]. The abrin content of the seeds is about 0.15% w/w and a dose as small as 0.1–1 μg/kg body weight is said to be fatal [3]. Common toxic manifestations develop after a latent period of around 3 days [3] and include nausea, vomiting, diarrhoea, gastrointestinal bleeding, focal necrosis of the kidneys and liver, haemagglutination, haemolysis, hypovolemic shock, retinal haemorrhages, central nervous system complications, and death even after 14 days. Symptoms may persist for even more than 10 days [4]. The mortality rate is usually around 5% [5]. The case we are reporting is an intracranial complication of basal ganglia haemorrhage, which was not previously described in association with *A. precatarius*.

2. Case Presentation

A previously well, 17-year-old, unmarried, Sinhalese school girl presented after deliberate consumption of four seeds of *A. precatarius* plant from her garden (Figures 1 and 2). Following a family dispute, she had chewed and swallowed those unaware of the fatal outcome. The following day, she had developed painful lower abdominal cramps with small-volume watery diarrhoea. The day after, she had mild chills without much diarrhoea. On the fourth day, abdominal cramps and small-volume mucoid to watery diarrhoea had returned and persisted, making her seek medical attention.

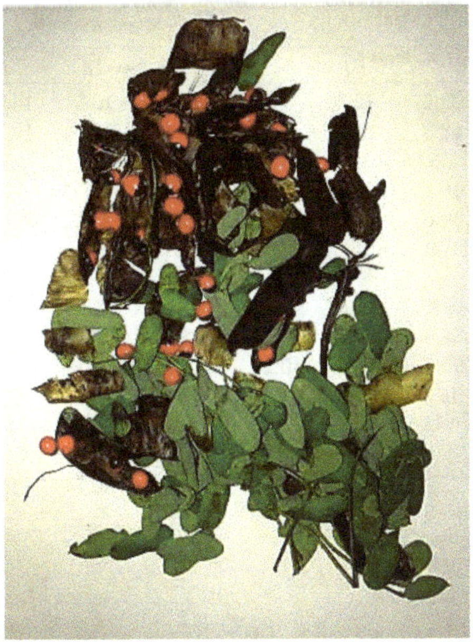

FIGURE 1: *A. precatarius* pod with seeds.

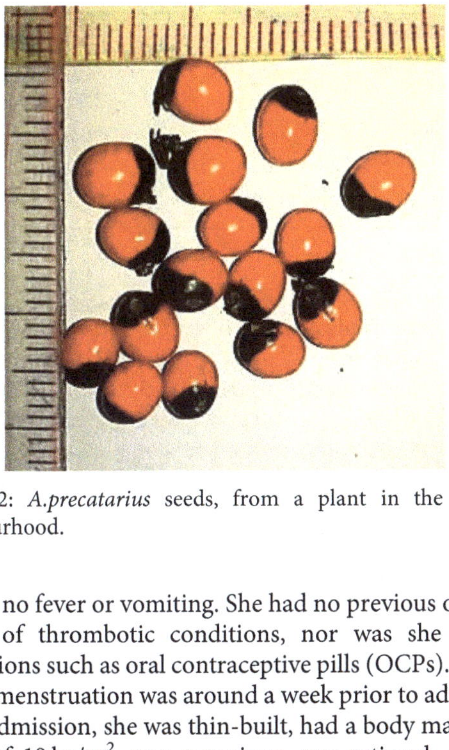

FIGURE 2: *A.precatarius* seeds, from a plant in the patient's neighbourhood.

She had no fever or vomiting. She had no previous or family history of thrombotic conditions, nor was she on any medications such as oral contraceptive pills (OCPs). Her last regular menstruation was around a week prior to admission.

At admission, she was thin-built, had a body mass index (BMI) of 19 kg/m^2, was conscious, was rational, and had stable vitals (core temperature of 37°C, pulse rate 110/minute, blood pressure-102/86 mmHg, respiratory rate of 29 breaths/minute and on-air arterial oxygen saturation (Sp_aO_2) of 99%. The rest of the examination was unremarkable apart from mild pallor, voluntary guarding, and tenderness of the lower abdomen. Rectal examination did not reveal any blood. She was initially treated with opiate analgesics, hydrated with intravenous normal saline and oral rehydration solution, and empirical antibiotics (intravenous meropenem and intravenous metronidazole), to cover possible infective gastroenteritis.

On the fifth day morning, she complained of fresh per rectal bleeding mixed with stools, had a slight drop in blood pressure, and required a transfer to the intensive care unit for monitoring. Later that night, she also had spontaneous vaginal bleeding. Urine human chorionic gonadotropin (hCG) was negative and serum beta hCG was low (< 2.39 mIU/ml). An abdominopelvic ultrasound revealed a normal liver, normal kidney size (measuring 9 cm bilaterally) and echotexture, a small amount of free fluid in the pelvic cavity, a slightly bulky and cystic right ovary, and an endometrial thickness of 0.8 cm without any evidence of intrauterine or extrauterine pregnancy. She was given a single dose of intravenous tranexamic acid (500 mg) to reduce the bleed. A few minutes later, she developed a generalised tonic-clonic seizure lasting for more than ten minutes with abnormal flexing, fixing of gaze, stridor, and subsequent drop in the Glasgow Coma Scale (GCS) from 15 to 10 and Sp_aO_2 to 70%, warranting immediate intubation and ventilation. Her hydration, blood pressure, and oxygenation status were normal at the time of the seizure. There was no papilloedema, neck stiffness, or focal neurological signs. Apart from a mild hyponatremia, the rest of the metabolic parameters including blood sugar were normal. A noncontrast computed tomogram (NCCT) of the brain performed within a few hours of intubation did not reveal any haemorrhage or cerebral oedema. An urgent MRI could not be performed at that moment. Following a specialist neurology consultation, she was commenced on a five-day course of intravenous methylprednisolone, suspecting of *A. precatarius* induced demyelination, along with intravenous antiepileptics (midazolam, thiopentone sodium, phenytoin, and levetiracetam) and oral topiramate for refractory seizures.

Serial neurological examinations were conducted daily, while under sedation and being ventilated did not reveal any signs of focal neurology, papilloedema, pupillary abnormalities, or signs of meningism. However, she was noticed to have generalised flaccidity with intermittent, brief (about 10 seconds) episodes of tonicity and involuntary movements of the extremities, hyporeflexia, and episodes of involuntary blinking. Digital electroencephalogram (EEG) performed while ventilated but off sedation, revealed continuous polymorphic delta activity that is suggestive of moderate generalised cerebral dysfunction. Epileptiform discharges were not seen in the EEG. The patient's parents did not consent for a lumbar puncture. Table 1 gives the trend of biochemical investigations. Table 2 gives the trend in arterial blood gas parameters. Serial blood pictures were revealing evidence of inflammation and iron deficiency with recent bleeding without haemolysis. Stool for occult blood was positive even during the second week. Her thryoid stimulating hormone (TSH) was 0.659 mIU/L·0(0.4–4.0), and free thyroxine (T4) was 8.50 ng/dL (10.3–25.3). She had a negative antinuclear antibody (ANA), which was found out after undergoing the Coombss test and PCR for SARS RNA. However, she had a high d-dimer (value: 1.2 mg/L, reference < 0.2 mg/L). Urine had no protein or active sediment. Serial blood, urine, and endotracheal cultures were negative.

Table 1: Trend of blood or serum biochemical parameters.

Day	Reference range	5	6	7	8	10	12	14	18	20	24
WBC ($X10^3/\mu L$)	4.0–10.0	23.4	42.5	34.5	23.4	22.2	17.5	39.0	13.5	14.1	10.5
Neutrophil ($X10^3/\mu L$)	2.0–7.0	20.0	37.9	30.9	18.8	18.9	16.1	33.3	10.0	10.9	7.3
Lymphocyte ($X10^3/\mu L$)	0.8–4.0	1.4	0.7	1.3	1.5	1.2	0.8	2.7	1.9	1.9	2.2
Haemoglobin (g/L)	11.0–15.0	13.2	14.5	11.1	10.1	8.2	8.8	7.8	7.7	9.0	9.1
Haematoctit (%)	37.0–54.0	43.5	44.4	32.7	30.6	27.9	26.9	24.2	24.1	28.1	28.1
Platelet count (X 106/μL)	150–40	161	123	110	140	181	202	287	349	313	268
ESR (mm/1st hour)	< 15	5									30
Blood urea (mmol/L)	2.8–7.2	5.0	3.38	4.13	4.8	10.0	17.0	16.7	7.8	5.1	
Serum creatinine (μmol/L)	65–120	49.0	63.6	75.8	64.3	92.8	107.0	142.7	87.8	57.4	53.7
Serum magnesium (mmol/L)	(0.7–1.0)				0.87	0.77	0.47	0.79	0.61		0.53
Serum phosphorus (mmol/L)	(0.8–1.45)		1.05		0.77	0.27	1.22	1.42	1.62		1.77
Serum total calcium (mmol/L)	(2.1–2.55)		1.8		1.83	1.80	1.86	1.87	2.17		2.22
Serum potassium (mmol/L)	3.5–5.5	4.0	3.5	3.9	4.7	4.1	4.2	3.8	4.0	4.2	4.0
Serum sodium (mmol/L)	1.5–150	131	130	128	132	135	138	139	144	143	140
Urine potassium (mmol/L)			14.1		15.7						
Urine sodium (mmol/L)			172	168.6	139.0						
Urine osmolality (mOsm/L)	300–900		683	565	877						
Serum osmolality (mOsm/L)	275–295	268		270	294						
ALT(U/L)	< 34	23.4	11.4	11.8	25.1	40.1	49.4	57.0	45.6	75.7	59.3
AST (U/L)	< 31	35.5	20.0	30.5	63.0	68.6	56.6	61.2	46.8	62.0	43.0
GGT (U/L)		10.8			11.7		23.1	31.0	33.9		67.9
ALP (U/L)		56.3						59.8	67.4		84.8
Total bilirubin (μmol/L)	5.0–19.0	7.33			3.57	4.13	3.47	3.14	4.56		6.59
Direct bilirubin (μmol/L)	1.7–6.8	2.19			1.31	1.47	0.62	0.71	1.57		2.32
Total protein (g/dL)	6.6–8.3	5.7	4.9	3.9	3.7	3.5	4.0	4.9	6.3		7.6
Serum albumin (g/dL)							2.4	2.8	3.7		4.2
APTT (sec)	32–35	32.8		30.2	36.2	28.9	22.1	35.0	33.3	32.2	36.7
PT/INR	0.9–1.1	1.13	1.42	1.22	1.31	1.21	1.09	1.30	1.02	1.05	1.16
LDH (U/L)	< 225	224									
CPK (U/L)	< 145				1184						164

Table 2: trend of arterial biochemical parameters.

Day	5	6	8	9	10	12	14	17
pH	7.33	7.31	7.35	7.44	7.56	7.43	7.48	7.45
pCO2	27.8	32.5	34.8	25.2	29.2	34.5	30.2	36.3
pO2	60.4	69.0	84.9	133.9	198	52	123.6	82.4
HCO3−	14.5	16.5	19.2	17.3	21.0	22.9	22.5	27.1
Lactate	1.0	2.5	1.4	1.2	1.5	1.6	1.3	0.4

Active limb physiotherapy was offered. Measures were taken to prevent pressure sores, aspiration, and venous thromboembolism (pneumatic compression stockings and low molecular weight heparin). With no marked improvement in neurology following a five-day course of methylprednisolone, she was commenced on seven daily cycles of plasma exchange cycles (day 12 to day 17 of illness) with FFP cover, replacing 1800 ml of plasma in each session. Although her diarrhoea settled, she had stool occult blood positivity. She was extubated and sedatives were withheld completely on the 14th day of illness, following which she initially was able only to turn her head sideways and to turn her eyes laterally, spontaneously, and as well as on command. Neurological examination revealed flaccid limbs with proximal and distal weakness (grade 3/5), hyporeflexia, down-going plantar response, cognitive dysfunction manifested by amnesia and poor attention, drowsiness, and difficult phonation.

Magnetic resonance imaging (with T1W, T2W, FLAIR, DWI, GAD, MRV, and MRA sequences) performed on the 15th day of poisoning showed bilateral, symmetric, ill-defined, heterogenous T2 weighted (T2W), and fluid attenuated inversion recovery (FLAIR) showed heterogenous (high with patchy central low) signal abnormality in striato-capsular areas of basal ganglia with thalami sparing (Figures 3–5). The low-intensity areas seen in T2W and FLAIR sequences showed intermediate signal intensity in T1 weighted (T1W) and blooming on susceptibility weighted imaging (SWI), with no enhancement of contrast, suggesting evidence for bilateral, symmetrical haemorrhage with associated vasogenic oedema involving basal ganglia and internal capsule (Figures 6 and 7). Cerebral sulci, gyri, subcortical white matter, ventricular system, brainstem, and cerebellum were normal with preserved grey and white differentiation. Bilateral septal veins visualized on SWI are not opacified in contrast to magnetic resonance venography (MRV) favouring bilateral septal vein thrombosis (Figure 8). Bilateral internal cerebral veins and thalomostriate veins, great vein of Galen, and straight sinus were normal. The rest of the MRV did not show major dural venous sinus thrombosis. Magnetic resonance arteriography (MRA) was normal. Interval MRI in 1 week showed persistence of

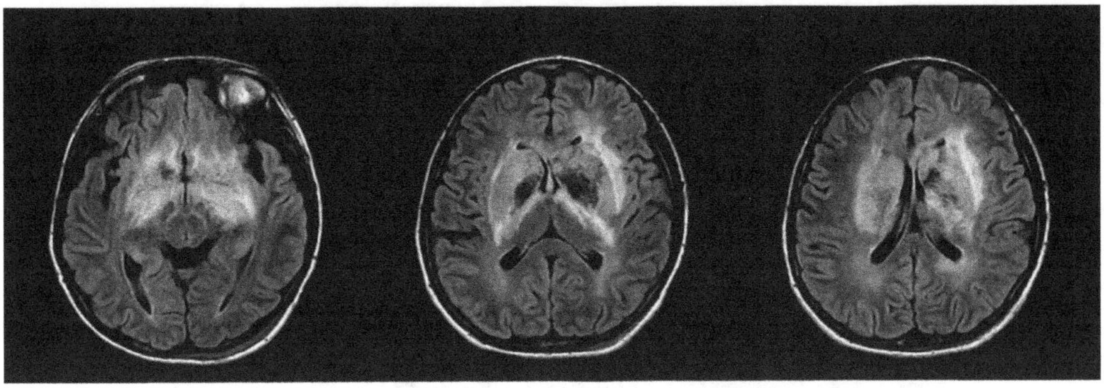

Figure 3: T2-FLAIR image, an axial section at basal ganglia.

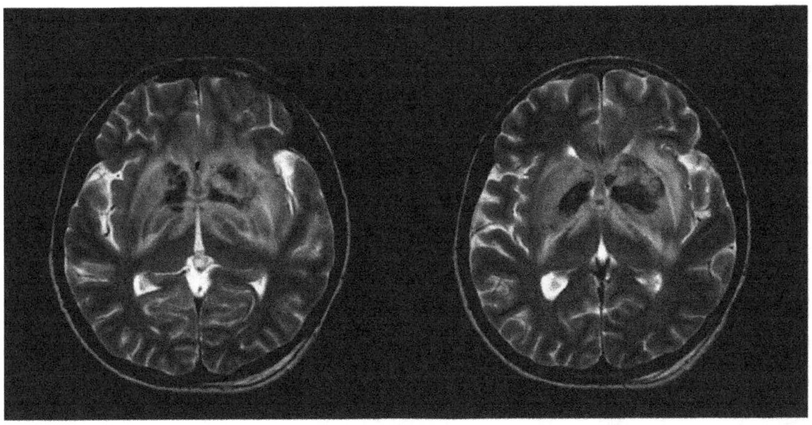

Figure 4: T2-W image, an axial section at basal ganglia.

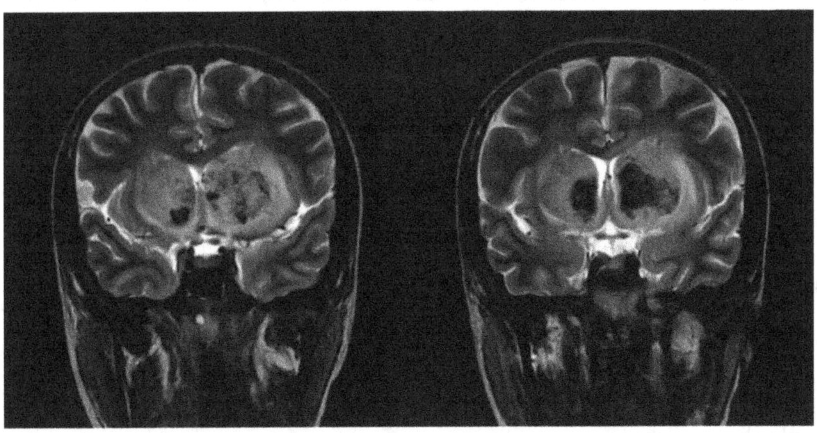

Figure 5: T2-W image, a coronal section at basal ganglia.

previously noted basal ganglia haemorrhage with no new intracerebral haemorrhage.

On day 18, she was in a normal ward, where physiotherapy, speech therapy, neurorehabilitation, nasogastric feeding, levetiracetam, and intravenous antibiotics were continued. Although she found difficulty in phonation and had impaired bladder sensation, there was a gradual improvement in comprehension, cognitive function, and limb power. She was discharged on the 24th day with oral levetiracetam and haemetinics and was emphasised on home-based physiotherapy and NG feeding. Modified Rankin Scale (MRS) was 4 on discharge. Oral feeding was commenced and the urinary catheter was removed 1-week postdischarge.

During a review at 1 month postdischarge, she was found to be alert, verbalising, scored 27/30 on the validated Sinhalese version Montreal Cognitive Assessment (MoCA) [6],

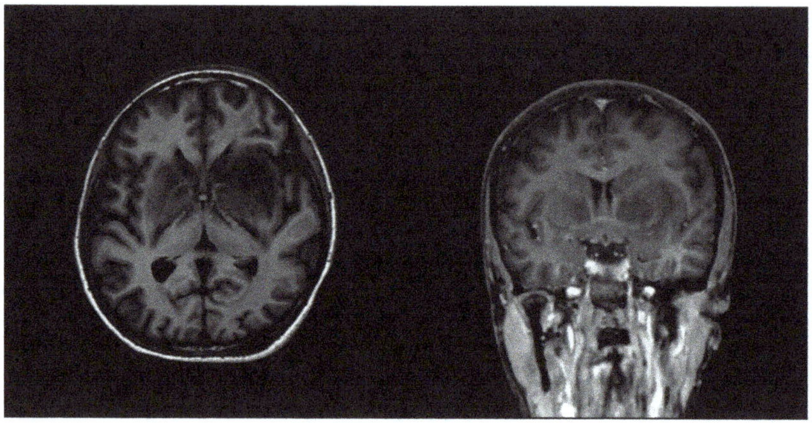

FIGURE 6: T1-W, an axial section and T1-W gadolinium contrast, a coronal section images at basal ganglia.

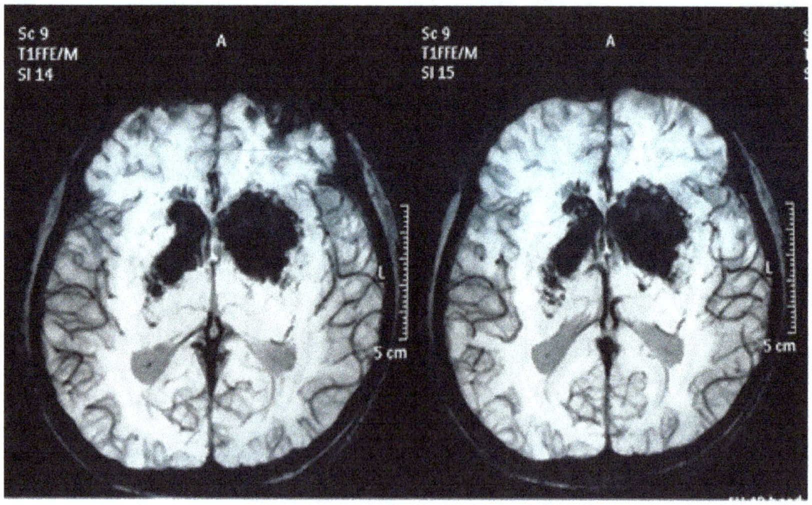

FIGURE 7: SWI image, an axial section at basal ganglia.

had improving limb functions except for a left-sided foot drop, and had an MRS of 1. Nerve Conduction Studies of the left lower limb only revealed evidence of a moderate partial common peroneal lesion at the fibular neck with active denervation and no reinnervation. She had lost weight (BMI 13.7 kg/m^2; midarm circumference of 17.5 cm), had minor nutritional insufficiencies (haemoglobin 9.6 g/dL, mean corpuscular volume 91 fL, vitamin D level 28.4 *n*g/ml, vitamin B12 level 262.2 pg/mL, serum ferritin 169.0 mg/mL, and serum iron 6.73 μmol/L), and had a patch of nonscarring alopecia. Antinuclear antibody level was nonsignificant (titre of 1 : 40). She had completely recovered functionally and cognitively at 2 months postdischarge. Nutritional supplementation was continued and levetiracetam was gradually tapered and omitted after 6 months but had to be recommenced at a low dose as seizures were recurring a few weeks after omission.

3. Discussion

Neurological consequences of abrin toxicity occur less frequently than gastrointestinal consequences. Reported neurological complications include headache, hallucinations, mydriasis, papilloedema, tetany, seizures, coma, and encephalitis-like syndrome [7, 8]. There are few cases of late-onset CNS immune-mediated demyelination, making us initially suspect it as the underlying pathological process in our patient [9–11]. CNS demyelination is due to abrin's immunomodulatory and immunostimulatory properties [12, 13]. Abrin-induced demyelination is reported to respond completely to methylprednisolone and plasma exchange [9–11]. A case of osmotic demyelination due to direct effects of abrin in the absence of serum sodium abnormalities was reported previously in a 2-year-old [14]. Thrombotic complications with abrin are sparsely reported. One case of superior sagittal sinus thrombosis attributed to dehydration from gastrointestinal loss, capillary leak syndrome, or from direct endothelial injury from abrin has been reported [15]. Abrin agglutinator causes haemagglutination. However, the exact effect of abrin on coagulation is unknown. Our patient had a normal coagulation profile despite bleeding and thrombosis occurring simultaneously.

MRI and MRV are the most sensitive tools in detecting early deep cerebral vein thrombosis (CVT) [16]. The

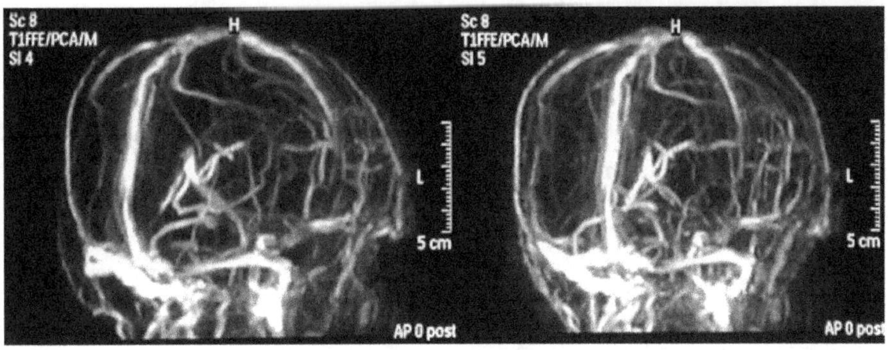

FIGURE 8: CT venogram.

difference in signal intensities of T1 and T2 weighted images may help to date the onset of thrombosis and subsequent vasogenic oedema and ischaemia [17]. Isolated thrombosis of bilateral septal veins is not frequently described. The bilateral septal veins, which drain the anterior basal ganglia, corpus callosum, and the deep medullary frontal white matter, begin at the lateral aspect of the anterior horns of lateral ventricles and then pass medially and inferior to the genu of the corpus callosum. These then turn posteriorly, traverse the septum pellucidum, and join with the thalamostiate veins behind the foramen of Monro to form the internal cerebral vein [18].

Abrin per se is described to induce endothelial injury leading to increased capillary permeability and vasogenic oedema [2, 19]. In this reported case, abrin's direct inhibitory effect on protein synthesis of the metabolically active basal ganglia may have resulted in tissue inflammation, ischaemic necrosis, and subsequent bleeding. Thrombosis of the thin calibre septal veins that traverse adjacent to the anterior basal ganglia may have occurred secondary to surrounding inflammation. Another possibility is that the direct endothelial injury by abrin activates the clotting cascade leading to bilateral septal vein thrombosis first, thereby leading to vasogenic and cytotoxic oedema, and later haemorrhage of the draining basal ganglia. The metabolically active basal ganglia are commonly targeted in other poisonings as well. Bilateral basal ganglia haemorrhages had been previously described due to carbon monoxide, methanol, ethylene glycol, and following scorpion sting [20–23]. Therefore, in the context of poisoning, MRI changes in our patient are likely to represent basal ganglia swelling which has subsequently undergone haemorrhagic transformation due to necrosis. The spatial resolution of MRV is not enough to reliably comment on septal vein thrombosis. Poor visualisation of septal veins on MRV/SWI is likely to be secondary to the mass effect of the swollen basal ganglia, rather than septal vein thrombosis.

Our patient had no diagnostic MRI evidence for acute haemorrhagic encephalomyelitis (AHEM) and acute demyelinating encephalomyelitis (ADEM). Nevertheless, she was initially managed for possible immune-mediated demyelination with methylprednisolone and therapeutic plasma exchange, until an MRI diagnosis was available. Although a partial neurological recovery was noticed with plasma exchange, much of the neurological and cognitive recovery occurred on its own with the passage of time, perhaps also supported by active neuro-rehabilitating care during the initial months. Plasma exchange may have had an effect in removing both the toxin and immune modulators. Untreated patients with deep CVT often develop features of raised intracranial pressure and brain herniation, which can lead to permanent residual disability and often death. However, in our patient prophylactic enoxaparin, which was given during the initial period, had to be discontinued due to persistent faecal occult bleeding and dropping haemoglobin levels. Our patient had no absolute indication to be screened for hereditary or autoimmune thrombophilias.

Till date, there is no antidote for abrin poisoning. Hence, treatment for abrin poisoning is largely supportive and symptomatic with the provision of intravenous fluids, correction of electrolyte imbalance, and correction of anaemia, as in our case. Gastric lavage, activated charcoal, and induced emesis may be used in the early hours after ingestion, but need to be administered with caution due to the necrotizing action of abrin [24]. Alkaline diuresis with sodium bicarbonate will prevent the precipitation of haemoglobin and its products in kidney tubules [5]. Aggressive treatment and monitoring are warranted for all patients even though there is a delay in presentation.

It is important to note that our patient was brought for medical care with three days of symptoms of abrin poisoning, reflecting the public unawareness of the grave consequences of the poisoning. Had she not come at the correct time, a fatality may not have been prevented. Hence, it is pertinent to create awareness on the harmful effects of such poisonous plants in the tropics. In countries such as the United States, where *A. precatarius* is not commonly grown, a legislature on restricting the labelling and import of *Abrus* and *Abrus* derived items have been effective [1].

4. Conclusion

The reported case depicts a unique and unusual neurological consequence of abrin poisoning. It is not very clear why abrin would predispose to both cerebral venous thrombosis and haemorrhage. Nevertheless, one needs to consider venous thrombotic and haemorrhagic causes in addition to the well-described demyelinating causes, when managing abrin-related central neurological manifestations such as seizures and coma. Magnetic resonance imaging and additional sequences are effective in differentiating these. Further studies may be needed to understand the effects of abrin on coagulation.

Consent

The consent for publication was obtained from the patient's biological mother.

References

[1] Ø Fodstad, J. V. Johannessen, L. Schjerven, and A. Pihl, "Toxicity of abrin and ricin in mice and dogs," *Journal of Toxicology and Environmental Health*, vol. 5, no. 6, pp. 1073–1084, 1979.

[2] H. Y. Chen, L. Y. Foo, and W. K. Loke, "Abrin and ricin: understanding their toxicity, diagnosis, and treatment," *Biological Toxins and Bioterrorism. Toxinology*, Springer, Berlin, Germany, 2015.

[3] K. J. Dickers, S. M. Bradberry, P. Rice, G. D. Griffiths, and J. A. Vale, "Abrin poisoning," *Toxicological Reviews*, vol. 22, no. 3, pp. 137–142, 2003.

[4] R. Fernando and Management of Poisoning, "National poisons information centre," *Colombo*, vol. 19, 1998.

[5] J. M. Arena, "Poisoning toxicity, symptoms treatments," *Poisonous Plants, Reptiles, Arthropods, Insects and Fish*, Charles C Thomas, Springfield, IL, USA, 1976.

[6] S. Karunaratne, R. Hanwella, and V. de Silva, "Validation of the Sinhala version of the montreal cognitive assessment in screening for dementia," *Ceylon Medical Journal*, vol. 56, no. 4, pp. 147–153, 2011.

[7] D. Subrahmanyan, J. M. Dks, and M. Raj, "An unusual manifestation of *Abrus precatorius* poisoning: a report of two cases," *Clinical Toxicology*, vol. 46, no. 2, pp. 173–175, 2008 Feb.

[8] B. Z. Horowitz, R. Castelli, A. Hughes, R. G. Hendrickson, R. C. Johnson, and J. D. Thomas, "Massive fatal overdose of abrin with progressive encephalopathy," *Clinical Toxicology*, vol. 58, no. 5, pp. 417–420, 2020.

[9] V. Sahni, S. K. Agarwal, N. P. Singh, and S. Sikdar, "Acute demyelinating encephalitis after jequirity pea ingestion (*Abrus precatorius*)," *Clinical Toxicology*, vol. 45, no. 1, pp. 77–79, 2007.

[10] R. Sahoo, A. Hamide, S. D. Amalnath, and B. S. Narayana, "Acute demyelinating encephalitis due to *Abrus precatorius* poisoning--complete recovery after steroid therapy," *Clinical Toxicology*, vol. 46, no. 10, pp. 1071–1073, 2008 Dec.

[11] E. C. Ninan and E. James, "Acute disseminated encephalomyelitis due to abrus precatorius poisoning a case report," *Saudi Pharmaceutical Journal*, vol. 27, no. 4, pp. 521–524, 2019.

[12] S. Tripathi and T. K. Maiti, "Immunomodulatory role of native and heat denatured agglutinin from *Abrus precatorius*," *The International Journal of Biochemistry & Cell Biology*, vol. 37, no. 2, pp. 451–462, 2005.

[13] V. Ramnath, G. Kuttan, and R. Kuttan, "Immunopotentiating activity of abrin, a lectin from *Abrus precatorius* Linn," *Indian Journal of Experimental Biology*, vol. 40, no. 8, pp. 910–913, 2002.

[14] S. Sarkar, K. Basu, J. Das, and S. Datta, "Abrus precatorius poisoning and central pontine myelinolysis," *Journal of Pediatric Neurosciences*, vol. 12, no. 4, pp. 353–355, 2017.

[15] K. V. Vinod, M. M. Thabah, T. Venkatesh, G. Thiruvikramaprakash, S. R. Kumar, and T. K. Dutta, "A rare cause of dural venous sinus thrombosis," *Neurology India*, vol. 61, no. 6, pp. 669-670, 2013.

[16] R. H. Ayanzen, C. R. Bird, P. J. Keller, F. J. McCully, M. R. Theobald, and J. E. Heiserman, "Cerebral MR venography: normal anatomy and potential diagnostic pitfalls," *AJNR. American journal of neuroradiology*, vol. 21, no. 1, pp. 74–78, 2000.

[17] P. J. Macchi, R. I. Grossman, J. M. Gomori, H. I. Goldberg, R. A. Zimmerman, and L. T. Bilaniuk, "High field MR imaging of cerebral venous thrombosis," *Journal of Computer Assisted Tomography*, vol. 10, no. 1, pp. 10–15, 1986.

[18] E. K. Miyawaki, R. B. Daroff, and M. J. Aminoff, "Cerebral veins and venous sinuses," in *Encyclopedia of the Neurological Sciences*Academic Press, Cambridge, MA, USA, 2014.

[19] M. M. Patil, S. V. Patil, A. S. Akki, B. Lakhkar, and S. Badiger, "An arrow poison (Abrus precatorius) causing fatal poisoning in a child," *Journal of Clinical and Diagnostic Research*, vol. 10, no. 3, pp. SD03–4, 2016.

[20] A. Dower, S. Camp, M. Cheik-Hussein, and G. Samandouras, "Bilateral basal ganglia haemorrhage secondary to carbon monoxide poisoning," *International Journal of Case Reports in Medicine*, vol. 2016, pp. 1–7, Article ID 448564, 2016.

[21] G. Ganguly, A. Banerjee, S. Mukherjee, S. K. Das, and B. Maity, "Bilateral basal ganglia haemorrhage--uncommon manifestation of methanol poisoning," *Journal of the Association of Physicians of India*, vol. 44, no. 11, pp. 834-835, 1996.

[22] P. Corr and M. Szolics, "Neuroimaging findings in acute ethylene glycol poisoning," *Journal of Medical Imaging and Radiation Oncology*, vol. 56, no. 4, pp. 442–444, 2012.

[23] A. Majumdar, V. Atam, S. A. Ansari, S. Kumar, and A. Bhardwaj, "Basal ganglia hemorrhage secondary to scorpion sting: a fatal presentation," *Egypt Journal of Neurology Psychiatry Neurosurgery*, vol. 56, no. 1, p. 65, 2020.

[24] V. V. Pillay, "Current views on antidotal therapy in managing cases of poisoning and overdose," *Journal of the Association of Physicians of India*, vol. 56, pp. 881–892, 2008.

19

Duodenal Neuroendocrine Tumour Presenting as GABA B Receptor Autoimmune Encephalitis

Dhanashree Peddawad and Manoj K. Singh

Department of Neurology, Continental Hospital, Nanakrumguda, Financial District, 500032 Hyderabad, India

Correspondence should be addressed to Dhanashree Peddawad; dhanashree27j@gmail.com

Academic Editor: Peter Berlit

GABA B receptor antibody positive autoimmune encephalitis is rarely seen in clinical practice. It is usually associated with small cell lung carcinoma, and occasionally with neuroendocrine tumour (NET) of lung. GABA B receptor antibody can be associated with other autoimmune antibodies like antinuclear antibody and antibody to Glutamic acid decarboxylase. We present a case with GABA B receptor autoimmune encephalitis associated with neuroendocrine tumour of the duodenum with special emphasis on correlation between immunostaining of the tumour and presence of GABA B receptor antibody.

1. Introduction

GABA B receptor antibody positive encephalitis other than small cell lung cancer & neuroendocrine tumour (NET) of lung has not been described in literature. Small cell lung cancer and neuroendocrine tumors have common immuno-histochemistry markers. It suggests that neuroendocrine tumors irrespective of their localization can be associated with GABA B receptor autoimmune encephalitis. It also suggests patho-physiological association of these immuno-histochemistry markers with GABA B antibody.

1.1. Case History. Seventy years male brought with complaints of left lower limb parasthesia of one hour duration followed by acute onset altered sensorium which started 12 hours prior to presentation to the emergency room. Altered sensorium remained for about 72 hours during hospital course from the time of onset. There were no features suggestive of motor seizures. He did not have fever, headache, vomiting, loss of consciousness, trauma, or fall.

1.2. Past History. He was diagnosed of having hypothyroidism, hypertension, diabetes for last 15 years and Parkinson disease for last 10 years. He was receiving 50 ug of Eltroxin every day. Patient was in euthyroid state on medication. He was receiving combination of Vildagliptin and Metformin 500 mg twice a day after meals for last 6 years. Patient never had episodes of hypoglycemia in past. He was prescribed combination of Levodopa (100 mg) and Carbidopa three times in a day. His modified Hoehn and Yahr scale was 2.5. Two and half years ago, patient had 5 kg weight loss in 4 weeks associated with watery diarrhea and was diagnosed to have well differentiated para—duodenal neuroendocrine tumor. CT abdomen and pelvis then revealed 5.0×3.8 cms heterogeneously enhancing partially necrotic exophytic mass lesion from D2 duodenum. There was no infiltration of adjacent structures or evidence of metastasis or lymph node involvement. Whole body FDG PET scan confirmed paraduodenal mass. Ga68DOTA-NOC scan and CT guided Biopsy were also done two and half years ago. Ga68DOTA-NOC scan revealed well defined DOTA avid heterogeneously intensely enhancing mass lesion in right sub-hepatic region, abutting the proximal lateral wall of D2 segment of duodenum, situated posterior to hepatic flexure of colon suggestive of neuroendocrine tumour (Figure 1a). CT guided biopsy revealed well differentiated neuroendocrine tumor (Figures 1b & 1c). Immunohistochemistry stains for synaptophysin, chromogranin, CD56 and neuron specific enolase were positive. (Figures 1d–1g). Serum Chromogranin A level was 155.70 ng/mL ($N < 39$ ng/mL).

1.3. Clinical Findings. His vital signs including pulse rate, blood pressure, oxygen saturation were normal. Pulse rate

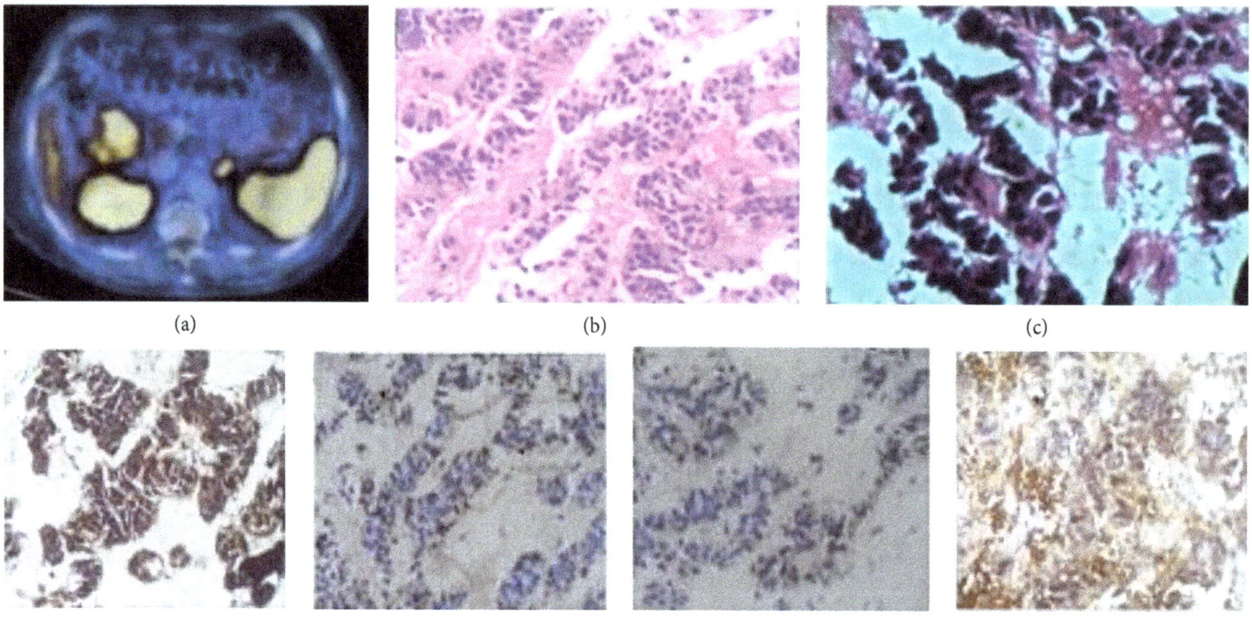

FIGURE 1: (a) Ga68DOTA-NOC—5 × 4 × 5 cm well defined DOTA avid heterogeneously intensely enhancing mass lesion in the right sub-hepatic region, abutting the proximal lateral wall of D2 segment of duodenum, situated posterior to hepatic flexure of colon s/o NET, (b) H & E Stain, (c) CT guided biopsy—Ribbons of small oval cells seperated by vascular channels. Cells have eosinophilic granular cytoplasm and relatively large dark nucleus. Cells and nuclei are uniform in size. No mitosis seen. Focal necrosis seen. Lower row images show positive stains by immunohistochemistry in our patient, (d) Synaptophysin, (e) Chromogranin, (f) CD56, and (g) Neuron specific enolase.

was 84/min regular, blood pressure was 130/80 mmHg and oxygen saturation of 98% on room air. On examination he was found to have aphasia and disorientation. He could not comprehend speech of others and was repeating same words and sentences. Patient was in confusional state but was not aggressive. He could not recognize his family members. There was no cranial neuropathy. He was having mild rigidity in right upper and lower limbs. Power was normal in all limbs. Deep tendon reflexes were depressed in upper limbs and absent in lower limbs. Sensory examination could not be done as patient was not able to comprehend verbal commands. But he was responding to pain stimuli. He could stand and walk without support. Right hand mild rest tremors were present. We did not observe any intentional tremors as he tried to pick objects while carrying out examination.

2. Diagnostic Assessment

2.1. Investigations. Laboratory tests showed hemoglobin 9 gm% and ESR 70 mm/hr. Blood sugar level checked by family member at home was 240 mg/dL. Blood sugar was rechecked by emergency doctor immediately after arriving to emergency room and it was 234 mg/dL. Fasting blood glucose and glycosylated hemoglobin levels were 136 mg/dL and 7.5, respectively. Complete blood count, liver, renal function tests, electrolytes, arterial blood gas analysis, serum ammonia, thyroid function test, anti TPO antibody, Antinuclear antibody, CSF routine study and HSV PCR were normal. MRI brain did not show any significant findings. EEG showed theta background slowing and right temporal spikes.

2.2. Differential Diagnosis. Differential diagnosis considered in our case were acute stroke, metabolic encephalopathy including Wernickes encephalopathy & electrolyte imbalance, brain tumor, intoxication, nonconvulsive status epilepticus, viral encephalitis, thyroid autoimmune encephalitis, other autoimmune encephalitis, and paraneoplastic encephalitis. Acute stroke was ruled out as there was no diffusion restriction and angiography was normal. MRI was not suggestive of Wernickes encephalopathy. There was no space occupying lesion on MRI. There were no features of viral or limbic encephalitis on MRI brain. Thyroid antibody titers were negative. All metabolic parameters including sodium, calcium, and magnesium were within normal limits. MRI did not show any signs of anoxia or hypoglycemia. There was no history or physical findings suggestive of any toxin consumption. Possibility of nonconvulsive status epilepticus was considered. Continuous EEG monitoring done which showed occasional focal spikes in right temporal region. But absence of continuous epilptiform activity ruled out the possibility of NCSE.

In view of presence of neuroendocrine tumor, possibility of paraneoplastic autoimmune encephalitis was considered. He underwent CT chest with CT abdomen and pelvis which showed same size of paradodenal mass. CT did not reveal any lung lesion or mass.

Our case fulfilled diagnostic criteria for paraneoplastic autoimmune encephalitis proposed by Gutelkin [1]. Our case had (i) aphasia, short term memory loss and confusional state, suggesting involvement of limbic system; (ii) an interval of two & half years between onset of neurological symptoms and cancer diagnosis; (iii) exclusion of other cancer-related complications (metastasis, infection, metabolic, and nutritional deficits, cerebrovascular disorder or side-effects of therapy); (iv) EEG showing spike wave activity in right temporal lobe.

Paraneoplastic antibody panel were sent in CSF sample. Paraneoplastic antibodies Amphiphysin, CV2.1, PNMA2 (Ma2/Ta), ANNA-1/Hu, ANNA-2/Ri, PCA-1//Yo were negative. Autoimmune antibodies AMPA1 and 2, GABA B receptor antibody, LGI-1, CASPR2, and NMDA were tested using HEK293 assay in serum and CSF sample. GABA B receptor antibody was tested positive in serum. HEK293 assay is immunofluorescent method in which human embryonic kidney cells are transfected with GABA B receptor which show reactivity with CSF/serum of patient with limbic encephalitis and polyclonal antibody to GABA B receptor. Both activities are merged. Control sample does not show reactivity to patients CSF/serum sample but shows reactivity to polyclonal antibody to GABA B receptor.

GABA B receptor autoimmune encephalitis cases reported in past had similar symptoms of limbic encephalitis in elderly patients with malignancies like small cell carcinoma of lung or rarely neuroendocrine tumor of lung [2–4]. According to prior case series there are cases with normal MRI brain and acellular CSF with normal protein sugar levels [2–4].

2.3. Treatment. Patient did not receive any antiviral or antibiotic treatment at any point during hospital course. Patient received five doses of one gram intravenous methylprednisolone which was started 36 hours after the onset of symptoms. He stopped repeating same words or sentences and his short term memory improved. He became oriented to time place and person and started recognizing his relatives. He showed complete recovery three days after admission. Other treatment modalities like IVIG or plasma exchange were considered and discussed with patients family at the beginning of pulse therapy. As patient showed complete clinical improvement after pulse steroid therapy and did not have any recurrence, plasma exchange, or IVIG were not considered later.

2.4. Follow up. Patient was found symptom free during five months of follow up. Repeat GABA B receptor antibody test in serum after five months of discharge was negative. Patient was receiving tablet Imatinib 400 mg once a day and also injection Octreotide 30 mg intramuscularly once a month since last two years. Tumor symptoms were under control on this treatment. There was no watery diarrhea, weight loss, or flushing since the onset of therapy. He also did not have relapse in encephalitic symptoms after discharge.

3. Discussion

Our case (i) Fullfill the criteria for paraneoplastic limbic encephalitis [1]; (ii) had serum GABA B receptor antibody; (iii) with paraduodenal well differentiated neuroendocrine tumor and; (iv) showed complete recovery after IV methylprednisolone course. According to prior case series [2–5], GABA B receptor antibody encephalitis is most commonly seen in small cell carcinoma of lung. There are occasional cases of lung neuroendocrine tumor presenting as GABA B receptor positive autoimmune encephalitis. Small cell lung cancer and neuroendocrine tumors have common immunohistochemistry markers [6]. To best of our knowledge neuroendocrine tumor of gastrointestinal tract has not been seen with GABA B receptor autoimmune encephalitis. Our case of GABA B receptor autoimmune encephalitis had histologically proven duodenal neuroendocrine tumor. It suggests that neuroendocrine tumors, irrespective of their localization are associated with GABA B receptor autoimmune encephalitis. Also as per our case, histopathology of even well differentiated NET can lead to paraneoplastic manifestation. These patients may not present with obvious symptoms of malignancy and may be missed without thorough clinical and radiological evaluation. Though surgical removal is not done routinely in well differentiated neuroendocrine tumors, it is important to consider removal of tumor in case of paraneoplastic manifestations.

Small cell lung cancer and neuroendocrine tumours have common immunohistochemistry markers [6]. Our case of neuroendocrine tumour of duodenum stained positive for different immunohistochemical markers (Figures 1d–1g). Considering common immunohistochemical staining in small cell lung carcinoma and neuroendocrine tumor, it can be inferred that there is common origin of GABA B receptor antibody from one of the neuroendocrine markers like synaptophysin, chromogranin, neuron specific enolase, or CD56.

Disclosure

Dhanashree Peddawad reports no disclosures. Manoj K. Singh reports no disclosures.

References

[1] S. H. Gultekin, "Paraneoplastic limbic encephalitis: neurological symptoms, immunological findings and tumour association in 50 patients," *Brain*, vol. 123, no. 7, pp. 1481–1494, 2000.

[2] A. Boronat, L. Sabater, A. Saiz, J. Dalmau, and F. Graus, "GABA B receptor antibodies in limbic encephalitis and anti-GAD–associated neurologic disorders," *Neurology*, vol. 76, pp. 795–800, 2011.

[3] R. Höftberger, M. J. Titulaer, L. Sabater et al., "Encephalitis and GABA B receptor antibodies. Novel findings in a new case series of 20 patients," *Neurology*, vol. 81, pp. 1500–1506, 2013.

[4] E. Lancaster, M. Lai, X. Peng et al., "Antibodies to the GABA receptor in limbic encephalitis with seizures: case series and characterization of the antigen B," *The Lancet Neurology*, vol. 9, no. 1, pp. 67–76, 2010.

[5] J. Dalmau and M. R. Rosenfeld, "Autoimmune encephalitis update," *Neuro-Oncology*, vol. 16, no. 6, pp. 771–778, 2014.

[6] E. Thunnissen, A. C. Borczuk, D. B. Flieder et al., "The use of immunohistochemistry improves the diagnosis of small cell lung cancer and its differential diagnosis. An international reproducibility study in a demanding set of cases," *Journal of Thoracic Oncology*, vol. 12, no. 2, pp. 334–346, 2017.

20

A Patient with Double-Negative VGKC, Peripheral Nerve Hyperexcitability and Central Nervous System Symptoms: A Postinfectious Autoimmune Disease

Birte Eikeland

Primary Health Clinic, A. Bergs vei 31, 5089 Bergen, Norway

Correspondence should be addressed to Birte Eikeland; birte.eikeland@gmail.com

Academic Editor: Peter Berlit

Research in the last few years has indicated that most voltage-gated potassium channel- (VGKC-) complex antibodies without leucine-rich glioma-inactivated protein 1 or contactin-associated protein-like 2 antibody specificity lack pathogenic potential and are not clear markers for autoimmune inflammation. Here we report on a patient with double-negative VGKC who developed severe peripheral nerve hyperexcitability, central nervous system symptoms with agitation and insomnia, dysautonomia, and systemic symptoms with weight loss, itch, and skin lesions. The disease started acutely one month after an episode of enteroviral pericarditis and responded well to immunotherapy. The patient is presumed to have developed a postinfectious immunotherapy-responsive autoimmune disease. In the setting of anti-VGKC positivity, it seems likely that anti-VGKC contributed to the pathogenesis of the patient's symptoms of nerve hyperexcitability and that the disease was caused by an acquired autoimmune effect on the neuronal kinetics of VGKC. It is still unknown whether or not there are unidentified extracellular molecular targets within the VGKC-complex, i.e., a novel surface antigen and a pathogenic antibody that can cause affected individuals to develop a peripheral nerve hyperexcitability syndrome. This case highlights the fact that less well-characterized autoimmune central and peripheral nervous system syndromes may have infectious triggers.

1. Introduction

Peripheral nerve hyperexcitability (PNH) is the term used to describe a group of disorders characterized clinically by muscle cramps, muscle twitching (fasciculations or myokymia), muscle stiffness, and pseudomyotonia (delayed muscle relaxation after contraction). Some patients also experience paresthesias and numbness, implying sensory nerve involvement. PNH includes a spectrum of rare disorders, ranging from the dramatic presentation of neuromyotonia or Morvan syndrome, i.e., coexistence of PNH, dysautonomia, and central nervous system (CNS) symptoms, to more benign variants such as cramp-fasciculation syndrome. The etiology can be genetic, particularly mutations in the voltage-gated potassium channel (VGKC), focal nerve injury, demyelination, toxin-induced, or autoimmune. The PNH syndromes were first associated with VGKC-complex antibodies in 1995 [1]. Initially, these autoantibodies were thought to target epitopes of the VGKC, thereby affecting neuronal excitation and causing spontaneous repetitive discharges arising at or near the motor nerve terminal. However, it is now recognized that most of these autoantibodies target proteins that are linked to the VGKC as a functional complex. These proteins include leucine-rich glioma-inactivated 1 protein (LGI1), which is thought to be restricted to the CNS, and contactin-associated protein-like 2 (Caspr2), which is expressed in both the peripheral nervous system and the CNS.

Furthermore, there is now evidence showing that a substantial proportion of patients with VGKC-complex immunoglobulin G seropositivity are double-negative, i.e., lack specificity for LGI1 and Caspr2 IgG, suggesting that other molecular targets of the VGKC-complex remain to be discovered [2]. However, recent research has found that almost all serum samples from double-negative patients show no binding to the surface of live neurons in culture, implying an absence of pathogenic neuronal surface antibodies [3]. Therefore, the clinical significance of isolated anti-VGKC-complex antibodies has been questioned. It is now thought that VGKC positivity in the absence of antibodies to LGI1 and Caspr2 is not a clear marker for autoimmune neuronal inflammation [4]. Here we report on a double-negative patient with severe peripheral nerve hyperexcitability and CNS symptoms who appears to have developed an autoimmune disease for which immunotherapy was effective.

2. Case Report

A 42-year-old Norwegian woman presented in November 2006 with a low-grade fever and severe left-sided chest wall pain that was felt to be pericardial in nature. She was otherwise in good health apart from Raynaud's phenomenon and seronegative Sjögren's syndrome. Her erythrocyte sedimentation rate and C-reactive protein were slightly elevated and her enterovirus antibody titer was positive at 128 (normal, <20). She was diagnosed with viral pericarditis.

One month later, she developed generalized body pain that was accompanied by fasciculations, painful cramps, burning sensations, and hyperalgesia that was so severe that she could not wear a watch, bra, or tight-fitting clothes. She reported painful swallowing and marked skin discoloration was noted on the extensor surfaces of the knees and elbows. There was no joint swelling. She then developed proximal muscle weakness in the thighs and became bed-bound. Blood tests for antinuclear antibody (ANA) and its subgroups were negative. The erythrocyte sedimentation rate and C-reactive protein and creatine kinase levels were normal. No muscle biopsy, neuroimmunology blood tests, or neurophysiological evaluation were performed at that time. She was treated with prednisone 40 mg and weaned over approximately 6 months but without significant benefit. The diagnosis was an immunological reaction with muscle involvement triggered by a viral infection.

The patient slowly improved over a period of 3 years. However, in the autumn of 2009, she started to develop further symptoms, including weight loss, anxiety, difficulty lifting her arms, and inability to drive a car. In the spring of 2010, she developed a tonic-dystonic posture and had difficulty relaxing her shoulders. She also developed severe insomnia and facial flushing with rosacea. Her insomnia was treated with a benzodiazepine that triggered a psychotic reaction during which she became manic, could not sleep, was prone to frequent bouts of singing, and was easily distracted. Eventually, this led to a psychiatric hospitalization during which she was diagnosed to have a somatoform disorder.

The psychotic reaction lasted for 6 weeks and was followed by a severe somatic exacerbation. During the course of a week, she developed torticollis-like head movements, myoclonic-like jerks in her right arm and leg, fluctuating flexion contractures in her elbows, dyspnea caused by both episodes of laryngospasm and chest muscle stiffness, and purplish skin discoloration on her hands and feet. During the subsequent weeks, she developed total body stiffness, palmar flexion contractures of her wrists and fingers, and ankles and toes that were fixed in plantar flexion. She was admitted to the neurology department but underwent limited testing. Needle electromyography (EMG) was essentially normal. Nerve conduction studies indicated F-wave hyperexcitability in the tibial nerve (see Figure 1) but were misinterpreted as normal. Repetitive nerve stimulation was not performed to look for afterdischarges. However, she did have positive ANA and ribonucleoprotein results with nonspecific inflammation and some atrophy in a biopsy from the right deltoid muscle. Unfortunately, she was suspected of malingering and her symptoms were considered to be psychogenic. Therefore, she was again diagnosed to have a somatoform disorder.

Over the next couple of years, she was essentially bed-bound because of her generalized muscle stiffness and contractures. Her symptoms gradually resolved spontaneously, and by 2014, she could walk 3-4 km. However, excessive physical activity at this time triggered a new relapse, which resulted in debilitating disease and the patient becoming bedridden again for about a year.

Her VGKC antibody titer was first measured (by radioimmunoassay, Euroimmun AG, Lübeck, Germany) in May 2015 and found to be positive at 100 pmol/l. She continued to have positive ANA and ribonucleoprotein tests. She was positive for SS-B at this time but later became negative. Other investigations included a comprehensive paraneoplastic evaluation and tests for antiglutamate, anti-GABA, glycine receptor antibodies, Caspr2, and LGI1, all of which were negative. An MRI scan of the brain and an analysis of cerebrospinal fluid were normal. In December 2015, she was readmitted to the neurology department as an inpatient because of her ongoing symptoms. She was presumed to have an autoimmune disorder and started on intravenous immunoglobulin (IVIg) 2 g/kg administered at a daily dosage of 30 g for 5 days, for a total dose of 150 g. She responded well to this treatment, which was repeated at the same dosage in March 2016 and June 2016.

In July 2016, she was referred to a well-regarded clinic in the US where nerve conduction studies confirmed normal sensory and motor conduction responses. Needle EMG showed slightly larger motor units in the distal muscles, which raised the question of motor involvement, but no neuromyotonia, cramps, fasciculations, or myokymic discharges were seen. An autonomic reflex screen was normal, including the Quantitative Sudomotor Axon Reflex Test. The Thermoregulatory Sweat Test revealed sweating abnormalities with hypohidrosis in the areas of worst pain, specifically the lateral aspects of the legs, thighs, and arms, consistent with small fiber neuropathy (see Figure 2). Laboratory investigations with markers for diffuse autoimmunity revealed a ribonucleoprotein level of >8, which was positive. On paraneoplastic peri-inflammatory evaluation, her anti-VGKC value was 0.01 nmol/l, which was within the normal range. This was 4 weeks after treatment with 150 g of IVIg and likely reflected the good response to treatment. LGI1 and Caspr2 were negative and there was mild

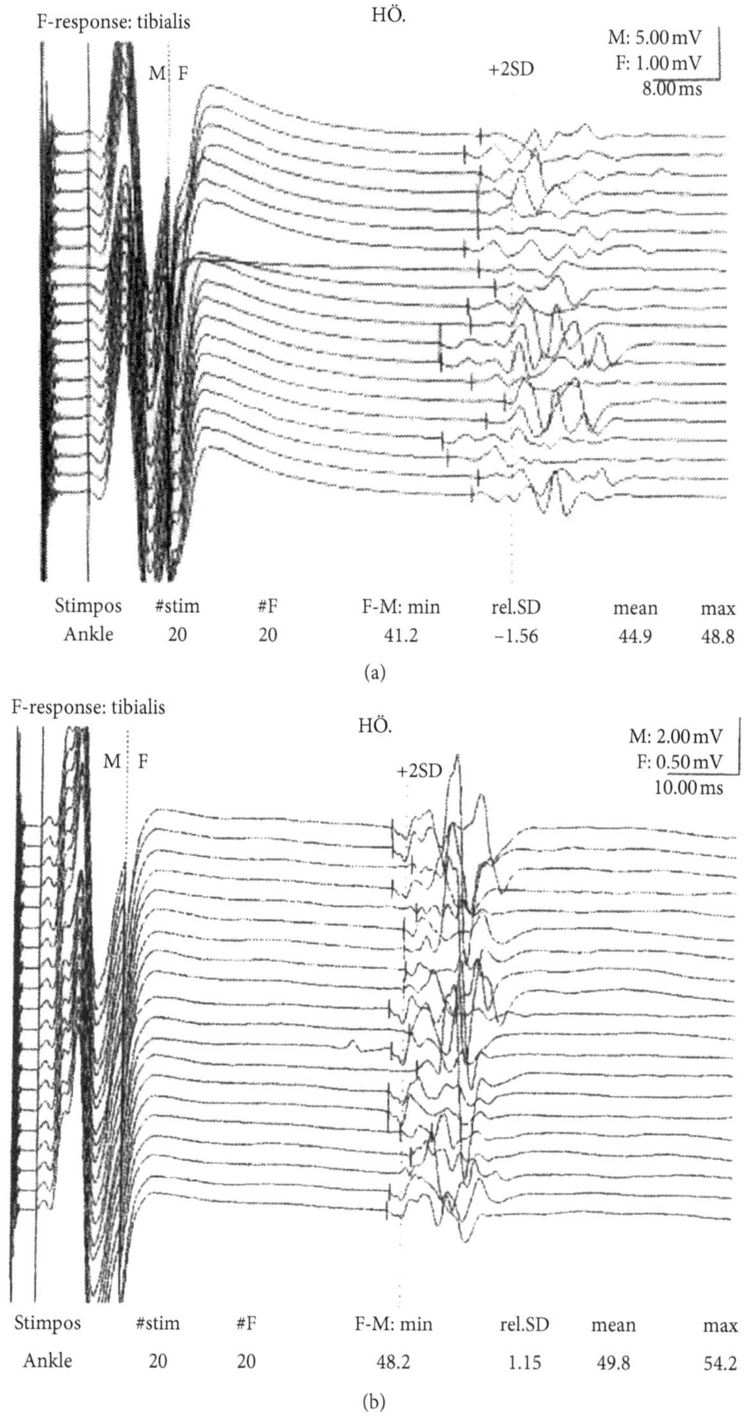

Figure 1: Nerve conduction studies in 2010 (a) indicating F-wave hyperexcitability in the tibial nerve with reduced minimal latency of 41.2 ms, a polyphasic appearance, and persistence. Nerve conduction studies in 2015 (b) showing a normalized minimal latency of 48.2 ms.

immunofluorescent cerebellar staining. The diagnosis was immunotherapy-responsive VGKC-associated autoimmunity with multiple immune-inflammatory markers.

Further ancillary tests were performed. Serum tested weakly positive for staining live-cell hippocampal neurons in one test at the Nuffield Department of Clinical Neurosciences (Oxford, UK). Immunohistochemistry of brain tissue showed fine granular to smooth fluorescence of the hippocampus and the molecular layer on rat cerebellum 1 : 100 and monkey cerebellum 1 : 32 (Euroimmun AG). Antibodies to subunits of the VGKC channel itself (anti-KCNA 1, 2, and 6) were negative, as was contactin 2 (Euroimmun AG). Paranodal/nodal testing with Caspr1, contactin 1, neurofascin 155, and neurofascin 186 was also negative (Euroimmun AG). Excitability tests using the QTRAC threshold-tracking software were normal. However, needle

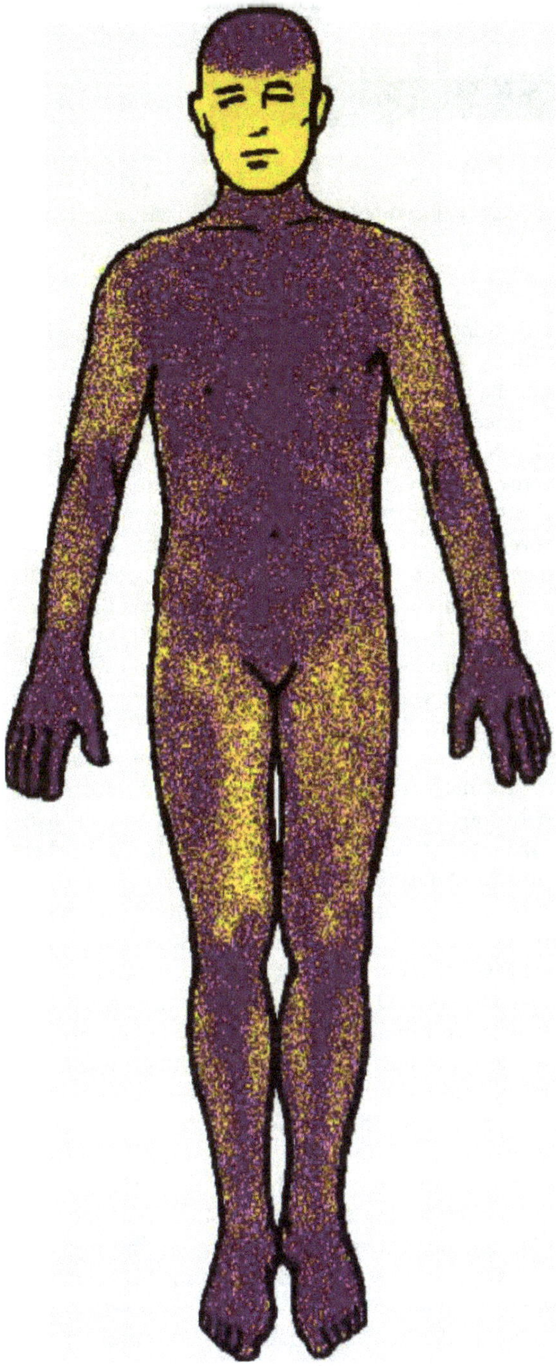

FIGURE 2: Thermoregulatory Sweat Test. Skin areas in yellow indicate reduced or absent sweat output consistent with small fiber neuropathy.

EMG revealed abnormal spontaneous activity in the form of fibrillation potentials, complex repetitive discharges, and myotonic discharges in the abductor pollicis brevis and extensor digitorum brevis muscles (Figure 3).

Treatment with IVIg was continued after she was correctly diagnosed in 2016. At first, 30 g of IVIg was administered every fourth week (0. 1 g/kg/week). However, her VGKC titer increased again from 10 pmol/l to 98 pmol/l. Therefore, the doses of IVIg were increased to 60–90 g every fourth week (0.2–0.3 g/kg/week). Serial anti-VGKC titers were ≤100 pmol/l but were never again found to be as low as 10 pmol/l. IVIg has been continued in this patient and she now seems to be dependent on this immunotherapy. Although she is still symptomatic, her autoimmune disease is now considered to be in remission. Her functioning and quality of life have improved markedly, given the previous severity of her symptoms and the lengthy course of the illness. She has much less pain and stiffness and a higher exercise tolerance, which has allowed her to resume her daily activities, including ambulation and part-time work. Her response to treatment is very similar to that in another report on a patient who developed VGKC autoimmunity (negative for both Caspr2 and LGI1) after exposure to aerosolized porcine neural tissue [5].

3. Discussion

This patient presented with a complex constellation of nerve hyperexcitability symptoms over a period of 10 years before she was diagnosed to have VGKC-associated autoimmune syndrome and treatment with IVIg was initiated. Several of her symptoms are reportedly rare in patients with this type of autoimmune channelopathy, i.e., respiratory distress caused by both laryngospasm and chest muscle stiffness, generalized persistent muscle contractions resulting in stiffness and an extended body posture, generalized pain of neuropathic character, painful swallowing, and facial flushing with rosacea.

Her symptoms were similar to those found in Morvan syndrome, with co-occurrence of CNS symptoms, peripheral nerve hyperexcitability, and autonomic dysfunction. She also had several of the core symptoms [6] described in the clinical spectrum of Caspr2 antibody-associated disease but did not present with Caspr2 or LGI1 positivity. However, Irani et al. [7] reported that 3 of 29 patients with Morvan syndrome did not have Caspr2 or LGI1 positivity and suggested that some patients may have antibodies against other VGKC-complex (or uncomplexed) antigens. There are no clear triggers for Morvan syndrome [8], although a series of 4 patients described in India in 2017 suggested a possible viral trigger [9], as suspected in our patient.

The symptoms and signs in this patient could also be consistent with a diagnosis of autoimmune pain, which is rare and typically presents with additional neurological manifestations [10]. Chronic pain is also a syndromic manifestation of VGKC-complex autoimmunity, and hyperexcitability of nociceptive pathways is implicated [11]. There is a significant association between Caspr2 and pain, but the antigenic VGKC-complex molecule has not been identified in most patients. However, VGKC-complex antibodies are not often found in complex regional pain syndrome [11], despite the occurrence of both pain and autonomic disturbance in patients with the disorder. Our patient presented with a severe pain syndrome and autonomic dysfunction with blue feet, so complex regional pain syndrome could have been a differential diagnosis.

Stiff person syndrome is another diagnosis to consider in this case. Manifestations of this autoimmune movement

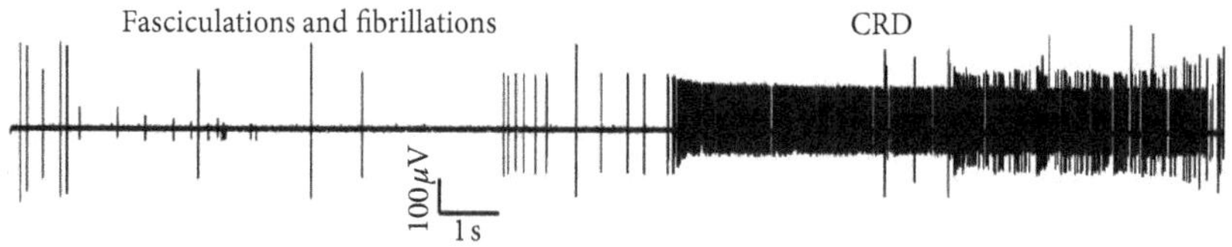

Figure 3: Needle electromyogram showing spontaneous activity in the right abductor pollicis brevis muscle with fasciculations, fibrillations, and complex repetitive discharge at 90–120 Hz.

disorder are truncal and limb stiffness with superimposed spasms. Our patient presented with both limb and total body stiffness and respiratory problems caused by chest muscle stiffness. Nevertheless, most patients with Stiff person syndrome have autoantibodies specific for GAD65 and also some for glycine receptor antibodies. Our patient tested negative for both of these types of autoantibodies.

This patient's disease started acutely after an episode of enteroviral pericarditis. The initial muscle symptoms with severe pain, proximal weakness in the lower limbs, and inflammation-related redness of the skin over the extensor surfaces of the knees and elbows could have suggested a viral myositis. Later she was found to be positive for ANA and ribonucleoprotein. This nonneurological autoimmunity, together with the premorbid history of Raynaud's phenomenon and seronegative Sjögren's syndrome, suggests a possible overlap with a connective tissue disease and cross-disease autoantibodies. Furthermore, our patient was identified as belonging to a group of patients with VGKC who are not positive for LGI1 and Caspr2 but tend to have multiple other immune-inflammatory markers. It is likely that immunotherapy-responsive VGKC-IgG-positive patients without LGI1 and Caspr2 autoantibodies have either coexisting or other immune-inflammatory processes without known primary autoimmunity targets.

Our patient's first positive VGKC antibody result in May 2015 was 100 pmol/l, which is a low titer. Hart et al. [12] found no correlation between the antibody titer and the severity of the clinical features in patients with peripheral nerve hyperexcitability. However, her anti-VGKC titer was not measured in 2010 when she presented with debilitating disease and she was diagnosed incorrectly to have a somatoform disorder. Given the rarity and phenotypic heterogeneity of this autoimmune channelopathy, our patient's case is an example of how such atypical neurological presentations can be dismissed as a functional disorder [13]. As a consequence, immunotherapy with IVIg was delayed for 10 years. This raises the questions of whether or not severe disease could have been avoided and if earlier immunotherapy would have resulted in a full clinical recovery in this patient.

Almost all her relapses and exacerbations were triggered by physical activity, as reported by Hart et al. [12], who found that exercise triggered all motor features of peripheral nerve hyperexcitability in most of their patients. Myokymia/fasciculations in the foot and fasciculations in the knee and finger provided clinical evidence of peripheral motor nerve hyperexcitability in our patient, as illustrated in the video clips in Supplementary Materials (video S1 showing fasciculations in the finger, video S2 showing myokymia/fasciculations in the foot, and video S3 showing fasciculations in the knee).

Needle EMG recordings in 2019 revealed abnormal spontaneous activity suggestive of hyperexcitability. Earlier EMG studies did not show any spontaneous discharges. However, Hart et al. [12] found that the extent of the electrophysiological abnormality did not relate to the clinical severity of muscle hyperactivity, and a single EMG study is liable to spatial as well as temporal sampling error. Nerve conduction studies performed in 2010 showed reduced minimal F-wave latency in the tibial nerve suggestive of hyperexcitability (see Figure 1). In 2004, Nobrega et al. [14] investigated the F-waves of 100 healthy individuals to establish normative data for clinical use. Their minimal latency value for the tibial nerve was 47.0 ± 4.1 ms, and our patient's minimal latency was reduced to 41.2 ms. In 2015, when our patient was clinically better, nerve conduction studies were repeated and the minimal latency for the tibial nerve was normal at 48.2 ms. Hyperexcitability features are often found in the EMG when F-waves are abnormal; in this patient, only one F-wave showed hyperexcitability and the EMG was more or less normal (with only slightly larger motor units and some units having a polyphasic appearance). F-wave hyperexcitability can be seen in the presence of continuous muscle activity, as in peripheral nerve hyperexcitability/neuromyotonia, but there are very few case reports in the literature documenting this phenomenon [15, 16].

Excitability testing with the threshold-tracking software QTRAC did not reveal any pathological findings, but the distal portion of the motor nerve is not investigated with threshold tracking. The likely locus for the generation of spontaneous discharges in patients with autoimmune peripheral nerve hyperexcitability is at the motor nerve terminal or intramuscular arborization area [12, 17]. The motor nerve terminal is relatively unprotected by the blood-nerve barrier and is potentially more vulnerable to antibody-mediated autoimmune attack.

The Thermoregulatory Sweat Test revealed sudomotor abnormalities with generalized hypohidrosis suggestive of a small fiber neuropathy (see Figure 2) and the Quantitative Sudomotor Axon Reflex Test was negative. These findings are compatible with a preganglionic sudomotor lesion. VGKCs also localize to the presynaptic nerve terminals, and the pathophysiology of peripheral nerve hyperexcitability is dysfunction of VGKCs. Other manifestations of autonomic dysfunction were the patient's facial flushing with rosacea and blue discoloration of the feet, most likely as a result of cutaneous dysautonomia. Hyperhidrosis was temporarily present. Dysautonomia is a prominent feature of Morvan syndrome. This patient's autonomic involvement started at the same time as her CNS symptoms with profound insomnia and agitation, which are very similar to the cardinal symptoms found in Morvan syndrome.

The question arises as to why an autoimmune etiology is most likely in this case. The patient had an underlying immunological profile with Raynaud's phenomenon and seronegative Sjögren's syndrome. Importantly, her illness was preceded by enteroviral pericarditis one month before the acute onset of her nerve hyperexcitability symptoms. She subsequently developed nonneurological autoimmunity with positive ANA and ribonucleoprotein, as well as a transiently positive SS-B. In 2010, she presented with both a movement disorder and psychiatric symptoms; a psychiatric presentation together with a movement disorder is a strong indicator of a possible autoimmune component [18]. Serum tested weakly positive for staining live-cell hippocampal neurons, suggesting the possibility of an extracellular pathogenic antibody [19, 20]. Our patient had a good clinical response to IVIg that was accompanied by a reduction in her anti-VGKC titer, which confirms that her disease was genuinely immunotherapy-responsive. Overall, the clinical picture and ancillary tests substantiate an autoimmune etiology for this patient's presenting neurological symptoms.

4. Conclusion

This patient presented with a clinical phenotype of severe nerve hyperexcitability symptoms with both CNS and peripheral nervous system involvement. In the setting of anti-VGKC positivity, it seems likely that anti-VGKC contributed to the pathogenesis of her nerve hyperexcitability. This finding is in contrast with recent research, indicating that almost all double-negative VGKC-complex antibodies lack pathogenicity and are not a clear marker for autoimmune inflammation. However, the decision whether or not to treat a patient for a suspected autoimmune disease should be guided by clinical reasoning including ancillary testing. Factors contributing to the autoimmune etiology and diagnosis in this patient were the preceding enteroviral infection, acute/subacute onset of muscle symptoms, psychiatric symptoms presenting at the same time as a movement disorder, positivity of markers for diffuse autoimmunity, positive staining of live hippocampal cells, and a clinical response to IVIg.

Acknowledgments

The author thanks Sigrid Svalheim MD, PhD, and Marion Boldingh MD, PhD, from the Department of Neurology, Rikshospitalet, Oslo, and Brit Haver, Professor Emeritus in Psychiatry, for their valuable comments during the preparation of the manuscript. The author also thanks Editage (http://www.editage.com) for English language editing.

References

[1] P. Shilito, "Acquired neuromyotonia: evidence for autoantibodies directed against K^+ channels of peripheral nerves," *Annals of Neurology*, vol. 38, no. 5, pp. 714–722, 1995.

[2] C. J. Klein, V. A. Lennon, P. A. Aston et al., "Insights from LGI1 and CASPR2 potassium channel complex autoantibody subtyping," *JAMA Neurology*, vol. 70, no. 2, pp. 229–234, 2013.

[3] B. Lang, M. Makuch, T. Moloney et al., "Intracellular and non-neuronal targets of voltage-gated potassium channel complex antibodies," *Journal of Neurology, Neurosurgery & Psychiatry*, vol. 88, no. 4, pp. 353–361, 2017.

[4] A. Van Sonderen, M. W. J. Schreurs, M. A. A. M. de Bruijn et al., "The relevance of VGKC positivity in the absence of LGI1 and Caspr2 antibodies," *Neurology*, vol. 86, no. 18, pp. 1692–1699, 2016.

[5] J. W. Meeusen, V. A. Lennon, and C. J. Klein, "Immunotherapy-responsive pain in an abattoir worker with fluctuating potassium channel-complex IGG," *Neurology*, vol. 79, no. 17, pp. 1824-1825, 2012.

[6] A. Van Sonderen, H. Ariño, M. Petit-Pedrol et al., "The clinical spectrum of Caspr2 antibody-associated disease," *Neurology*, vol. 87, no. 5, pp. 521–528, 2016.

[7] S. R. Irani, P. Pettingill, K. A. Kleopa et al., "Morvan syndrome: clinical and serological observations in 29 cases," *Annals of Neurology*, vol. 72, no. 2, pp. 241–255, 2012.

[8] S. R. Irani and A. Vincent, "Voltage-gated potassium channel-complex autoimmunity and associated clinical syndromes," *Handbook of Clinical Neurology*, vol. 133, pp. 185–197, 2016.

[9] R. Singh, P. Das, U. Kaur et al., "Morvan's syndrome–is a pathogen behind the curtain?" *Neurological Sciences*, vol. 39, no. 11, pp. 1965–1969, 2018.

[10] M. Xu, D. L. H. Bennett, L. A. Querol et al., "Pain and the immune system: emerging concepts of IgG-mediated autoimmune pain and immunotherapies," *Journal of Neurology, Neurosurgery & Psychiatry*, vol. 91, no. 2, pp. 177–188, 2020.

[11] C. J. Klein, V. A. Lennon, P. A. Aston, A. McKeon, and S. J. Pittock, "Chronic pain as a manifestation of potassium channel-complex autoimmunity," *Neurology*, vol. 79, no. 11, pp. 1136–1144, 2012.

[12] I. K. Hart, P. Maddison, J. Newsom-Davis, A. Vincent, and K. R. Mills, "Phenotypic variants of autoimmune peripheral nerve hyperexcitability," *Brain*, vol. 125, no. 8, pp. 1887–1895, 2002.

[13] S. Shribman, R. Patani, J. Deeb, and A. Chaudhuri, "Voltage-gated potassium channelopathy: an expanding spectrum of clinical phenotypes," *BMJ Case Reports*, vol. 2013, no. 1, Article ID bcr2012007742, 2013.

[14] J. A. M. Nobrega, D. S. Pinheiro, G. M. Manzano, and J. Kimura, "Various aspects of F-wave values in a healthy population," *Clinical Neurophysiology*, vol. 115, no. 10, pp. 2336–2342, 2004.

[15] J. S. Kass, J. H. Button, and F. Y. Chiou-Tan, "F-wave hyperexcitability in Isaac syndrome," *American Journal of Physical Medicine & Rehabilitation*, vol. 87, no. 4, p. 339, 2008.

[16] M. Tanosaki, M. Baba, H. Miura, M. Matsunaga, and K. Arimura, "Reversible F-wave hyperexcitability associated with antibodies to potassium channels in Isaacs' syndrome," *European Journal of Neurology*, vol. 6, no. 1, pp. 95–98, 1999.

[17] M. C. Kiernan, I. K. Hart, and H. Bostock, "Excitability properties of motor axons in patients with spontaneous motor unit activity," *Journal of Neurology, Neurosurgery & Psychiatry*, vol. 70, no. 1, pp. 56–64, 2001.

[18] H. Prüss and B. R. Lennox, "Emerging psychiatric syndromes associated with antivoltage-gated potassium channel complex antibodies," *Journal of Neurology, Neurosurgery & Psychiatry*, vol. 87, no. 11, pp. 1242–1247, 2016.
[19] P. Waters, P. Pettingill, and B. Lang, "Detection methods for neural autoantibodies," *Handbook of Clinical Neurology*, vol. 133, pp. 147–163, 2016.
[20] M. Van Coevorden-Hametee, M. J. Titulaer, M. W. Schreurs, E. de Graaff, P. A. E. Sillevis Smitt, and C. C. Hoogenraad, "Detection and characterization of autoantibodies to neuronal cell-surface antigens in the central nervous system," *Frontiers in Molecular Neuroscience*, vol. 9, p. 37, 2016.

21

Paraneoplastic Opsoclonus Myoclonus in a Patient with Pancreatic Adenocarcinoma

Divine C. Nwafor,[1] Ashley B. Petrone,[2] Joseph M. Collins,[3] and Amelia K. Adcock[4]

[1]*Department of Neuroscience, School of Medicine, West Virginia University, Morgantown, WV, USA*
[2]*Department of Pathology, Anatomy and Laboratory Medicine, School of Medicine, West Virginia University, School of Medicine, Morgantown, WV, USA*
[3]*Department of Radiology, Mayo Clinic Arizona, Scottsdale, AZ, USA*
[4]*Department of Neurology, School of Medicine, West Virginia University, Morgantown, WV, USA*

Correspondence should be addressed to Amelia K. Adcock; akadcock@hsc.wvu.edu

Academic Editor: Isabella Laura Simone

Opsoclonus myoclonus syndrome (OMS) is an extremely rare neurological syndrome typically affecting as few as 1 in 10,000,000 people annually. OMS is characterized by the presence of involuntary, saccadic eye movements, as well as ataxia, including gait incoordination, rigidity, and tremor. The origin of OMS is unclear, but a significant percentage of OMS cases are indicative of an underlying malignancy, most commonly neuroblastoma and small cell lung cancer. Here we describe an adult patient with OMS, who was ultimately diagnosed with a small ductal adenocarcinoma of the pancreas. To our knowledge, this is the third published report of an association between OMS and pancreatic malignancy, and the only case where the pancreatic malignancy was detected prior to metastasis or autopsy at death. This case report highlights the importance of careful, aggressive malignancy screening with OMS, as the pancreatic duct cut-off sign may be overlooked if pancreatic malignancy is not suspected.

1. Introduction

Opsoclonus myoclonus syndrome (OMS) is an extremely rare autoimmune neurological syndrome typically affecting as few as 1 in 10,000,000 people annually. The etiology of OMS is thought to be paraneoplastic (e.g., malignancies) or nonparaneoplastic (e.g., idiopathic, parainfectious) in origin [1–3]. The clinical presentation of OMS is characterized by the presence of involuntary and saccadic eye movements, as well as ataxia, including gait incoordination, rigidity, and tremor. The pathogenesis of OMS remains unclear; however, it has been proposed that it could be the result of dysfunctional motor neurons, specifically pontine omnipause neurons and/or cerebellar Purkinje cells [4]. Twenty to forty percent of OMS cases in adults and children are indicative of an underlying malignancy [2, 5, 6]. The tumors most frequently associated with OMS in children and adults are neuroblastoma and small cell lung cancer (SCLC), respectively [7]. We describe an adult patient with OMS, who was ultimately diagnosed with ductal adenocarcinoma of the pancreas. To our knowledge, this is the third published report of an association between OMS and pancreatic malignancy, and the only case where the pancreatic malignancy was detected prior to metastasis or autopsy at death [8, 9].

2. Case Presentation

Here we describe, a 72-year-old female with a history of hypothyroidism, hyperlipidemia, hypertension, and 50 pack years of smoking, who presented to an outside facility with a 30-pound weight loss, severe nausea, emesis, mild imbalance which graduated to bedbound instability, and involuntary body "shakes" progressing over 6 months. Initial investigations at an outside facility, including contrast enhanced-MRI imaging of the entire neuroaxis, EEG, colonoscopy, and basic hematologic and chemistry panels, were all normal. The only initial abnormal findings were as follows: esophagogastroduodenoscopy (EGD) revealed possible gastritis, thyroid

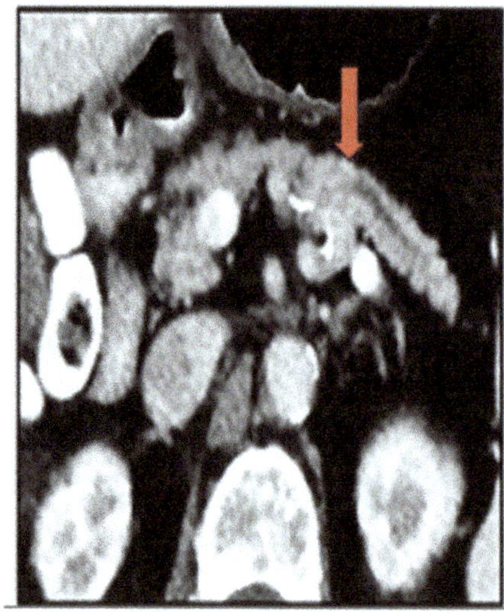

Figure 1: Axial abdominal CT-scan showing dilatation of the pancreas and duct cut-off sign (red arrow).

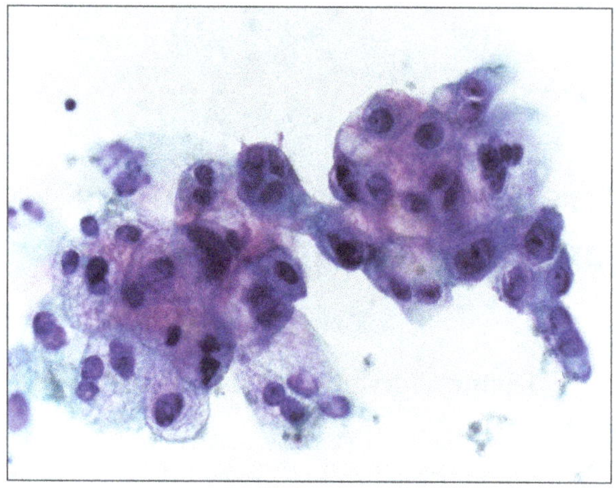

Figure 2: Endoscopic ultrasound (EUS) fine needle biopsy of pancreas revealed adenocarcinoma with mucinous features.

stimulating hormone was mildly elevated (9 U/mL), and anti-thyroid peroxidase antibody was elevated at 50 mg/L. She was evaluated by a psychiatrist who prescribed sertraline, as well as recommended relaxation techniques; however, her family requested further evaluation, and she was transferred to our institution. On physical exam, she had disorganized high amplitude conjugate horizontal movements of her eyes which persisted with eye closure, severe truncal ataxia that prevented her from sitting up without support, and distinct abdominal myoclonus. Otherwise, her neurological exam, including detailed mental status exam testing, was unremarkable.

Symptomatic and empiric therapy with lorazepam, levetiracetam, and a 5-day course of high dose IV methylprednisolone was immediately initiated. Further work-up revealed a lymphocytic pleocytosis in her cerebrospinal fluid (CSF) of 25 WBCs, with an otherwise unremarkable profile. Cytology was negative for malignancy and flow cytometry demonstrated a T cell dominant inflammatory process believed to be reactive. Paraneoplastic panel was negative in the CSF; however, voltage-gated potassium channel antibodies (VGKC) were detected in her serum (0.05 nmol/L; normal <0.02 nmol/L). Notably, the CSF VGKC assay was not yet available in our laboratory at the time of this patient's evaluation. Review of outside duodenal biopsy slides obtained during EGD was consistent with acute *H. Pylori* infection.

Computed tomography (CT) of the chest was normal. A subtle pancreatic duct cut-off sign was noted on abdominal CT, suggestive of a pancreatic mass (Figure 1). Subsequent MRI and endoscopic ultrasound-guided fine needle biopsy confirmed a ductal adenocarcinoma of the body of the pancreas (Figure 2). The patient underwent laparoscopic distal pancreatectomy and splenectomy, and a ductal adenocarcinoma, histologic grade 3/4 measuring 1.8 x 1.7 x 1.5 cm, in the body of the pancreas was removed. Negative operative margins were achieved, and all resected lymph nodes were negative for metastasis. Acutely following surgical resection, she experienced marked resolution of OMS symptoms. Upon taper and discontinuation of levetiracetam, some of her initial symptoms returned, including slight tremor and gait instability; however, the opsoclonus did not recur. Repeat serum paraneoplastic panel demonstrated VGKC normalization. She was initiated on single agent cisplatin-based chemotherapy and appeared to be responding well; however, she unfortunately died 7 months later, due to recurrent lung infections and pulmonary compromise.

3. Discussion

While the cellular origin of OMS is unclear, the cause of this dysfunction is likely autoimmune in nature. Although classic cases of OMS describe anti-Ri antibody (otherwise known as anti-neuronal nuclear autoantibody type 2 or ANNA2) as the biological culprit, the presence of several other anti-neuronal and surface antibodies has been confirmed, and these antibodies may be the mediators of motor neuron dysfunction that causes OMS [2, 4, 10–12]. VGKC, for example, the surface antibody in our patient, is a complex linked to the neuronal cell surface, and it is typically associated with limbic encephalitis or Morvan's syndrome, defined by neuropsychiatric symptoms and muscle hyperexcitability [13, 14]. To our knowledge, this is the first reported case of adult onset OMS associated with VGKC.

In both children and adults, OMS is often an indicator of an occult malignancy. In children, OMS is most commonly associated with neuroblastoma; however, in adults, OMS indicates the presence of cancer of the lung, breast, ovary, thyroid, or Hodgkin's Lymphoma [2, 15]. There is no current diagnostic test for OMS because the antigen responsible for initiating OMS has not been identified yet. Hence, the diagnosis of OMS is often clinical. The presence of involuntary, saccadic eye movements, ataxia, gait incoordination, rigidity, and tremor, and the detection of surface or onconeural antibodies in serum or CSF are extremely useful in diagnosing paraneoplastic OMS [15]. However, it is also common for OMS symptoms to be observed prior to cancer diagnosis, as was the case in our patient.

Treatment of OMS relies heavily on understanding the pathogenesis of the disease process. In the case of occult malignancy OMS, removal of the tumor, immunotherapy, and symptomatic management can be beneficial, especially if they are initiated in the early stages of symptom presentation, rather than once deficits are well established [16, 17]. The resolution of our patient's opsoclonus, improvement of her ataxia, and normalization of her neuronal antibodies following resection further support the hypothesis that her OMS was of paraneoplastic origin.

This patient is unique in that she presented with typical symptoms of OMS, yet her symptoms were caused by an underlying pancreatic adenocarcinoma, rather than a more commonly associated malignancy (e.g., lung cancer, breast cancer, and neuroblastoma). Importantly, her preclinical paraneoplastic symptoms provoked an aggressive malignancy screen, revealing pancreatic dilatation with a duct cut-off sign on CT. Upon resection, the patient's tumor was only 18 mm in greatest diameter. At this small size, the pancreatic mass is a subtle finding on CT and MRI and is only perceptible due to its obstruction of the main pancreatic duct, due to an abrupt duct cut-off sign [18, 19]. Presence of a duct cut-off sign should therefore prompt the clinician to pursue a more invasive malignancy search, as in our case with endoscopic biopsy.

Taken together, we highlight a rare case of OMS with an unusual presentation manifested as a result of pancreatic malignancy. Not only is this association with pancreatic cancer atypical, this case emphasizes and reviews the importance of the duct cut-off sign as an indicator for underlying pancreatic malignancy and highlights the next appropriate step to ensure accurate structural evaluation when the duct cut-off sign is observed in a patient with paraneoplastic neurological symptoms.

References

[1] K. Glatz, H.-M. Meinck, and B. Wildemann, "Parainfectious opsoclonus-myoclonus syndrome: High dose intravenous immunoglobulins are effective," *Journal of Neurology, Neurosurgery & Psychiatry*, vol. 74, no. 2, pp. 279-280, 2003.

[2] J. P. Klaas, J. E. Ahlskog, S. J. Pittock et al., "Adult-onset opsoclonus-myoclonus syndrome," *JAMA Neurology*, vol. 69, no. 12, pp. 1598–1607, 2012.

[3] J. N. Kaviness, P. A. Forsyth, D. D. Layton, and T. J. McPhee, "The movement disorder of adult opsoclonus," *Mov Disord*, vol. 10, no. 1, pp. 22–27, 1995.

[4] D. S. Zee and D. A. Robinson, "A hypothetical explanation of saccadic oscillations," *Annals of Neurology*, vol. 5, no. 5, pp. 405–414, 1979.

[5] K. B. Digre, "Opsoclonus in adults: report of three cases and review of the literature," *JAMA Neurology*, vol. 43, no. 11, pp. 1165–1175, 1986.

[6] L. Bataller, F. Graus, A. Saiz, and J. J. Vilchez, "Clinical outcome in adult onset idiopathic or paraneoplastic opsoclonus-myoclonus," *Brain*, vol. 124, no. 2, pp. 437–443, 2001.

[7] F. Blaes, M. Jauss, J. Kraus et al., "Adult paraneoplastic opsoclonus-myoclonus syndrome associated with antimitochondrial autoantibodies," *Journal of Neurology, Neurosurgery & Psychiatry*, vol. 74, no. 11, pp. 1595-1596, 2003.

[8] S. Galgano and S. Royal, "Primary pancreatic neuroblastoma presenting with opsoclonus-myoclonus syndrome," *Radiology Case Reports*, vol. 11, no. 1, pp. 36–40, 2016.

[9] A. Aggarwal and D. Williams, "Opsoclonus as a paraneoplastic manifestation of pancreatic carcinoma," *Journal of Neurology, Neurosurgery & Psychiatry*, vol. 63, no. 5, pp. 687-688, 1997.

[10] F. A. Luque, H. M. Furneaux, R. Ferziger et al., "Anti-Ri: An antibody associated with paraneoplastic opsoclonus and breast cancer," *Annals of Neurology*, vol. 29, no. 3, pp. 241–251, 1991.

[11] S. J. Pittock, C. F. Lucchinetti, and V. A. Lennon, "Anti-neuronal nuclear autoantibody type 2: Paraneoplastic accompaniments," *Annals of Neurology*, vol. 53, no. 5, pp. 580–587, 2003.

[12] T. Armangué, L. Sabater, E. Torres-Vega et al., "Clinical and immunological features of opsoclonus-myoclonus syndrome in the era of neuronal cell surface antibodies," *JAMA Neurology*, vol. 73, no. 4, pp. 417–424, 2016.

[13] J. Dalmau and M. R. Rosenfeld, "Paraneoplastic syndromes of the CNS," *The Lancet Neurology*, vol. 7, no. 4, pp. 327–340, 2008.

[14] A. Mckeon and A. Mckeon, "Paraneoplastic and other autoimmune disorders of the central nervous system," *The Neurohospitalist*, vol. 3, no. 2, pp. 53–64, 2013.

[15] F. Graus et al., "Recommended diagnostic criteria for paraneoplastic neurological syndromes," *Journal of Neurology, Neurosurgery & Psychiatry*, vol. 75, no. 8, pp. 1135–1140, 2004.

[16] F. Keime-Guibert, F. Graus, A. Fleury et al., "Treatment of paraneoplastic neurological syndromes with antineuronal antibodies (Anti-Hu, Anti-Yo) with a combination of immunoglobulins, cyclophosphamide, and methylprednisolone," *Journal of Neurology, Neurosurgery & Psychiatry*, vol. 68, no. 4, pp. 479–482, 2000.

[17] S. Vernino, B. P. O'Neill, R. S. Marks, J. R. O'Fallon, and D. W. Kimmel, "Immunomodulatory treatment trial for paraneoplastic neurological disorders," *Neuro-Oncology*, vol. 6, no. 1, pp. 55–62, 2004.

[18] P. Tummala, O. Junaidi, and B. Agarwal, "Imaging of pancreatic cancer: an overview," *Journal of Gastrointestinal Oncology*, vol. 2, no. 3, pp. 168–174, 2011.

[19] R. W. Prokesch, L. C. Chow, C. F. Beaulieu, R. Bammer, and R. B. Jeffrey Jr., "Isoattenuating pancreatic adenocarcinoma at multidetector row CT: secondary signs," *Radiology*, vol. 224, no. 3, pp. 764–768, 2002.

22

Nilotinib-Induced Dystonia and Cognitive Deficits in a Neurologically Normal Patient with Chronic Myeloid Leukemia

Justine Chan, Paarth Shah, and Guillermo Moguel-Cobos

Department of Neurology, Barrow Neurological Institute, St. Joseph's Hospital and Medical Center, Phoenix, AZ, USA

Correspondence should be addressed to Guillermo Moguel-Cobos; samantha.soto@barrowneuro.org

Academic Editor: Massimiliano Filosto

Nilotinib is a tyrosine kinase inhibitor used to treat patients with chronic myeloid leukemia (CML). This agent is also being studied in neurodegenerative disorders including Parkinson disease. Studies have shown that nilotinib may decrease the accumulation of parkin substrates and decrease the loss of dopaminergic cells. The use of nilotinib in neurologic disorders is relatively new, and little information about this use has been published. We report on a patient receiving nilotinib for CML. The patient had no previous neurologic deficits, and developed intermittent dystonic posturing of the left upper extremity and cognitive impairment after she began nilotinib treatment. The mechanisms behind this adverse effect are not clear; however, her symptoms began after nilotinib was introduced, decreased with dose reduction, stopped with its cessation, and re-emerged when the medication was restarted. To our knowledge, this is the first reported patient with neurologic symptoms secondary to nilotinib use.

1. Introduction

Nilotinib is a tyrosine kinase inhibitor used to treat patients with chronic myeloid leukemia (CML) by deactivating the Philadelphia chromosome, which contains the fusion gene *BCR-ABL*. The *BCR-ABL* gene is also present in patients with Parkinson disease (PD) [1]. Over-activation of tyrosine kinase may indicate increased oxidative stress, which may play a role in the loss of dopaminergic neurons contributing to the pathogenesis of PD. Nilotinib has been studied in PD patients because it may decrease the accumulation of parkin substrates and decrease the loss of dopaminergic cells. We report on a patient receiving nilotinib for CML who developed intermittent dystonic posturing of the left upper extremity and cognitive impairment. To our knowledge, this is the first reported patient with neurologic symptoms believed to be secondary to nilotinib use.

2. Case Presentation

A 38-year-old woman, with a history of CML, presented for evaluation of abnormal movements that began several months prior. Clinical examination showed speech difficulty, cognitive deficits, intermittent left upper extremity dystonic posturing (elevation, adduction and flexion of arm and hand, fist posturing) and head tilting to the left. The remainder of her neurologic examination was normal.

She had been diagnosed with CML 3 years previously and was initially treated with imatinib, but she was later transitioned to nilotinib 300 mg twice a day because of lack of response to imatinib. Within a few weeks of starting nilotinib, her neurologic symptoms appeared. Months later, nilotinib was discontinued, and her neurologic symptoms resolved. She remained free from neurologic symptoms until nilotinib was restarted at a lower dose (150 mg twice daily), then the neurologic symptoms returned again after a few weeks. A further reduction of nilotinib dose to 150 mg once daily resulted in significant amelioration of her symptoms, and she remains this way clinically.

Results from magnetic resonance imaging of the patient's brain with and without contrast, electroencephalography, a serum paraneoplastic panel, and cerebrospinal fluid analysis while she was on the higher dose of nilotinib (ie, 300 mg twice daily) were normal. Neuropsychological testing, performed while the patient was on the higher dose of nilotinib, showed mild cognitive impairment with frontal lobe and executive function deficit. Results of FDG positron emission tomography (PET) when she was on the lower dose (150 mg twice daily) were also normal. Also noted were impairments in her semantic verbal fluency and verbal processing speed, and she exhibited intermittent dysarthric speech.

3. Discussion

This patient with CML had no previous neurologic deficits but developed neurologic symptoms after she began treatment with nilotinib. The mechanisms behind this adverse effect are not clear, but her symptoms began after medication was introduced, decreased with dose reduction, stopped with its cessation, and re-emerged when the medication was restarted.

Nilotinib is a selective breakpoint cluster region-Abelson (BCR-ABL) tyrosine kinase inhibitor developed for CML patients who are resistant to treatment with imatinib [1, 2]. Nilotinib is more potent and selective than imatinib, has improved brain penetration, and is considered one of the most effective drugs for treatment of CML today [2]. The Abelson nonreceptor tyrosine kinase (c-Abl) is vital for physiologic cellular processes, including regulation of the cell cycle and DNA repair [1, 3, 4].

Parkinson disease is a neurodegenerative disorder characterized by loss of dopaminergic neurons in the substantia nigra neurons and accumulation of alpha synuclein protein. PD models have suggested that overactivation of c-Abl tyrosine kinase phosphorylation leads to loss of the ligase activity of parkin and thus leads to mitochondrial dysfunction and the accumulation of toxic substrates and synuclein [3–5]. Mouse models of PD have shown that nilotinib clears both brain and blood alpha-synuclein, whose gene encodes for alpha-synuclein, and it reverses the loss of tyrosine hydroxylase-positive neurons [6]. c-ABL is also activated in 1-methyl-4-phenyl-1,2,3,6-tetrahydropyridine (MPTP) mice [3]. Evidence from MPTP models of PD has suggested that nilotinib reduces c-ABL activation and further prevents dopamine neuron loss by reducing the parkin substrate, PARIS, independent of reduction of tyrosine phosphorylation of parkin [3]. These animal models suggest a potential neuroprotective effect of nilotinib; however, this concept still needs to be evaluated in human studies. Nilotinib's importance in PD is believed to be due to its ability to penetrate the blood-brain barrier and degrade misfolded alpha-synuclein via autophagy, as well as to inhibit BCR-ABL and reduce oxidative stress, thus protecting dopamine neurons and leading to improvement in motor and cognitive outcomes [3, 5]. However, this theory has not been tested in those unaffected by PD, and our reported adverse effect of dystonia and cognitive deficits has not been previously associated with this tyrosine kinase inhibitor.

Pagan et al. [7] conducted a small study of 12 patients with PD dementia and dementia with Lewy bodies and found that nilotinib at small doses was safe and tolerated, with good cerebrospinal fluid penetration, and with some possible benefit in motor and cognitive outcomes. This study prompted a larger study by Pagan that is currently recruiting toward a goal of 60 patients to evaluate the safety, tolerability, and pharmacokinetics of nilotinib in patients with PD; this study is projected to end in 2023. The NILO-PD study is a Phase 2a randomized, double-blind, placebo-controlled cohort study looking at nilotinib in 135 patients at low doses in those with PD and its safety and tolerability. Secondary outcomes will assess cognitive and motor effects [8]. The nilotinib dosage used in these trials (150–300 mg/day) is much lower than the FDA-approved dosage for the treatment of CML (600–800 mg/day). Severe adverse effects have been reported for this drug when used for CML and have primarily consisted of cardiac symptoms [7].

While our patient had no symptoms of parkinsonism, it is possible that parkin substrates had accumulated and could have led to functional modifications of her basal ganglia, leading to dystonia. However, it is also likely that she experienced a symptomatic effect of nilotinib due to altered central nervous system dopamine levels as suggested by Pagan et al. [7]. At 150 mg/day and 300 mg/day dose, Pagan and colleagues found increased levels of cerebrospinal fluid homovanillic acid (a dopamine metabolite), suggesting a direct alteration of dopamine metabolism [7].

Other rare neurologic adverse effects that have been reported with BCR-ABL inhibitors include rapidly progressive vasculopathy as well as dasatinib-associated reversible demyelinating peripheral polyneuropathy [9, 10]. Nilotinib has been associated with progressive peripheral arterial disease and ischemic heart disease, and a few cases have been reported of intracranial vasculopathy, such as that described by Chen et al. [9], with an atypical case of rapid intravascular nonatherosclerotic arterial stenosis. That case report reviews varying etiologies that could explain nilotinib's prothrombotic state, including expression of cell adhesion molecules that promote a pro-atherogenic phenotype [9]. This is certainly a possible explanation of symptoms in our case. A 4-vessel cerebral angiogram should have been performed, but was not in our patient. As noted, the brain FDG PET revealed normal glucose metabolism globally and, although this procedure can be used as a test for blood flow and metabolism, the lack of a cerebral angiogram is certainly a limitation to our case report. Given that our patient had no sensory deficits, an electromyography and nerve conduction study were not conducted. It is important to be mindful that medications that cause a peripheral neuropathy are usually distal, symmetric, and axonal, and cause a sensory neuropathy. However, there are rare cases of drug-induced peripheral neuropathy, such as that described by Ishida et al. [11].

Regarding our patient's cognitive changes, we theorize that it is related to nilotinib, on the basis of the timing of her symptoms in correlation with medication and the dose-dependent correlation of her symptoms. It is possible that alteration of dopamine levels may play a role in changes in cognition or clearance of intraneuronal phosphorylated tau and alpha synuclein by nilotinib itself [12]. As mentioned above, on one hand, a cerebral blood flow limitation is also another possibility for our patient's symptoms. On the other hand, the small clinical study by Pagan also suggests cognitive improvement with low doses of this tyrosine kinase inhibitor.

Another limitation of this report is that nilotinib levels in the cerebrospinal fluid were not directly measured to provide a correlation with the patient's symptoms. In addition, no measurements of cerebrospinal fluid disease-related biomarkers such as alpha synuclein were taken.

4. Conclusions

Nilotinib is currently used in CML patients to deactivate BCR-ABL kinase. In PD, nilotinib is thought to act by reducing harmful parkin substrates, thus preventing dopaminergic neuron cell loss. We report the first case known to demonstrate nilotinib causing intermittent dystonic posturing, dysarthric speech, and cognitive impairment in a neurologically normal patient. The pathophysiology underlying this adverse effect is most likely associated with disruption of the alternate protein kinases that are responsible for the proliferation and transduction of normal signals through the basal ganglia or by a direct effect on dopamine levels. As nilotinib is further studied for its usefulness in PD, we believe that its adverse effect profile and dosage should be carefully considered in a randomized, double-blind trial that includes a placebo group. This is important, as c-ABL inhibitors such as nilotinib may have a role in treating other neurodegenerative diseases, such as Alzheimer disease, and human tauopathies given c-ALB over-activation has been implicated in the pathogenesis of these neurodegenerative diseases [13].

Abbreviations

CML: Chronic myeloid leukemia
MPTP: 1-methyl-4-phenyl-1,2,3,6-tetrahydropyridine
PD: Parkinson disease.

Authors' Contributions

Justine Chan, MD; manuscript preparation, writing of draft, review, and critique. Paarth Shah, MD; manuscript preparation, writing of draft, review, and critique. Guillermo Moguel-Cobos, MD; manuscript preparation, writing of draft, review, and critique.

Acknowledgments

We thank Dr. Anthony E. Lang (Toronto Western Hospital Research Institute, Toronto, Canada) and Dr. José Obeso (University of Navarra Medical School and Clinica Universitaria in Pamplona, Spain) for guiding and for criticizing constructively our paper. The authors thank the staff of Neuroscience Publications at Barrow Neurological Institute for assistance with manuscript preparation.

References

[1] A. K. Kakkar, H. Singh, and B. Medhi, "Old wines in new bottles: repurposing opportunities for Parkinson's disease," *European Journal of Pharmacology*, vol. 830, pp. 115–127, 2018.

[2] R. K. Wyse, P. Brundin, and T. B. Sherer, "Nilotinib-differentiating the hope from the hype," *Journal of Parkinson's Disease*, vol. 6, no. 3, pp. 519–522, 2016.

[3] A. I. Abushouk, A. Negida, R. A. Elshenawy et al., "c-Abl inhibition; a novel therapeutic target for Parkinson's disease," *CNS & Neurological Disorders–Drug Targets*, vol. 17, no. 1, pp. 14–21, 2018.

[4] S. Z. Imam, Q. Zhou, A. Yamamoto et al., "Novel regulation of parkin function through c-Abl-mediated tyrosine phosphorylation: implications for Parkinson's disease," *Journal of Neuroscience*, vol. 31, no. 1, pp. 157–163, 2011.

[5] S. S. Karuppagounder, S. Brahmachari, Y. Lee, V. L. Dawson, T. M. Dawson, and H. S. Ko, "The c-Abl inhibitor, nilotinib, protects dopaminergic neurons in a preclinical animal model of Parkinson's disease," *Scientific Reports*, vol. 4, no. 1, Article ID 4874, 2014.

[6] M. L. Hebron, I. Lonskaya, and C. E. Moussa, "Tyrosine kinase inhibition facilitates autophagic SNCA/alpha-synuclein clearance," *Autophagy*, vol. 9, no. 8, pp. 1249–1250, 2013.

[7] F. Pagan, M. Hebron, E. H. Valadez et al., "Nilotinib effects in Parkinson's disease and dementia with lewy bodies," *Journal of Parkinson's Disease*, vol. 6, no. 3, pp. 503–517, 2016.

[8] T. Simuni, B. Fiske, K. Merchant et al., "A phase 2A study of nilotinib in patients with advanced and early Parkinson's disease: study design (abstract)," *International Congress*, vol. 33, no. 2, 2018.

[9] C. J. Chen, B. J. Sorace, A. Shakeri et al., "Tyrosine kinase inhibitor induced rapidly progressive vasculopathy after intracranial stent placement," *Journal of Neurointerventional Surgery*, vol. 10, no. 11, e28 pages, 2018.

[10] D. Sanford, M. MacDonald, M. Nicolle, and A. Xenocostas, "Development of myasthenia gravis in a patient with chronic myeloid leukemia during treatment with nilotinib," *Hematology Reports*, vol. 6, no. 2, p. 5288, 2014.

[11] T. Ishida, N. Akagawa, T. Miyata et al., "Dasatinib-associated reversible demyelinating peripheral polyneuropathy in a case of chronic myeloid leukemia," *International Journal of Hematology*, vol. 107, no. 3, pp. 373–377, 2018.

[12] T. Guttuso Jr, K. L. Andrzejewski, D. G. Lichter, and J. K. Andersen, "Targeting kinases in Parkinson's disease: a mechanism shared by LRRK2, neurotrophins, exenatide, urate, nilotinib and lithium," *Journal of the Neurological Sciences*, vol. 402, pp. 121–130, 2019, Epub 2019/05/28.

[13] S. D. Schlatterer, C. M. Acker, and P. Davies, "c-Abl in neurodegenerative disease," *Journal of Molecular Neuroscience*, vol. 45, no. 3, pp. 445–452, 2011.

23

Spontaneous Recovery of Penetrating Cervical Spinal Cord Injury with Physiotherapeutic Treatment: Case Report and Review of the Literature

Yao Christian Hugues Dokponou, Mamoune El Mostarchid, Housni Abderrahmane, Niamien Patrice Koffi, Miloudi Gazzaz, and Brahim El Mostarchid

Department of Neurosurgery, Mohammed V Military Teaching Hospital, Faculty of Medicine and Pharmacy Rabat, Rabat, Morocco

Correspondence should be addressed to Yao Christian Hugues Dokponou; dokponou2407@gmail.com

Academic Editor: Peter Berlit

Stab wounds to the cervical spine are less common than injuries from road accidents, sports injuries, and falls. The presence of vital, vascular, neural, respiratory, and digestive structures in the neck region mean that this kind of spinal injury is generally critical, and its management is a challenge. We report a unique case of a previously healthy 17-year-old adolescent admitted for quadriplegia secondary to a stab wound to the cervical spine at the C4C5 level. There was no surgical indication. The patient underwent physiotherapy. He showed spontaneous neurological improvement two weeks later and was able to sit on his own and to walk about three months of physical rehabilitation.

1. Introduction

Road accidents, falls, and gunshots are the leading causes of spinal cord injury. These may result from bone fragments impacting and compressing the spinal cord or from concussive shock waves generated by the impact of striking a vertebral body. Different types of injury have different motor recovery outcomes. The global incidence of spinal cord injury has been estimated to range between 15 and 40 individuals per million. Functional outcome is a primary concern for clinicians and patients and is dependent on neurological status [1–3].

Although relatively uncommon, penetrating neck trauma has the potential for serious morbidity and estimated mortality of up to 6%. Correct assessment and management of patients who have sustained a penetrating neck injury have been a controversial issue in the past [4, 5]. Controversy over the surgical treatment of stab wounds to the spinal cord persists, even regarding cases where neurological deficits are apparent.

We report a case of penetrating injury to the cervical spine. This case was unique in two aspects. First, the mechanism was exceptional, with a stab wound to the neck from which the knife had been removed prior to admission. Second, the patient showed spontaneous neurological improvement with physical therapy rehabilitation. After presenting this case, we discuss relevant comparative cases from the literature.

2. Case Presentation

A 17-year-old patient was admitted with quadriplegia secondary to a penetrating wound to the cervical spine. The patient reported an assault a few hours earlier resulting in a knife wound to his neck. According to witnesses, a free pocket knife was the assault weapon with the blade oriented vertically. Upon physical examination, he was found to be unable to walk or hold a sitting position. The knife wound entry point was on the right side of the posterior of his neck. Neurological examination found the patient to be alert, with

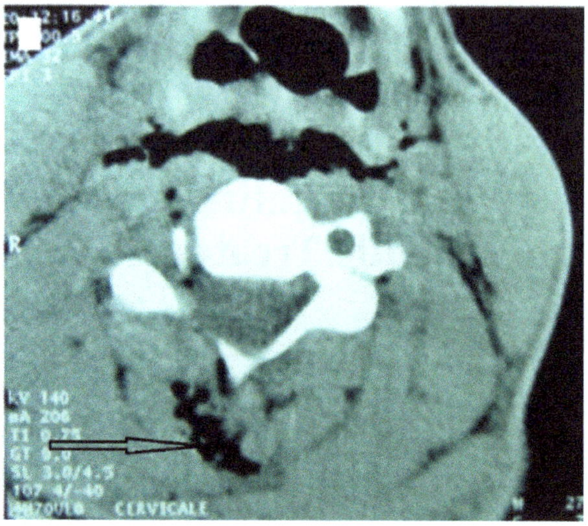

(a)

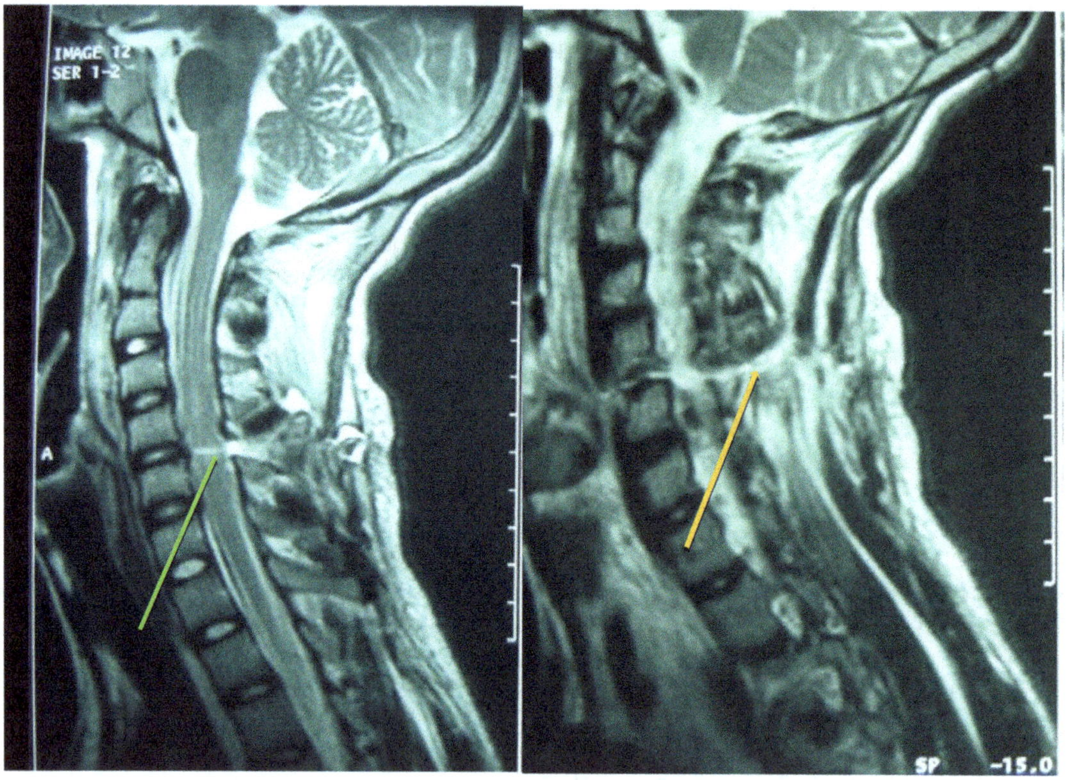

(b)

FIGURE 1: (a) CT scan, axial section at C4C5, showing hypodensity in the posterior left-sided soft tissue representing the knife track with its passage filled with air (black arrow). (b) MRI sagittal T2-weighted hyperintense signal of the spinal cord at C4C5 level sign of medullary contusion (green arrow), with the continuous posterior soft tissue hyperintense representing the knife track (yellow arrow).

a Glasgow Coma Scale score of 15, and hemodynamically stable. His blood pressure was 130/80 mm Hg, his heart rate was 80 beats/min^{-1}, his respiratory rate was 19 mn^{-1}, and his body temperature was 37°C. The osteotendinous reflexes were abolished with indifferent cutaneoplantar reflexes. Grade B of the ASIA impairment scale, sensory but no motor function is preserved below the cervical region at the admission. The patient's medical and family histories were unremarkable.

A computed tomography (CT) scan at 4 hours after the injury showed the path of the knife. This was filled with air, and there was no apparent injury to the visceral structures of the neck (Figure 1(a)). A magnetic resonance imaging (MRI) scan of the cervical spine at the admission (about 10 hours from the assault) also showed the knife track and revealed spinal cord contusion at the C4C5 level (Figure 1(b)). Routine laboratory tests of the patient's blood sample were normal.

Table 1: The management and outcomes of stab wounds to the cervical spinal cord reported in the literature.

First author	Stab wound to cervical spinal cord	Symptomatic	Conservative treatment	Surgical treatment	Outcome (worsened/improved)
Lin et al. [6], 2005	1 case	Yes	—	1 case	Improved
Kendall et al. [7], 1998	218 cases	Yes	—	218 cases	Improved
Barkana et al. [1], 1999	12 cases	Yes	5 cases	7 cases	Improved
Prichayudh et al. [8], 2015	64 cases	40 cases	24 cases	40 cases	Improved
Como et al. [9], 2005	45 cases	Yes	—	45 cases	Eight died
Kamaoui et al. [10], 2007	1 case	Yes	—	1 case	Improved
Dran et al. [11], 2005	2 cases	Yes	—	2 cases	Improved
Harrop et al. [12], 2001	12 cases	Yes	9 cases	3 cases	Three worsened
Wang et al. [13], 2012	1 case	Yes	—	1 case	Improved
Demetriades et al. [14], 1996	89 cases	Yes	—	31 cases	Improved
Ihalainen et al. [3], 2017	168 cases	Yes	142 cases	26 cases	Improved
Demetriades et al. [15], 1997	123 cases	Yes	—	14 cases	Improved

There were no secondary complications, such as meningitis or worsening of neurological deficits. The patient did not undergo surgery but benefited from a series of physical therapy, 30 sessions of 30 minutes each on daily basis aiming at functional recovery. The functional electrical stimulation was not used. The main physiotherapy treatment were muscles stretching, strengthening for elasticity and mobility. This allowed to reinforce the muscles and teach the patient the control and usage of his limbs. He showed spontaneous neurological improvement and regain the usage of his arms and hands as well as the lower limbs. The medical treatment was made of pain relievers (paracetamol + tramadol) and empirical antibiotic (third generation cephalosporins, rocephin 2 g/day for two weeks + metronidazole 500 mg twice a day for 10 days). After two weeks, he was able to sit unaided and walked at three months of physiotherapy.

3. Discussion

Our study finds that a patient with neurological deficit secondary to a penetrating spinal injury can be completely recovered with a constant and repeated series of physiotherapy rehabilitation treatment. There was no foreign material to be taking care of, no hemorrhage, no life-threatening sign, and no spinal stability lesion; therefore, no indication for surgery. But taking into account the patient's neurological status, following this spinal trauma, one might be tempted to carry out surgery for exploration and decompression.

We have reviewed other cases of penetrative spinal cord injuries to determine appropriate management and treatment. Our findings are discussed, and the cases identified are given in Table 1.

The initial management of penetrating spinal injury follows the standard principles of trauma care. Once the patient is hemodynamically stabilized and concomitant life-threatening injuries have been addressed, the spinal injury can be treated [16]. Radiological exploration of spinal cord injuries can find anything from severe damage to no harm at all and patients might or might not demonstrate neurologic deficits. This makes the choice of treatment challenging as it is difficult to determine whether or not a patient is a candidate for surgery. There are no clinical findings specific to, and always present in, patients with stab wounds to the spine. Barkana et al. [1] reviewed cases of cervical injury to the neck and found that 22% presented with life-threatening symptoms while others were asymptomatic. The thoracic spine is the most commonly affected area in spinal stab wounds, while such injuries to the cervical spine are rare.

Diagnostic imaging studies used with spinal injuries consist of a standard X-ray and a contrast CT scan. MRI scans are also recommended to define the extent of neural damage. However, with most knife wounds, the latter can only be performed postoperatively because of the metallic nature of the weapon [5]. However, in our case, the knife was not present, so we were able to perform an MRI immediately. The CT scan was not performed until later. MRI can be used to evaluate the damage to the spinal cord, including contusions, hematoma, and compression of extramedullary origin. In stab wounds, intramedullary injuries can include contusion, hematoma, and knife-track damage. A contusion appears as hypointense signals on T1-weighted images and hyperintense signals on T2-weighted images. Oxyhemoglobin reveals acute hemorrhage as isosignals or low-signal intensity on T2-weighted images. Knife-track lesions appear as linear high-signal intensity on T2-weighted images [10]. The MRI in our case showed the knife-track lesion and medullary contusion. Thus, the MRI is the modality of choice for the evaluation of penetrating injuries to the spinal canal in patients with neurological symptoms. Nevertheless, researchers who have reported early use of a CT scan of the cervical spine were able to ascertain that the continuity of the spinal cord had been severely disrupted by penetrative injury [6].

Most authors agree that, depending on the injury, the operative management of penetrating injuries to the cervical spine may focus on the prevention of cerebrospinal fluid fistula or consist of debridement of the devitalized tissues to minimize the chance of infection and decompression of the spinal cord and nerve roots by removing hematomas and bone fragments [17–20]. Burgess et al. [4] suggest that indications for immediate surgical exploration of penetrating neck injuries include airway compromise, massive subcutaneous emphysema, air bubbling through a wound, profuse active bleeding, refractory shock, evolving stroke, and rapidly expanding hematoma. The policy of mandatory surgical exploration for all injuries that breach the platysma is no longer widely practiced. Data from both retrospective and prospective case series support a conservative approach to the management of asymptomatic patients with negative results in physical examinations and imaging investigations. However, there is no evidence-based data in the literature for cases such as ours in which the patient is symptomatic, but physical examination and imaging results are negative. We chose not to operate on our patient, and he began to recover spontaneously from his tetraplegia. This suggests that some patients with neurological deficits may also respond to conservative treatment. Kendall et al. [7] reviewed 218 patients with penetrating neck injuries who underwent surgical exploration. They found that stab wounds had a 10% higher rate of negative exploration than injuries from a projectile. A systematic review and meta-analysis with a large sample is required to gather sufficient data to provide the basis for standardized protocol in the treatment of patients with penetrating injuries to the cervical spine.

4. Conclusions

Penetrating stab wounds to the cervical spine are uncommon, and the best protocol for their management is controversial. Nevertheless, we should not rush to operate on patients with penetrating spinal injuries, particularly when there is no obvious indication for surgery. This remains true even when neurological deficits are present.

In the absence of secondary complications, physiotherapy management should be the first-line treatment for penetrative injuries to the spine.

Consent

The patient gave his informed consent and verbal permission to publish his case.

Authors' Contributions

Yao Christian Hugues Dokponou conceptualized the study and wrote and edited the article. Mamoune El Mostarchid and Housni Abderrahmane wrote, reviewed, and edited the article. Niamien Patrice Koffi and Miloudi Gazzaz reviewed and edited the article. Brahim El Mostarchid supervised, validated, and reviewed the article.

References

[1] Y. Barkana, M. Stein, A. Scope et al., "Prehospital stabilization of the cervical spine for penetrating injuries of the neck-is it necessary?" *Injury*, vol. 31, no. 5, pp. 305–309, 2000.

[2] R. L. Waters, I. Sie, R. H. Adkins, and J. S. Yakura, "Injury pattern effect on motor recovery after traumatic spinal cord injury," *Archives of Physical Medicine and Rehabilitation*, vol. 76, no. 5, pp. 440–443, 1995.

[3] T. Ihalainen, I. Rinta-Kiikka, T. M. Luoto, E. A. Koskinen, A.-M. Korpijaakko-Huuhka, and A. Ronkainen, "Traumatic cervical spinal cord injury: a prospective clinical study of laryngeal penetration and aspiration," *Spinal Cord*, vol. 55, no. 11, pp. 979–984, 2017.

[4] C. A. Burgess, O. T. Dale, R. Almeyda, and R. J. Corbridge, "An evidence based review of the assessment and management of penetrating neck trauma," *Clinical Otolaryngology*, vol. 37, no. 1, pp. 44–52, 2012.

[5] A. Kettani, N. El Fatemi, Z. Belkhadir, A. Mosadik, M. Faroudy, and A. Sbihi, "Stab wound to the dorsal spine with partial transsection of the dura: case report and review of the literature," *Journal Européen des Urgences*, vol. 20, no. 1, pp. 11–14, 2007.

[6] P.-H. Lin, T.-Y. Chuang, S.-F. Liao, and H. Cheng, "Cervical spinal cord injury by unusual foreign body penetration," *Injury Extra*, vol. 36, no. 2, pp. 22–25, 2005.

[7] J. L. Kendall, D. Anglin, and D. Demetriades, "Penetrating neck trauma," *Emergency Medicine Clinics of North America*, vol. 16, no. 1, pp. 85–105, 1998.

[8] S. Prichayudh, J. Choadrachata-anun, S. Sriussadaporn et al., "Selective management of penetrating neck injuries using "no zone" approach," *Injury*, vol. 46, no. 9, pp. 1720–1725, 2015.

[9] J. J. Como, E. R. H. Sutton, M. McCunn et al., "Characterizing the need for mechanical ventilation following cervical spinal cord injury with neurologic deficit," *Journal of Trauma and Acute Care Surgery*, vol. 59, no. 4, pp. 912–916, 2005.

[10] I. Kamaoui, M. Maaroufi, M. Benzagmout, N. Sqalli Houssaini, S. Boujraf, and S. Tizniti, "MRI findings in spinal cord penetrating injury: three case reports," *Journal of Neuroradiology*, vol. 34, no. 4, pp. 276–279, 2007.

[11] G. Dran, D. Fontaine, S. Litrico, P. Grellier, and P. Paquis, "Plaie médullaire cervicale par arme blanche présentation de deux cas," *Neurochirurgie*, vol. 51, pp. 476–480, 2005.

[12] J. S. Harrop, A. D. Sharan, A. R. Vaccaro, and G. J. Przybylski, "The cause of neurologic deterioration after acute cervical spinal cord injury," *Spine*, vol. 26, no. 4, pp. 340–346, 2001, https://journals.lww.com/spinejournal/Abstract/2001/02150/The_Cause_of_Neurologic_Deterioration_After_Acute.8.aspx.

[13] Z. Wang, Y. Liu, Z. Qu, J. Leng, C. Fu, and G. Liu, "Penetrating injury of the spinal cord treated surgically," *Orthopedics*, vol. 35, no. 7, pp. e1136–e1140, 2012.

[14] D. Demetriades, J. A. Asensio, G. Velmahos, and E. Thal, "Complex problems in penetrating neck trauma," *Surgical Clinics of North America*, vol. 76, no. 4, pp. 661–683, 1996.

[15] D. Demetriades, D. Theodorou, E. Cornwell et al., "Evaluation of penetrating injuries of the neck: prospective study of 223 patients," *World Journal of Surgery*, vol. 21, no. 1, pp. 41–48, 1997.

[16] G. I. Jallo, "Neurosurgical management of penetrating spinal injury," *Surgical Neurology*, vol. 47, no. 4, pp. 328–330, 1997.

[17] R. B. Bell, T. Osborn, E. J. Dierks, B. E. Potter, and W. B. Long, "Management of penetrating neck injuries: a new paradigm for civilian trauma," *Journal of Oral and Maxillofacial Surgery*, vol. 65, no. 4, pp. 691–705, 2007.

[18] J. P. Meyer, J. A. Barrett, J. J. Schuler, and D. P. Flanigan, "Mandatory vs. selective exploration for penetrating neck trauma: a prospective assessment," *Archives of Surgery*, vol. 122, no. 5, pp. 592–597, 1987.

[19] J. A. Asensio, C. P. Valenziano, R. E. Falcone, and J. D. Grosh, "Management of penetrating neck injuries: the controversy surrounding zone II injuries," *Surgical Clinics of North America*, vol. 71, no. 2, pp. 267–296, 1991.

[20] B. H. Venger, R. K. Simpson, and R. K. Narayan, "Neurosurgical intervention in penetrating spinal trauma with associated visceral injury," *Journal of Neurosurgery*, vol. 70, no. 4, pp. 514–518, 1989.

Demyelinating Neurological Adverse Events following the use of Anti-TNF-α Agents: A Double-Edged Sword

Miral H. Gharib[1] **Mohamed Awni AlKahlout**[1] **Beatriz Garcia Canibano**[2] **Dirk Theophiel Deleu**[2] **Hani Malallah AlEssa**[1] **and Samar AlEmadi**[1]

[1]*Rheumatology, Department of Medicine, Hamad Medical Corporation, Doha, Qatar*
[2]*Neurology, Department of Medicine, Hamad General Hospital, Doha, Qatar*

Correspondence should be addressed to Miral H. Gharib; dr_miral_gharib@hotmail.com

Academic Editor: Dominic B. Fee

Background. Tumor necrosis factor antagonists (anti-TNF-α) are an established therapeutic option for several autoimmune and inflammatory bowel diseases. Despite their clinical effectiveness, neurological adverse events have been reported, and literature data suggest a potential role of anti-TNF-α in the induction of demyelination. *Case Presentation.* In this series, we present three cases of demyelination after the use of anti-TNF-α agents. The first case involved a 21-year-old man with HLA-B27 negative peripheral spondylarthritis who had been taking adalimumab for 2 years. He developed headache, urinary incontinence, and bilateral lower extremity numbness that progressed to the middle of the trunk for 2 days. Magnetic resonance imaging (MRI) showed multiple hyperintense enhancement lesions in the left paramedian anterior pons consistent with multiple sclerosis (MS). The second case included a 17-year-old woman who was on 2 years of adalimumab treatment for juvenile idiopathic arthritis and chronic anterior uveitis and developed new-onset dizziness and tremors. The clinical examination showed signs of cerebellar dysfunction. MRI findings were consistent with multiple sclerosis. The third case was a 34-year-old male who was on 5 years of infliximab treatment for ankylosing spondylitis when he developed left hand numbness and weakness. Cerebrospinal fluid (CSF) analysis and MRI findings were consistent with demyelination. Discontinuation of tumor necrosis factor antagonists (anti-TNF-α) resulted in resolution of the symptoms with no recurrence in the first case, but there was evidence of recurrence in the other 2 cases, where one was managed with rituximab and the second one improved with pulse steroid therapy. *Conclusion.* Despite the small number of patients, our series adds to the growing body of evidence supporting a causal link between anti-TNF-α agents and demyelination. Thus, we can conclude that on suspicion of any neurological side effects, early discontinuation of the TNF-α blockers and requesting urgent MRI scan to confirm the diagnosis is of utmost importance.

1. Introduction

Tumor necrosis factor-α (TNF-α) is a pleiotropic cytokine that plays a key role in host defense mechanisms and exhibits multifunctional proinflammatory properties [1]. It was found that the pathogenesis of many diseases, including rheumatoid arthritis, Crohn's disease, atherosclerosis, psoriasis, sepsis, diabetes, and obesity, has been associated with aberrant TNF-α development and TNF receptor signaling. Therefore, TNF-α and its receptor were proposed as a therapeutic target in the treatment of many diseases [2]. With great success in terms of efficacy and safety, anti-TNF-α agents have revolutionized the treatment of rheumatoid arthritis, ankylosing spondylitis, psoriasis, psoriatic arthritis, juvenile polyarticular rheumatoid arthritis, and inflammatory bowel disease. These agents act by abrogating the soluble TNF-α, thus preventing its binding on TNFR1/TNFR2 receptors [3, 4]. Currently, many anti-TNF-α agents have been licensed for treating certain inflammatory diseases including rheumatoid arthritis and inflammatory bowel disease. However, these agents are not without side effects. Aside from the usual presumed infectious difficulties, uncommon cases of neuroinflammatory demyelinating disorders, such as multiple sclerosis (MS), myelitis, and optic neuritis, have been documented with the use of anti-TNF-α, with a very low absolute risk below one in 1000 patients/year as recently shown in large Denmark and Sweden Cohort [5].

In our rheumatology division, around 500 patients are being treated with anti-TNF-α agents such as infliximab, adalimumab, and etanercept, which have been used widely specially in the treatment of rheumatoid arthritis, ankylosing spondylitis, and inflammatory bowel disease. However, their increasing use has revealed a variety of adverse events. We reported three cases of demyelination following the use of anti-TNF-α. The cases were diagnosed with MS based on McDonald's criteria (2017) for the diagnosis of multiple sclerosis [6]. These cases aimed at increasing the physician's awareness of the demyelinating adverse effect associated with anti-TNF-α therapy.

2. Case Presentation

Case 1: a 21-year-old Qatari gentleman was on adalimumab for HLA-B27-negative peripheral spondyloarthritis. After being kept on adalimumab for 2 years, he developed severe headache, urinary incontinence, and bilateral lower limb numbness, which progressed towards the middle of the trunk over several days. The neurological examination uncovered dysesthesias below the dermatome T4 associated with brisk tendon reflexes, while the remainder of the examination was normal. Lumbar puncture was not done, and the diagnosis of multiple sclerosis (MS) was established by the presence of multiple hyperintense lesions on brain MRI in the left paramedian anterior pons, left posterolateral medulla, and bilateral periventricular white matter, some of them involving the optic radiations. Similar lesions were identified in the right lateral aspect of corpus callosum splenium and in the cervical spinal cord at the level of C2-C3 level and a small area of T2 hyperintensity in the thoracic spinal cord at the T5 level as shown in Figures 1(a)–1(d). There was no family history of MS.

Complete resolution of neurological symptoms due to discontinuation of adalimumab was observed within one month. So, no pulse steroid was given, and MRI was not repeated. However, he developed abdominal pain with loose bloody motions, in which ileocolonoscopy and biopsy confirmed the diagnosis of Crohn's disease. Remarkably, we found that he had a significant family ancestry of inflammatory bowel disease. His inflammatory bowel disease and peripheral arthritis were well-controlled on ustekinumab (IL12/23 inhibitor), and a 4 years follow-up showed no relapses.

Case 2: a 19-year-old Qatari woman, who was on adalimumab for juvenile idiopathic arthritis and chronic anterior uveitis for 2 years, developed new-onset dizziness and hand tremors. Neurological examination showed impaired cerebellar function as evidenced by intention tremors, ataxia, dysmetria, and dysdiadochokinesia with normal tone, power, and sensation; reflexes were less brisk. She had no history of multiple sclerosis. MRI revealed multiple hyperintense white matter lesions especially in bilateral cerebellar peduncles, periventricular, subcortical and juxtacortical, brain stem, corpus callosum, and left anterior thalamus, and also, multiple patchy T2 hyperintensities are noted in the cervical and midthoracic spinal cord with foci of enhancement noted in the midthoracic spinal cord, in keeping with active lesions as shown in Figures 2(a) and 2(b). Her CSF analysis revealed the presence of CSF unique oligoclonal bands.

Discontinuation of adalimumab resulted in near-complete improvement in her symptoms; she was offered pulse steroid, but she declined and was shifted to methotrexate with good control of her arthritis and uveitis. Repeated MRI after one year showed regression of the previous lesions, but it showed newly detected lesions in different areas. Subsequently, patient was switched to rituximab to control her arthritis and demyelinating disease. A year later, another MRI was done, and it showed stable appearance of the previous demyelinating lesions with no signs of disease activity.

Case 3: a 34-year-old man was diagnosed with ankylosing spondylitis 7 years ago in his home country. He was initially treated with sulfasalazine and nonsteroidal anti-inflammatory drugs. After two years, he was started on infliximab to control his disease activity. Five years after infliximab initiation, he developed unexplained left hand numbness and weakness. A diagnosis of multiple sclerosis was made based on MRI findings and CSF analysis which were done at his home country. Infliximab was discontinued, and he received IV pulse steroid for five days with complete recovery; but two years later, he developed another attack with diplopia, left leg numbness, and weakness and again was treated with IV pulse steroids with good recovery. 4 years later, he presented to our hospital with a third attack of left facial numbness; MRI done at our center to confirm the diagnosis showed numerous bilateral variable-sized, different-shaped plaques of high signal intensity on T2WI/FLAIR involving mainly in the brain and spinal cord associated with left deep periventricular frontal and left cerebellar peduncle enhanced plaques as shown in Figures 3(a)–3(e). The cerebrospinal fluid revealed oligoclonal, while the rest of the parameters were within the normal limits.

He was treated with IV pulse dose steroids 1 g for 5 days with complete recovery. He was kept on NSAIDS for his ankylosing spondylitis and was recommended to start rituximab as a disease-modifying treatment to control multiple sclerosis. The patient left to his home country and was lost to follow-up.

3. Discussion

The development of CNS demyelination with anti-TNF-α therapy has been shown in several reports from various countries [5, 7, 8]. It is unclear, however, whether these demyelinating events are coincidental or whether they are causally associated with the use of TNF-α antagonists [7]. Clinical trials of TNF-α blockers in patients with MS showed an increase in demyelinating events [9], in addition to the complete remission of symptoms after withdrawal of this agent [5, 7] and temporal relation, as well as the rechallenge phenomenon that was demonstrated in many cases [10–13] favor a causal association.

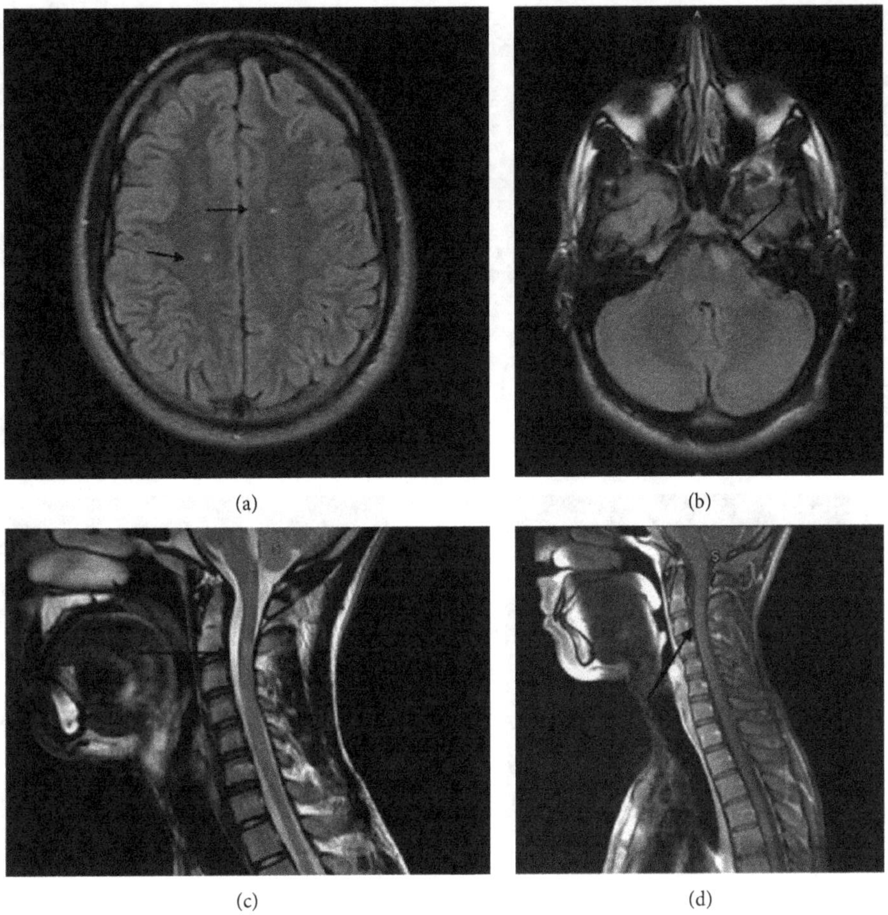

FIGURE 1: (a) There are few small foci of T2 and FLAIR hyperintensity noted in the periventricular white matter (bilaterally), perpendicular to the ventricular margin. (b) There is a small area of T2 and FLAIR hyperintensity noted in the left paramedian anterior pons. ((c), (d)) There is a small area of T2 hyperintensity with corresponding postcontrast enhancement noted in the cervical spinal cord at the C2-C3 level.

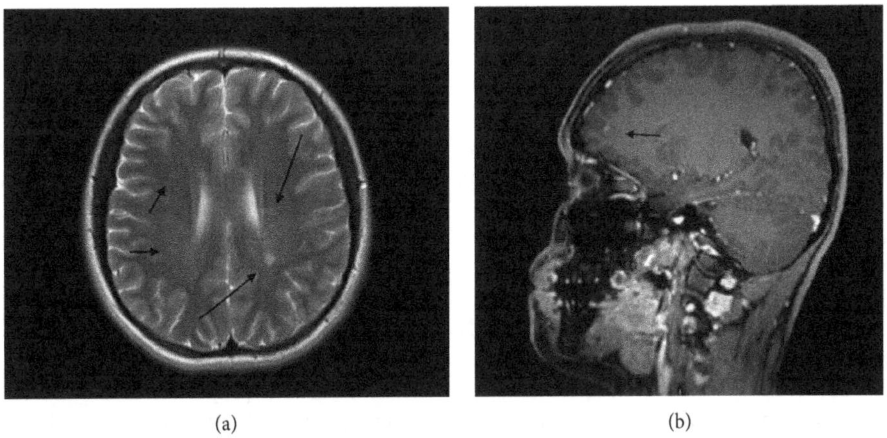

FIGURE 2: (a) There are multiple periventricular, subcortical, and juxtacortical white matter foci of T2 and FLAIR hypersignal in both cerebral hemispheres, brain stem, bilateral middle cerebellar peduncles, corpus callosum, and left anterior thalamus. (b) There is focal enhancement noted in the left peritrigonal white matter lesion.

On the other hand, one wonders whether this correlation is simply the unmasking of a preexisting MS or the onset of new demyelinating diseases [5, 7, 8]. Interestingly, some authors identified the demyelination of the CNS in asymptomatic patients before the initiation of anti-TNF-α therapy, which suggests that TNF-α blockers may unmask preexisting MS as well as provoking new-onset demyelination [5].

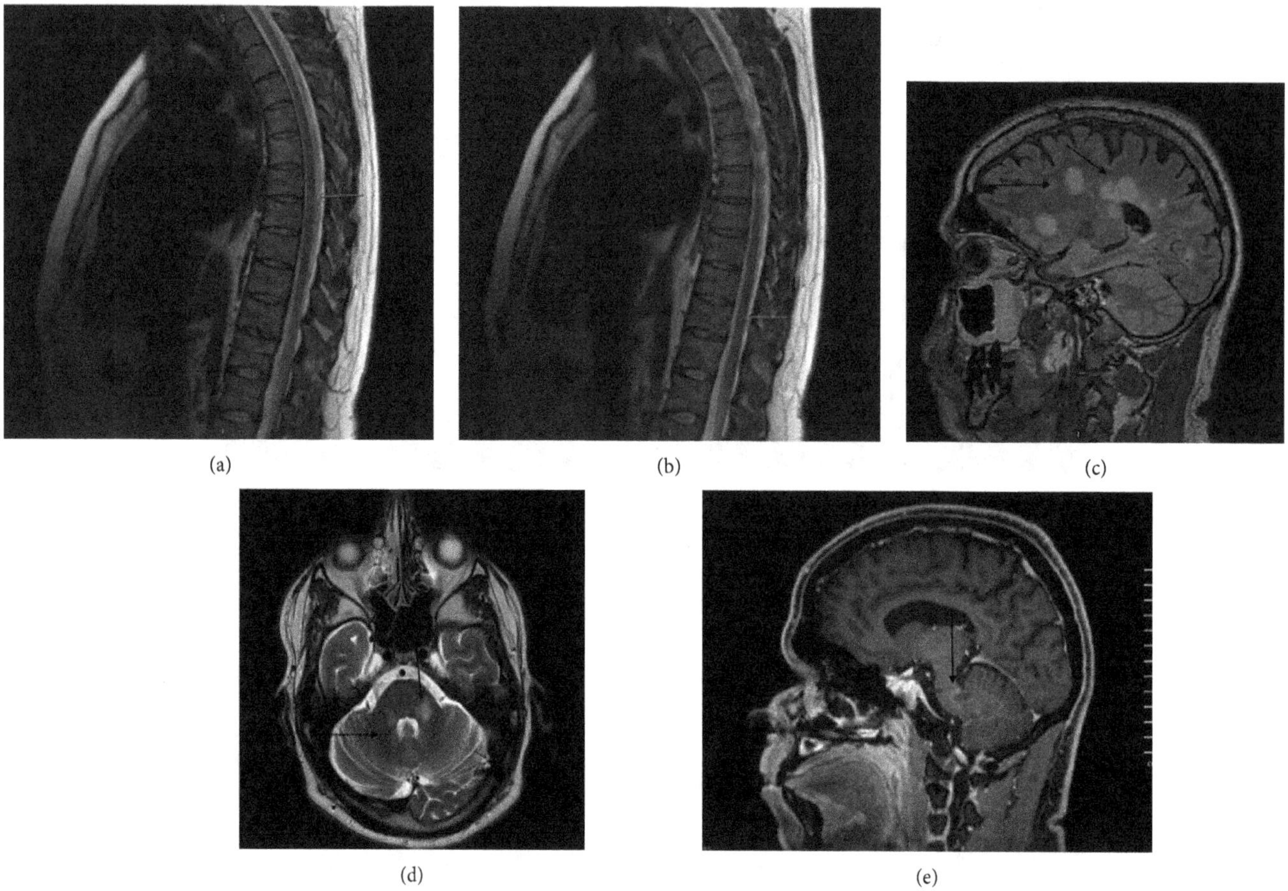

FIGURE 3: ((a), (b)) There are at least 2 definite high signal intensity plaques on the sagittal T2W1 seen at D6-7, D9-10 levels (arrow). ((c), (d)) Numerous bilateral variable-sized, different-shaped plaques of high signal intensity on T2W1/FLAIR seen mainly in the deep white matter at periventricular location and centrum semiovale, perpendicular callososeptal lesions, cerebellar peduncles, and cerebellar white matter. (e) Incomplete ring enhancement lesions seen in the left deep periventricular frontal lobe and left cerebellar peduncle.

The mechanisms underlying demyelination predisposition or demyelination exacerbation in patients treated with anti-TNF-α agents are not fully understood, and several theories have been suggested. One of these theories is called lack of entry theory, which suggests that TNF-α blockers cannot penetrate the intact blood-brain barrier (BBB) to suppress demyelination, but they can enhance demyelination through increased ingress of peripheral autoreactive T cells into the CNS [8]. This theory provides a possible explanation for the failure of anti-TNF-α blockers in reducing demyelination and for their effect on aggravating MS. However, they cannot adequately explain the new onset of demyelination, as in our cases.

The time between exposure to TNF-α blockers and the onset of symptoms varies widely between different reports. In the report by Kemanetzoglou et al. [8], the time between exposure to TNF-α blockers and the onset of symptoms ranged between 3 days and 6 years, while Mohan et al. [11] found that the time between exposure and the onset of symptoms was between 1 week and 15 months. As noted in our series, the time between the initiation of TNF-α blocker and the development of symptoms ranged between 2 years as in cases 1 and 2 and 5 years as in case 3, which falls within the range of 3 days to 6 years that was mentioned above.

As noted in our series and other reports [5, 7, 8], the discontinuation of TNF-α blockers led to a complete remission of symptoms. Relapses of demyelination after remission have been reported by many authors [14, 15] as well as in case 3 of our series, which could be explained by the common spontaneous relapsing-remitting episodes of MS. However, despite discontinuation of treatment, demyelination disorders may persist, indicating that anti-TNF-α agents may activate the demyelination mechanism, which further develops independently [15]. Our small number of cases despite the increased use of TNF-α blockers is reassuring and similar to other recently published data from the British registry [16]. Another question to be answered is whether demyelination during anti-TNF-α agents actually meets the criteria for MS diagnosis or whether it constitutes a different MS-like syndrome. From our study, it is recommended to avoid the use of TNF-α blockers in patients with own history or family history of MS or any other demyelinating disease. In case of development of any new neurological symptoms, the patient needs a thorough neurological examination, and once demyelination is confirmed, anti-TNF blockers should be withdrawn. In addition to those with a family history of demyelination, those with a family history of autoimmune disease might also be at higher risk of developing demyelinating events as in our first case, even in the absence of TNF-α blockers due to shared common gentic and environmental triggers [17].

4. Conclusion

Despite the small number of patients, our series adds to the growing body of evidence supporting a causal link between anti-TNF-α agents and demyelination, which clinicians should be aware of. On expectation of any neurological side effects, early discontinuation of TNF-α blockers and requesting urgent MRI scan to confirm the diagnosis is of utmost importance.

Abbreviations

Anti-TNF-α:	Tumor necrosis factor antagonists
MRI:	Magnetic resonance imaging
MS:	Multiple sclerosis
CSF:	Cerebrospinal fluid
BBB:	Blood-brain barrier.

Consent

Written informed consent was obtained from the participants.

References

[1] L. B. Silva, A. P. dos Santos Neto, S. M. A. S. Maia et al., "The role of TNF-α as a proinflammatory cytokine in pathological processes," *The Open Dentistry Journal*, vol. 13, no. 1, pp. 332–338, 2019.

[2] N. Parameswaran and S. Patial, "Tumor necrosis factor-α signaling in macrophages," *Critical Reviews in Eukaryotic Gene Expression*, vol. 20, no. 2, pp. 87–103, 2010.

[3] J. Lin, D. Ziring, S. Desai et al., "TNFα blockade in human diseases: an overview of efficacy and safety," *Clinical Immunology*, vol. 126, no. 1, pp. 13–30, 2008.

[4] M. P. Karampetsou, S. N. C. Liossis, and P. P. Sfikakis, "TNF-antagonists beyond approved indications: stories of success and prospects for the future," *QJM*, vol. 103, no. 12, pp. 917–928, 2010.

[5] T. I. Kopp, B. Delcoigne, E. V. Arkema et al., "Risk of neuroinflammatory events in arthritis patients treated with tumour necrosis factor alpha inhibitors: a collaborative population-based cohort study from Denmark and Sweden," *Annals of the Rheumatic Diseases*, vol. 79, no. 5, pp. 566–572, 2020.

[6] A. J. Thompson, B. L. Banwell, F. Barkhof et al., "Diagnosis of multiple sclerosis: 2017 revisions of the McDonald criteria," *The Lancet Neurology*, vol. 17, no. 2, pp. 162–173, 2018.

[7] E. Andreadou, E. Kemanetzoglou, C. Brokalaki et al., "Demyelinating disease following anti-TNFa treatment: a causal or coincidental association? Report of four cases and review of the literature," *Case Reports in Neurological Medicine*, vol. 2013, pp. 1–9, 2013.

[8] E. Kemanetzoglou and E. Andreadou, "CNS demyelination with TNF-α blockers," *Current Neurology and Neuroscience Reports*, vol. 17, no. 4, p. 36, 2017.

[9] No Authors Listed, "TNF neutralization in MS: results of a randomized, placebo-controlled multicenter study. The lenercept multiple sclerosis study group and the university of British columbia MS/MRI analysis group," *Neurology*, vol. 53, no. 3, pp. 457–465, 1999.

[10] A. Kim and N. Saffra, "A case report of adalimumab-associated optic neuritis," *Journal of Ophthalmic Inflammation and Infection*, vol. 2, no. 3, pp. 145–147, 2012.

[11] N. Mohan, E. T. Edwards, T. R. Cupps et al., "Demyelination occurring during anti-tumor necrosis factor? therapy for inflammatory arthritides," *Arthritis & Rheumatism*, vol. 44, no. 12, pp. 2862–2869, 2001.

[12] M. Tanno, I. Nakamura, S. Kobayashi, K. Kurihara, and K. Ito, "New-onset demyelination induced by infliximab therapy in two rheumatoid arthritis patients," *Clinical Rheumatology*, vol. 25, no. 6, pp. 929–933, 2006.

[13] M. Gomez-Gallego, J. Meca-Lallana, and A. Fernandez-Barreiro, "Multiple sclerosis onset during etanercept treatment," *European Neurology*, vol. 59, no. 1-2, pp. 91–93, 2008.

[14] M. C. Fernández-Espartero, B. Pérez-Zafrilla, A. Naranjo, C. Esteban, A. M. Ortiz, and J. J. Gómez-Reino, "Demyelinating disease in patients treated with TNF antagonists in rheumatology: data from BIOBADASER, a pharmacovigilance database, and a systematic review," *Seminars in Arthritis and Rheumatism*, vol. 40, no. 4, pp. 330–337, 2011.

[15] R. Seror, C. Richez, C. Sordet et al., "Pattern of demyelination occurring during anti-TNF-α therapy: a French national survey," *Rheumatology*, vol. 52, no. 5, pp. 868–874, 2013.

[16] T. R. P. Taylor, J. Galloway, R. Davies, K. Hyrich, and R. Dobson, "Demyelinating events following initiation of anti-TNFα therapy in the British society for rheumatology biologics registry in rheumatoid arthritis," *Neurology-Neuroimmunology Neuroinflammation*, vol. 8, no. 3, Article ID e992, 2021.

[17] A. Alonso, M. A. Hernán, and A. Ascherio, "Allergy, family history of autoimmune diseases, and the risk of multiple sclerosis," *Acta Neurologica Scandinavica*, vol. 117, no. 1, pp. 15–20, 2008.

25

Into a Shaking Limbo: Case Report of a Nonneoplastic Limbic Encephalitis with Faciobrachial Dystonic Seizures and Parkinsonism

Vijay Renga

Department of Neurology, Dartmouth Hitchcock Medical Center, Geisel School of Medicine at Dartmouth, One Medical Center Drive, Lebanon, NH 03756, USA

Correspondence should be addressed to Vijay Renga; drvijayrenga@gmail.com

Academic Editor: Majaz Moonis

This case report describes a rare but classic presentation of a non-paraneoplastic, antibody-mediated limbic encephalitis. The clinical course did put us in a limbo as it evolved from seizure to Parkinsonism and then from metastasis to stroke, before it finally announced itself by its pathognomonic finding. Knowledge of this rare condition is important as early identification and treatment can change the course.

1. Case Scenario

A 63-year-old male was referred to us for an urgent evaluation of new onset left-sided shaking spells for two weeks. He felt that his left side was clenching up suddenly at times. Sometimes he had a choking sensation with short vocalization. Things that he would be holding in his left hand could be thrown away during these spells. By the time he realizes it happening, the spell would be over.

He had a history of renal calculi and experienced hematuria recently. His physician suspected seizures from brain metastases due to possible renal cancer. A CT scan of the head and abdomen was arranged, and the patient was started on carbamazepine. The medicine reduced the frequency of the events but did not stop it. CT head showed pansinusitis without evidence of any metastases. CT abdomen revealed renal stones.

In Neurology clinic, he had few episodes characterized by sudden, involuntary jerking of his left arm. Each of these episodes caught him by surprise. He had Parkinsonism features, more so on the left side with increased tone, bradykinesia, and hyper-reflexia. We were concerned that these spells represented alien limb phenomenon which is typically seen in cortico-basal syndrome. Segmental myoclonus and dystonic spells were also in differentials.

To capture and characterize these spells, he was hospitalized for VEEG monitoring. Multiple spells were captured which had no epileptiform correlates. An MRI of his brain without contrast showed only sinusitis. CSF was unremarkable with 1 cell, protein of 42, and glucose of 88.

A repeat MRI brain with contrast was then obtained. This showed two tiny enhancing lesions, one in the right motor strip (Figure 1) and the other in the left parietal region, suspicious for metastases.

Outpatient malignancy workup was done with PET scan of the brain and whole body and paraneoplastic panel. PET scan of the body found no primary malignancy. PET scan of the brain showed hyperactivity in the left temporal region, suspicious for epileptic activity (Figure 2). Clinical seizures were on the left side, which did not correlate with this finding. His seizure episodes worsened, and he was started on levetiracetam in addition to increased dose of carbamazepine.

Few days later, he was admitted with generalized rashes from carbamazepine and antiepileptics were changed. He was evaluated by Dermatology, ENT, Oncology, and Gastroenterology for any potential malignancy, and none was

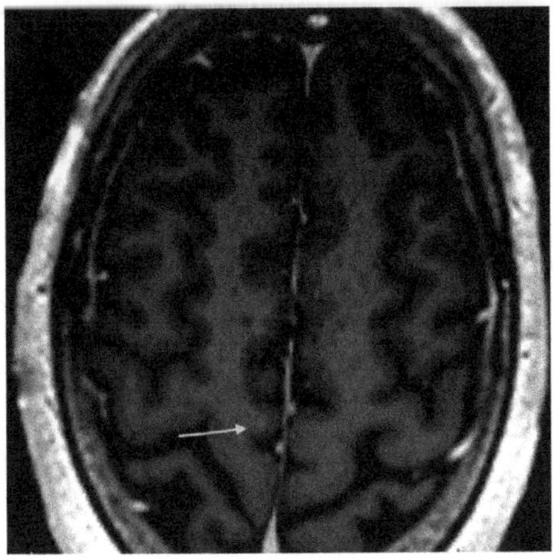

FIGURE 1: MRI Brain: T1 post-contrast sequence with an arrow pointing to an enhancing lesion over the right motor strip.

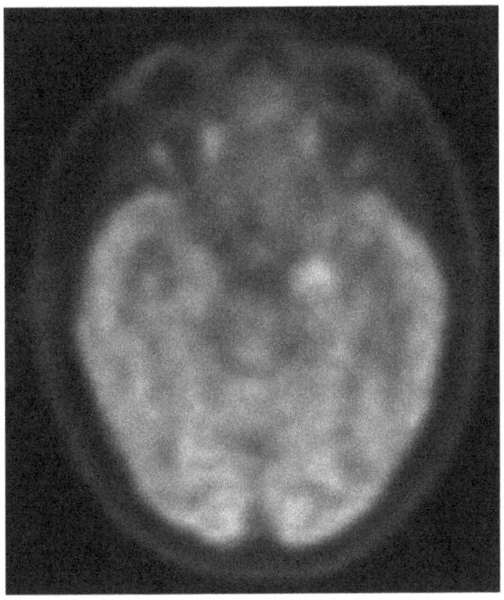

FIGURE 2: PET scan of brain showing increased activity in the left mesial temporal region.

detected. We repeated video-EEG monitoring and MRI brain. Video-EEG again captured multiple spells without epileptiform correlate. Seizures became difficult to control with multiple AEDs.

Repeat MRI showed new scattered embolic infarcts in the left hemisphere (Figure 3) with disappearance of previously seen enhancing lesions that were thought to be metastases. Radiology determined that strokes were possibly misinterpreted as metastases because of the enhancement in the acute phase. Strokes were considered as a potential cause of his seizure at this point. He had extensive stroke workup with vascular imaging, echocardiogram, telemetry, hypercoagulability panel, and vascular doppler, all of which were negative for a cause.

Seizure semiology changed at this point with new right-sided facial spasms and simultaneous arm shaking on the right side, which now correlated with previous PET findings of a left sided process. A diagnosis of paraneoplastic limbic encephalitis was considered. His seizures evolved into the

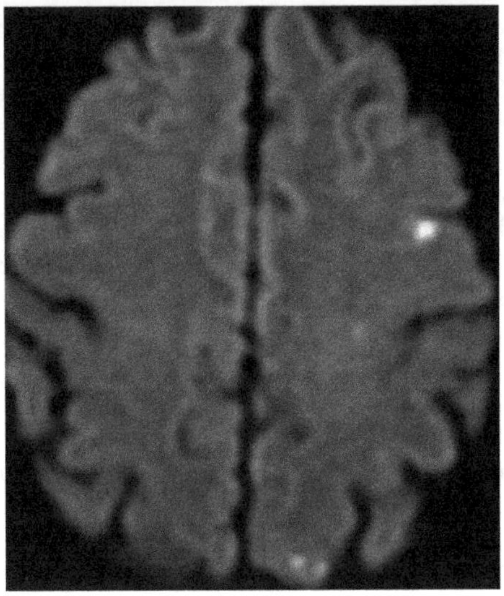

FIGURE 3: Diffusion MRI sequence showing embolic appearing regions of restricted diffusion (bright white spots) in the left hemisphere.

characteristic "Faciobrachial dystonic" appearance previously described in LG1/VGKC antibody-related limbic encephalitis.

Empiric trial of steroids was started and seizures got controlled. He was discharged on oral prednisone and two antiepileptic medications. Few weeks later, his serum paraneoplastic panel came positive for both LG1 and VGKC antibodies while the CSF panel was negative for the same. Caspr2-IgG was negative.

On the clinic follow-up, his seizures had completely abated and he was tapered off steroids. The Parkinsonism features seen during earlier visits also resolved. He continued to have some memory changes.

1.1. Final Diagnosis

(1) Nonneoplastic limbic encephalitis secondary to VGKC/LG1 antibodies.

(2) Embolic strokes of indeterminate etiology

2. Discussion

Voltage-gated potassium channel antibodies have been described in nonmalignancy-related limbic encephalitis since the 1990s [1]. Over a decade later, newer antibodies associated with VGKC were characterized. These include (1) leucine-rich glioma protein (LG1) antibodies and (2) contactin-associated protein-like 2 (Caspr2) antibodies. The LGI proteins are secreted by neurons and modulate synaptic excitability. Mutations causing defective LG1 proteins are associated with epilepsy syndromes. Antibodies to LG1 proteins can cause limbic encephalitis. This is the second most common form of antibody-associated limbic encephalitis, after NMDA receptor antibody-related encephalitis [2]. These tend to be clinically less severe than NMDARAb-related encephalitis. Different scenarios can occur with VGKC antibody positive syndromes. These include (1) patients with only VGKC antibody positivity (2) those with VGKC and LG1 positive (as in our patient), and (3) VGKC and Caspr2 positive. Clinical features may give a clue to the underlying antibody type. The VGKC and LG1 positive patients tend to have limbic encephalitis. Memory and behavioral changes are common. Parkinsonism can be seen with striato-limbic encephalitis. While it is not widely reported in association with LG1/VGKC-related encephalitis, this was noted in our patient. A variety of other manifestations including hyponatremia, behavioral disorders, and cognitive issues have been described [3]. Faciobrachial dystonic seizures is the hallmark feature of LG1 antibody-related limbic encephalitis, even though partial and generalized seizures can coexist [4]. Faciobrachial dystonic seizures are rapid and short lasting seizures with facial twitching and involuntary arm jerking. These may not have an epileptic correlate. Semiology is very characteristic and can help diagnose the condition long before the paraneoplastic antibodies are resulted [5]. The lead time can help gain control over the seizure with appropriate treatment.

Caspr2 protein is more widespread and distributed in nerve membranes of peripheral and central nervous systems [3]. Caspr2 antibodies are seen in conditions like Morvan or Isaac's syndrome and associated with peripheral nerve hyperexcitability with fasciculations, muscle spasm, and neuromyotonia along with cognitive changes and seizures [6]. Our patient was Caspr2 negative and did not have any peripheral hyperexcitability related symptoms.

Both these forms of limbic encephalitis respond to steroids or immunotherapy. Relying on the CSF paraneoplastic panel alone could have resulted in a "missed-diagnosis" as serum antibody is more sensitive for LG1 Ab-related limbic encephalitis.

3. Conclusion

(i) VGKC antibody-related limbic encephalitis is commonly a *non-paraneoplastic* limbic encephalitis. In addition to VGKC antibodies, antibodies to LG1 and Caspr2 are now available. Clinical manifestations differ based on the antibody type.

(ii) VGKC with LG1 antibodies are associated with the *pathognomonic faciobrachial dystonic seizures*, which may not have an epileptiform correlate.

(iii) *Striato-limbic encephalitis* with Parkinsonism, while not classically described with VGKC/LG1 antibodies can be seen in this syndrome.

(iv) It is important to test *both serum and CSF paraneoplastic panel antibodies* as either can be false negative. Serum LG1 antibodies are more sensitive than CSF antibodies.

(v) This condition usually *responds to steroids and immunotherapy.*

References

[1] C. E. Bekircan-Kurt, E. Derle Çiftçi, A. T. Kurne et al., "Voltage gated calcium channel antibody-related neurological diseases," *World Journal of Clinical Cases*, vol. 3, no. 3, pp. 293–300, 2015.

[2] A. van Sonderen, M. Petit-Pedrol, J. Dalmau, and M. J. Titulaer, "The value of LGI1, Caspr2 and voltage-gated potassium channel antibodies in encephalitis," *Nature Reviews Neurology*, vol. 13, no. 5, pp. 290–301, 2017.

[3] M. Wang, X. Cao, Q. Liu, W. Ma, X. Guo, and X. Liu, "Clinical features of limbic encephalitis with LGI1 antibody," *Neuropsychiatric Disease and Treatment*, vol. 13, pp. 1589–1596, 2017.

[4] G. d'Orsi, T. Martino, A. Lalla, M. T. D. Claudio, E. Carapelle, and C. Avolio, "Faciobrachial dystonic seizures expressed as epileptic spasms, followed by focal seizures in anti-LGI1 encephalitis: a video-polygraphic study," *Epileptic Disord*, vol. 20, no. 6, pp. 525–529, 2018.

[5] S. R. Irani, A. W. Michell, B. Lang et al., "Faciobrachial dystonic seizures precede Lgi1 antibody limbic encephalitis," *Annals of Neurology*, vol. 69, no. 5, pp. 892–900, 2011.

[6] E. Lancaster, "The diagnosis and treatment of autoimmune encephalitis," *Journal of Clinical Neurology*, vol. 12, no. 1, p. 1, 2016.

A Case of Tick-Borne Paralysis in a Traveling Patient

Kevin Ha, Kathryn Lewis, Vandan Patel, and Jennifer Grinceri

University of California, Riverside, School of Medicine, USA

Correspondence should be addressed to Kevin Ha; kevin.ha@medsch.ucr.edu

Academic Editor: Isabella Laura Simone

Background. Tick paralysis is a neurotoxic tick-borne illness that causes ascending paralysis and may lead to respiratory failure. Patients often undergo extensive testing and prolonged hospitalization before the proper diagnosis is reached. *Case Presentation.* An 88-year-old man with dementia and dyslipidemia presented with new onset gait instability and was admitted for suspected cerebellar stroke. Exam was significant for the inability to perform tandem gait. Investigations included comprehensive metabolic panel, complete blood count, and noncontrast CT scan; none of them found any evidence of acute pathology. Two days into admission, a tick with surrounding erythema was found on the patient's left lateral chest during bathing. Dramatic improvement in truncal ataxia was noted following tick extraction. *Discussion.* Clinical suspicion of tick paralysis is often low due to the rarity of the condition. Although it is imperative to rule out acute cerebral or cerebellar pathology, a thorough skin examination should be performed on admission in any patient with new onset ataxia and ascending paralysis. This can lead to early diagnosis, conservation of resources, and the avoidance of subjecting patients to invasive testing.

1. Introduction

Tick paralysis is a rare neurotoxic response to the envenoming by an adult female tick endemic to North America and the eastern coast of Australia. The most common presentation is an ascending paralysis, preceded by a nonspecific prodromal phase marked by fatigue, fever, and generalized weakness. Full recovery of paralysis is often reported within 24-48 hours of tick removal [1]. Although rare, untreated tick paralysis carries a 10% mortality rate, secondary to respiratory failure. Risks of paralysis developing after tick bite are correlated with milligram of toxin-per-kilogram of patient as well as the time between attachment and tick removal. Therefore, most reports of tick paralysis are of young girls whose long hair provides camouflage for feeding ticks. We present a rare case of tick paralysis in an active elderly male visiting the desert.

2. Case Report

An 88-year-old male with dementia, dyslipidemia, and status after cochlear implantation presented to a community hospital after new onset gait instability. The patient was on a road trip from Wisconsin when he developed an inability to walk at dinner after arriving in the Coachella Valley, approximately 100 miles east of Los Angeles. The patient was unable to ambulate and experienced worsening instability in his trunk. History was negative for atrial fibrillation, transient ischemic attacks, and strokes. The patient's only medications were an 81 mg daily aspirin and simvastatin. Given his progressive truncal ataxia, the patient was admitted for suspected cerebellar stroke.

On exam, the patient was alert and oriented to person, place, and time without sensory or cranial nerve deficits. Strength was 5/5 in all limbs. Exam was remarkable for ataxia of the trunk with unstable gait. Patient was unable to perform tandem gait. Laboratory findings for complete metabolic panel and complete blood count were unremarkable. A noncontrast CT was done, revealing stable age-related atrophy without evidence of acute ischemia or hemorrhage. Complete evaluation for cerebellar stroke was limited, as MRI could not be done due to cochlear implantation. The patient was then admitted for further management and workup of ataxia given concern for stroke.

Two days into admission, a tick with surrounding ecchymosis was found on the patient's left lateral chest wall during bathing (Figures 1 and 2). Upon further questioning, he

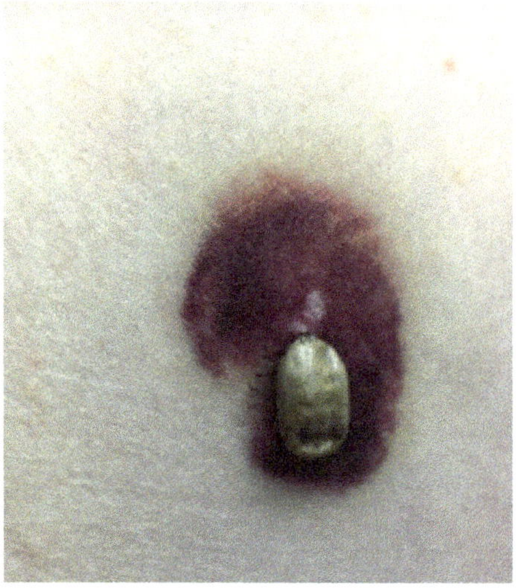

FIGURE 1: Engorged female tick with surrounding ecchymosis on the left axilla.

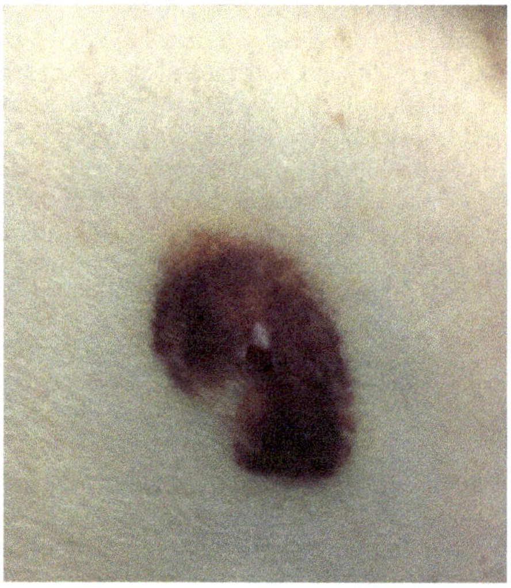

FIGURE 2: Left axilla ecchymosis status after tick extraction.

reported hotel stays and visited national parks throughout his travels. He denied animal exposures, camping, and use of insect repellant. Following tick removal, truncal ataxia dramatically improved. The patient worked with physical therapy for an additional two days and was then safely discharged without ataxia.

3. Discussion

There are over 60 identified species of ticks whose toxins can cause paralysis. The ability to cause paralysis is dependent on the type of tick–soft versus hard, host species, life cycle stage, and sex. For example, the tick identified in this case, *Dermacentor variabilis*, is a hard tick in which the female can only cause paralysis [2]. In the United States, the most reported species is the *Dermacentor* tick, often found in wooded regions of the Rocky Mountains and Pacific Northwest. Ticks often remain dormant under leaves during winter months and become active in the spring, with incidents of tick bites being highest from March to July. Bites are often painless, and ticks may hook onto their hosts for up to ten days [1, 3, 4]. In the process of feeding, neurotoxins from the salivary glands of ticks may be released into the host. It is hypothesized that the toxins produced by ticks, or holocyclotoxin, act similarly to botulinum toxins by blocking the presynaptic release of acetylcholine into the synaptic cleft causing delays to nerve conduction [1, 3–5]; however, there are multiple proposed methods of paralysis unique to different species which may be used in combination or alone [2].

Tick paralysis may be broken up into two distinct stages: prodromal and proper paralysis. The prodromal period often appears within 36 hours and presents with nonspecific flu-like symptoms, headache, and tingling. If the tick remains attached, the proper paralysis phase begins (often by day four) with ataxia followed by weakness to the lower extremities. Eventually, the paralysis ascends, causing lower-motor-neuron signs of flaccid paralysis to all extremities and quadriplegia [1, 3, 4]. Cranial nerve involvement has been reported, with patients presenting with ophthalmoplegia, facial weakness, and bulbar palsy [6]. Although rare, untreated tick paralysis carries a 10% mortality rate, secondary to respiratory failure [1, 3].

Diagnosis of tick paralysis is made via complete physical examination of the skin. Once identified, ticks are removed by grasping the tick as close to the skin surface while avoiding squeezing additional toxins. Full recovery of paralysis has been reported within 24-48 hours of tick removal with repeat nerve conduction study showing amplitude values and conduction time returning to normal [1]. Given that Lyme Disease is caused by the *Borrelia burgdorferi* bacteria transmitted by the *Ixodes scapularis* tick, considerations of travel history to the Northeast US, tick morphology, and symptoms such as target rashes, arthralgia, and heart block should be considered as Lyme Disease requires both tick removal and introduction of oral or IV antibiotics. In this case, we identified the tick causing paralysis to be *D. variabilis* based on geographic predominance [7]. Our group did not attempt to identify the tick species while in the hospital by morphology or direct assay. However, we argue that there is benefit to identifying encountered ticks in future cases for tracking purposes as well as for research that is being done to provide antiparalysis vaccines [2].

More often, tick paralysis is often misdiagnosed as Guillain-Barre Syndrome (GBS), as both diseases present with an ascending paralysis [3]. As a result, clinicians may spend time ordering spirometry, CSF analysis, nerve conduction studies, and intravenous gamma globulin G as a treatment for the ascending paralysis. Interestingly, both tick paralysis and GBS demonstrate similar nerve conduction studies of decreased amplitudes of compound muscle action potentials and diminished nerve conduction velocities [3, 8]. Tick paralysis lacks the fevers or autonomic dysfunction that should point a clinician away from a GBS diagnosis. Other diseases incorrectly worked up include botulism, encephalomyelitis, and stroke [3, 9].

Unfortunately, the literature suggests that detection of ticks in patients presenting with ascending paralysis is often not made during the initial assessment but instead later in the hospital course by the patient's family members, nursing staff, or other providers. This finding is often after an extensive workup for a wide array of diseases was already performed, prolonging the time of attachment to detection and removal of the tick. Given that tick paralysis is dependent on both milligram of toxin-per-kilogram of host as well as time of attachment, delay in care is both an inefficient use of resources and potentially dangerous to patient care [1, 3, 4].

4. Conclusion

Tick paralysis is poorly surveilled in the United States with one meta-analysis reporting only fifty well documented cases of tick paralysis between 1946 and 2006 [3]. Patients presenting with symptoms of ascending paralysis in endemic areas or recent travel to endemic areas should prompt clinicians to do a thorough skin examination for ticks before working up other etiologies. A stroke rule-out was both time sensitive and necessary in our patient given his symptoms of acute onset weakness; however, tick paralysis was low on our list of differentials demonstrated by the delay in obtaining the patient's recent travel history and more thorough skin examination. This case further illustrates the importance of proper history taking, physical examination, and consideration of tick paralysis as a differential in patients presenting with ascending paralysis.

Disclosure

This case was presented in abstract form at the American College of Physicians National Conference for Clinical Vignettes-Medical Students in Philadelphia, Pennsylvania by contributing author Ms. Kathryn Lewis on April 13, 2019.

References

[1] K. Borawski, S. Pancewicz, P. Czupryna, J. Zajkowska, and A. Moniuszko, "Tick paralysis," *Przeglad Epidemiologiczny*, vol. 72, pp. 17–24, 2018.

[2] R. Pienaar, A. Neitz, and B. Mans, "Tick paralysis: solving an enigma," *Veterinary Sciences*, vol. 5, no. 2, article 53, 2018.

[3] J. H. Diaz, "A comparative meta-analysis of tick paralysis in the United States and Australia," *Clinical Toxicology*, vol. 53, no. 9, pp. 874–883, 2015.

[4] J. A. Edlow, "Tick paralysis," *Current Treatment Options in Neurology*, vol. 12, no. 3, pp. 167–177, 2010.

[5] B. J. Mans, R. Gothe, and A. W. Neitz, "Biochemical perspectives on paralysis and other forms of toxicoses caused by ticks," *Parasitology*, vol. 129, no. 7, pp. S95–S111, 2004.

[6] P. Grattan-Smith, "Clinical and neurophysiological features of tick paralysis," *Brain*, vol. 120, no. 11, pp. 1975–1987, 1997.

[7] Centers for Disease Control and Prevention, "Geographic distribution of ticks that bite humans," https://www.cdc.gov/ticks/geographic_distribution.html.

[8] A. V. Krishnan, C. S. Lin, S. W. Reddel, R. Mcgrath, and M. C. Kiernan, "Conduction block and impaired axonal function in tick paralysis," *Muscle & Nerve*, vol. 40, no. 3, pp. 358–362, 2009.

[9] M. Uguz, N. Mendil Erdogan, and E. Eken, "Tick-induced facial palsy," *Turkish Journal of Parasitology*, vol. 39, no. 3, pp. 248–251, 2015.

Recurrent Hodgkin's Disease Presenting as a Clinically Isolated Cavernous Sinus Syndrome

Aayesha Jalaluddin Soni and Edward Bernard Lee-Pan

Department of Neurology, University of Cape Town, Cape Town, South Africa

Correspondence should be addressed to Aayesha Jalaluddin Soni; ajsoni008@gmail.com

Academic Editor: Peter Berlit

Background. Hodgkin's disease involving the central nervous system is uncommon and is usually seen in patients with uncontrolled systemic disease or those who have had multiple episodes of recurrent disease. Common symptoms of intracranial Hodgkin's disease are motor and/or sensory deficits, headache, papilloedema, coma, and seizures. The rarity of Hodgkin's disease presenting with intracranial involvement is marked, but patients presenting with cavernous sinus syndrome is even rarer. Despite its rarity, the presence of a cavernous sinus syndrome in a patient with a known history of Hodgkin's disease warrants full utilization of modern diagnostic techniques in terms of investigation. *Case Presentation.* A 34-year-old woman, known with previous Hodgkin's lymphoma and now in remission for the past 7 years, presented with signs and symptoms suggestive of a left cavernous sinus syndrome. She was otherwise systemically well with no other complaints. Extensive investigations revealed no obvious cause for the cavernous sinus syndrome. A CT chest revealed subclinical axillary lymphadenopathy, which on excisional biopsy confirmed recurrent Hodgkin's disease. The patient's sole clinical presentation of her recurrent disease was the cavernous sinus syndrome, with no other clinically obvious systemic signs or symptoms to suggest a relapse. This was treated with steroids, and clinical improvement was noted; she was referred to oncology for extensive chemotherapy. *Conclusions.* Whilst there is a paucity of literature around this topic, it must be remembered by the clinician that cavernous sinus syndrome may be the sole clinical presentation of recurrent Hodgkin's disease. Even though it is reported that lymphomatous involvement in the brain usually occurs late in the disease process, this case is evidence that cavernous sinus syndrome may precede other systemic signs and symptoms. Recognising this possibility will ensure a rigorous search for Hodgkin's disease, an early and effective diagnosis, and a better prognosis in affected patients.

1. Background

Hodgkin's disease (HD) involving the central nervous system (CNS) is uncommon and is usually seen in patients with uncontrolled systemic disease or those who have had multiple episodes of recurrent disease. [1] There have been no identifiable risk factors for HD presenting with intracranial involvement. Whether at initial presentation or at relapse, the occurrence of intracranial HD without overt evidence of disease elsewhere is very rare. Whilst the literature acknowledges the rarity of HD presenting with CNS symptoms (especially in contrast to non-Hodgkin's disease which frequently presents in the CNS), patients presenting with cavernous sinus syndrome (CSS) is even rarer. There are only 2 other documented adult patients with HD in remission who presented with recurrence in the cavernous sinus [2] and no adult cases of primary HD presenting with isolated CSS. All of our knowledge on the topic is limited to isolated case reports in patients with salient features. Our patient presented clinically with a CSS only and no other systemic signs or symptoms to suggest a relapse of HD.

2. Case Presentation

A 34-year-old woman presented with an 8-day history of a progressively worsening left-sided headache, originating around her eye and radiating backwards. She also reported six days of worsening horizontal diplopia on binocular

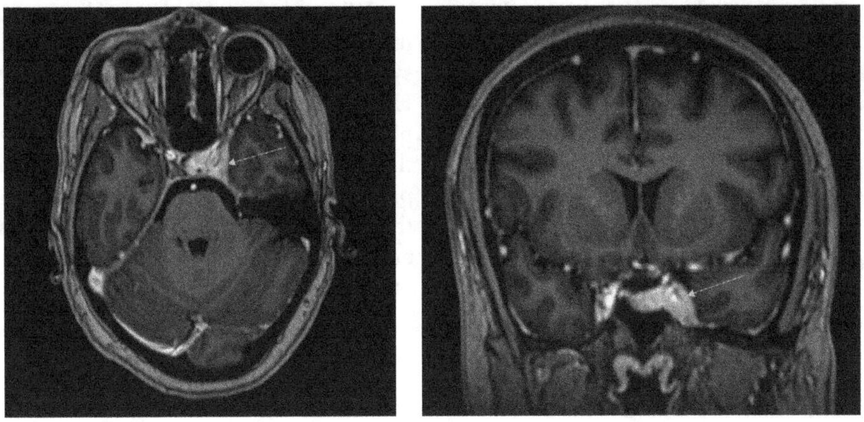

(a) (b)

FIGURE 1: T1-weighted postcontrast MRI brain showing abnormal enhancement of the left cavernous sinus (arrows) in the axial and coronal views, respectively.

TABLE 1: Different aetiologies of cavernous sinus syndrome.

Aetiology	Division	Example
Infection	Fungal Viral	Mucomycosis, phycomycosis Herpes zoster virus opthalmicus
Tumours	Within cavernous sinus Compressive tumours	Meningioma, schwanomma Pituitary adenomas, chordomas, chondrosarcomas, metastatic lesions
Vascular	Aneurysms Carotid-cavernous fistulas Cavernous sinus thrombosis	Cavernous segment aneurysm, intramural intracranial aneurysm Direct and indirect fistulas
Trauma		Any base of skull fracture which involves the cavernous sinus
Inflammation	Sarcoid Tolosa–Hunt syndrome	

vision and more recent nausea. There were no other constitutional symptoms.

She has a ten pack-year smoking history, with otherwise sober social habits. On past medical history, she was previously treated for Hodgkin's lymphoma (HL), achieving remission in 2009. She was diagnosed with HL stage IIA in May 2007 and was treated with six cycles of ABVD chemotherapy, followed by DHAP chemotherapy and involved-field radiation therapy. In February 2009, she suffered a relapse of her HL which was treated with six cycles of OPEC chemotherapy. A PET scan after this treatment revealed no further active disease. There was no neurological involvement during either of these presentations. She then had yearly follow-up appointments with the oncology team until she was discharged in 2014 and considered to be in remission. Since then, she remained asymptomatic.

On examination, she was a healthy-looking young lady with no remarkable abnormalities noted on general, respiratory, or cardiovascular exam. Of note, there were no palpable lymph nodes globally. Neuro-ophthalmic examination revealed normal visual acuity and visual fields, and fundoscopy was normal, with no evidence of proptosis or chemosis. Neurological examination on admission revealed a left abducens nerve palsy and left-sided trigeminal sensory loss in the first and second divisions. The rest of the neurological exam was initially normal; however, within days of her admission, her symptoms progressed to involve the oculomotor nerve on the left as well. This was accompanied with worsening pain, consistent with involvement of the left cavernous sinus.

In terms of investigations, an extensive blood work-up revealed only a slightly raised ESR of 26 on admission. A full blood count, renal and liver function panel, thyroid function, beta D glucan, HIV and syphilis screen, hepatitis screen, and autoimmune screen were all normal and negative. A lumbar puncture revealed normal cerebrospinal fluid testing including cytology and flow cytometry. An MRI brain confirmed the presence of abnormal enhancement and expansion of the left cavernous sinus and paracavernous dura extending to the orbital apex and posteriorly to the tentorial insertion (Figure 1). The neurosurgical team was reluctant to perform a biopsy of the cavernous sinus before further systemic work-up had been performed. A CT of the neck, chest, abdomen, and pelvis revealed subclinical clustered right axillary lymphadenopathy (maximum diameter 15 mm) as the only finding. A mammogram noted the axillary lymph node complex, but was otherwise normal. Excisional biopsy of the right axillary lymph nodes revealed scattered Reed–Sternberg cells with prominent macronucleoli, with positive CD30 and CD15 noted on immunohistochemistry of the atypical cells.

The patient was diagnosed with recurrent Hodgkin's lymphoma (nodular sclerosing). She received intravenous steroids for the treatment of her left cavernous sinus syndrome which resolved clinically within five days and was referred to oncology for further management, which she is currently awaiting. A repeat MRI brain was not performed following clinical improvement.

3. Discussion and Conclusions

Cavernous sinus syndrome (CSS) is defined as ophthalmoplegia, chemosis, proptosis, Horner syndrome, or trigeminal sensory loss secondary to pathologic changes in or around the cavernous sinus [1]. Due to the fact that several cranial nerves including the oculomotor, trochlear, abducens, and the ophthalmic and maxillary parts of the trigeminal nerve can be wholly or partially involved in this syndrome, there is a range of clinical signs that may be elicited. Nevertheless, the diagnosis can be made clinically with reasonable confidence in the presence of a combination of deficits of these cranial nerves. There are many causes, principally due to infectious or noninfectious inflammation, vascular, traumatic, and neoplastic processes (Table 1) [1].

Retrospective and prospective cohort studies suggest that CNS involvement occurs in 0.2% to 0.5% of patients with systemic HD [3]. In a review of 2 large series which included 780 and 2185 patients, the incidence of intracranial involvement of HD was reported as only 0.4% and 0.5%, respectively [3,4]. The main sites of brain involvement were the parenchyma (64%) and dura (19%) [5]. The mechanism of brain metastasis is either direct tumour extension through the skull bone or systemic haematogenous dissemination, with the latter being the most common [6].

The most common CNS symptoms of intracranial HD are motor and/or sensory deficits, headache, papilloedema, coma, and seizures [7].

CNS lesions in HD pose a diagnostic dilemma in view of the rare occurrence of brain involvement by Hodgkin's disease. Despite its rarity, the presence of CSS signs and symptoms in a patient with a known history of HD warrants full utilization of modern diagnostic techniques. The association of ICHD with lymph node, bone, and pulmonary sites indicates that the work-up of suspected ICHD should include a minimum of a careful history and physical examination, blood and cerebrospinal fluid testing, imaging of the brain, chest, abdomen and pelvis, and bone, or PET scans [4]. To note, there is a specific subset of patients who develop painful ophthalmoplegia due to a nonspecific inflammatory process in the region of the cavernous sinus and who are exquisitely responsive to steroid treatment [8]. These patients have a disease entity which has come to be known as Tolosa–Hunt syndrome. Although the pathogenetic basis of Tolosa–Hunt syndrome remains unknown, from a practical clinical standpoint, it can be regarded as a distinct entity which may be simulated by various other disorders and is a diagnosis of exclusion after a rigorous search for other causes [8]. Had this patient not received the extensive work-up as mentioned above, she could have been misdiagnosed as having Tolosa–Hunt syndrome.

Whilst there is a paucity of literature around this topic, it must be remembered by the clinician that cavernous sinus syndrome may be the sole clinical presentation of recurrent Hodgkin's disease. Even though it is reported that lymphomatous involvement in the brain usually occurs late in the disease process, this case is evidence that CSS may precede other systemic signs and symptoms. Recognising this possibility will ensure a rigorous search for HD, an early and effective diagnosis, and a better prognosis in affected patients.

Abbreviations

HD: Hodgkin's disease
CNS: Central nervous system
CSS: Cavernous sinus syndrome
ABVD: Adriamycin/ bleomycin/ vinblastine/ dacarbazine
DHAP: Dexamethasone/ high-dose aracytarabine/ platinol
OPEC: Vincristine/prednisolone/etoposide/chlorambucil
PET: Positron-emission tomography
ICHD: Intracranial Hodgkin's disease
ESR: Erythrocute sedimentation rate
HIV: Human immunodeficiency virus.

Consent

Written informed consent for publication of clinical details and any accompanying images was obtained from the patient.

Acknowledgments

The authors would like to acknowledge the patient for generously permitting the use of the data in this report.

References

[1] B. Aliglo, H. Ustun, A. Sonmez, H. Kaplan, F. I. Arikan, and Y. Dallar, "A rare presentation of central nervous system in a pediatric patient with Hodgkin disease cavernous sinus syndrome," *Journal of Pediatric Hematology/Oncology*, vol. 31, pp. 774–777, 2009.

[2] S. E. Kasner, S. L. Galetta, and D. J. Vaughn, "Cavernous sinus syndrome in Hodgkin's disease," *Journal of Neuro-Ophthalmology*, vol. 16, no. 3, pp. 204–207, 1996.

[3] C. Akyüz, B. Yalcin, İ. L. Atahan, A. Varan, M. T. Kutluk, and M. Büyükpamukçu, "Intracranial involvement in hodgkin's disease," *Pediatric Hematology and Oncology*, vol. 22, no. 7, pp. 589–596, 2005.

[4] M. D. Sapozink and H. S. Kaplan, "Intracranial Hodgkin's disease. A report of 12 cases and review of the literature," *Cancer*, vol. 52, no. 7, pp. 1301-1307, 1983.

[5] K. Hirmiz, A. Foyle, D. Wilke et al., "Intracranial presentation of systemic hodgkin's disease," *Leukemia and Lymphoma*, vol. 45, no. 8, pp. 1667–1671, 2004.

[6] M. Comert, N. Bassullu, E. Kaya, and A. Kocak, "Intracranial involvement in a patient with Hodgkin's lymphoma," *Singapore Medical Journal*, vol. 52, no. 9, pp. el80–e183, 2011.

[7] M. Demirkaya, B. Sevinir, O. Ozdemir, H. O. Nazlioğlu, and M. Okan, "Lymphoma of the cavernous sinus mimicking

tolosa-hunt syndrome in a child," *Pediatric Neurology*, vol. 42, no. 5, pp. 351–354, 2009.

[8] L. B. Kline and W. F. Hoyt, "Nosological entities?: the Tolosa-Hunt syndrome," *Journal of Neurology, Neurosurgery and Psychiatry*, vol. 71, no. 5, pp. 577–582, 2001.

Contrast-Induced Encephalopathy following Cerebral Angiography in a Hemodialysis Patient

Marija Bender[1] **Gojko Bogdan,**[2] **Dorijan Radančević,**[2] **and Nataša Pejanović-Škobić**[1]

[1]*University Hospital Mostar, Department of Neurology, Mostar, Bosnia and Herzegovina*
[2]*University Hospital Mostar, Department of Radiology, Mostar, Bosnia and Herzegovina*

Correspondence should be addressed to Marija Bender; marijabender@yahoo.com

Academic Editor: Shahid Nimjee

Contrast-induced encephalopathy (CIE) is a rare complication of contrast media use during angiographic procedures. With the growing use of endovascular interventions, this complication is likely to become more common. We present a case of a 46-year-old woman with hypertension, hypothyroidism, and chronic renal failure. She developed CIE following cerebral angiography for diagnosis of intracranial aneurysm. We had a high index of suspicion for CIE, excluded the most common differential such as stroke, and immediately started hemodialysis with a short course of corticosteroids. The disease runs a benign course, and neurological symptoms resolved completely after five days. We emphasize the need for increased awareness of CIE to make a valid diagnosis and to start supportive therapy as soon as possible.

1. Introduction

Contrast-induced encephalopathy (CIE) is a rare but well-known complication of contrast media use during angiographic procedures [1]. CIE was first reported in the 1960s [2]. The main features of this condition are transient cortical blindness, characterized by bilateral amblyopia or amaurosis, normal pupillary light reflexes, extraocular movements, and fundus [3]. Additional symptoms may include headache, memory loss, hemiparesis, aphasia, and reduction in higher mental function such as agraphia, loss of coordination, confusion, seizures, and coma [4]. Symptoms may begin during the procedure and up to 12 hours afterward, and they are usually self-limiting, resolving within 2–4 days of onset; rarely, complete recovery may take as long as few weeks [5, 6]. The disease typically runs a benign course; however, there have been reports of cases with persistent neurological deficit and even fatal outcome. Exact underlying mechanism of CIE remains unclear, and it likely relates to a transient breakdown of the blood-brain barrier with direct neurotoxicity of the contrast, which results in cerebral edema and alters neuronal excitability. This occurs most often in parieto-occipital lobes [7, 8]. Imaging in the form of CT or MRI scanning is essential to exclude this differential and confirm the diagnosis of CIE [5].

2. Case Report

A 46-year-old woman underwent cerebral angiography as a part of the diagnostic workup of an unruptured middle cerebral artery (MCA) aneurysm. An aneurysm of MCA, with a size of 15 mm × 12 mm, was detected on brain MRA during screening for headache. On admission, physical examination showed no signs of neurologic deficits. Her past medical history included hypertension, hypothyroidism, and polycystic kidney disease. Hemodialysis was initiated four years previously for chronic renal failure. She was a non-smoker. Hemodialysis was performed on the day before the procedure. Under local anesthesia, diagnostic DSA showed a middle cerebral artery saccular aneurysm, with the size of 16 mm × 13 mm × 9 mm. The procedure lasted 20 minutes. A total of 80 ml of nonionic, hypoosmolar contrast medium "Iopamiro 370" (Iopamidol) was used, which is a standard in our hospital. This was the patient's first exposure to contrast medium. The contrast material was injected into the left and right carotid artery, as well as in the right vertebral artery,

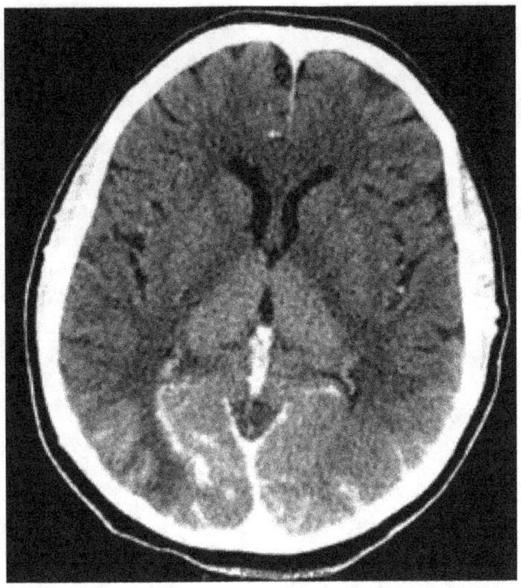

FIGURE 1: CT (axial) obtained one hour after DSA shows bilateral symmetrical contrast enhancement in parieto-occipital cortex and subarachnoid spaces, as well as in thalami.

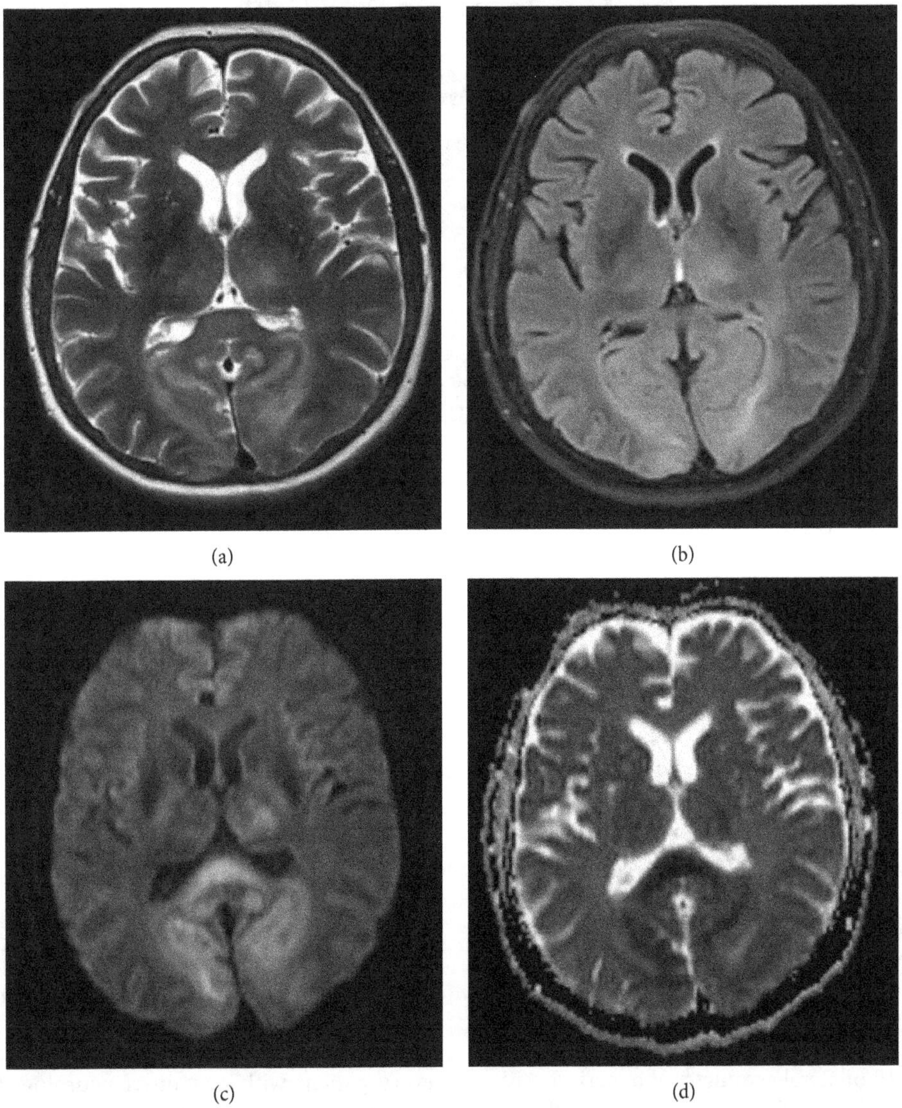

(a) (b)

(c) (d)

FIGURE 2: Brain MR (axial images) obtained 2 days after angiography. T2 and FLAIR images (a, b) show bilateral symmetrical hyperintensities in basal ganglia, in parieto-occipital cortex, and in splenium of corpus callosum. DWI and ADC images (c, d) demonstrate restricted diffusion in the same areas.

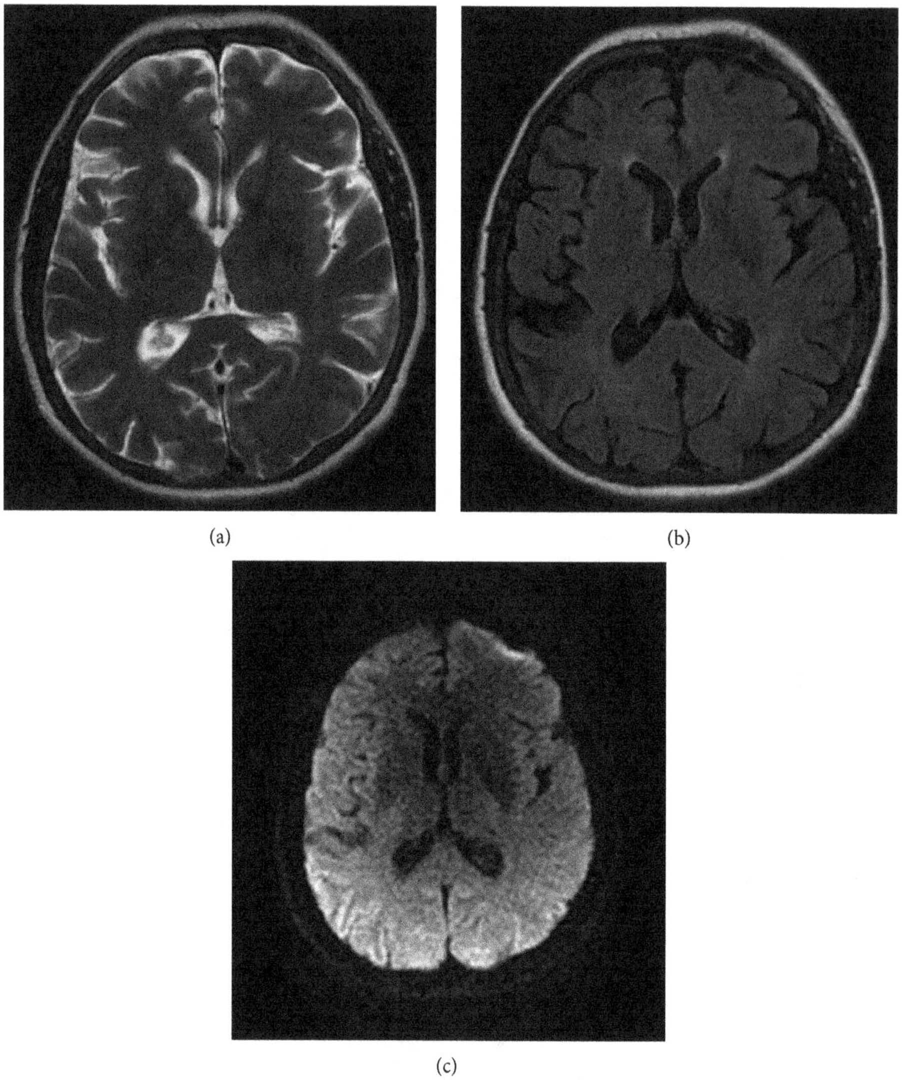

Figure 3: Follow-up brain MR-T2 (a), FLAIR (b), and DWI (c) axial images obtained in another facility 1 month after the initial MR shows complete resolution of the lesions.

with no side effects noted. During injection of the contrast material into the left vertebral artery, the patient complained of blurring of vision which deteriorated to near-total blindness within minutes. The pupils were equal in size and responsive to light. The rest of the neurological examination was normal. Approximately 1 hour after the procedure, the patient developed an episode of a generalized tonic-clonic seizure. An emergency CT brain scan was requested and revealed bilateral symmetrical contrast enhancement in parieto-occipital cortex and subarachnoid spaces, as well as in thalami (Figure 1). Based on the CT brain scan, the presumed diagnosis was contrast-induced encephalopathy and hemodialysis was quickly performed. Later on, over the next 24 hours, she was confused and agitated, with severe headache, vomiting, and no signs of improvement. A brain MRI, performed on second postprocedure day, demonstrated T2 and FLAIR bilateral symmetrical hyperintensities in basal ganglia, in parieto-occipital cortex, and in splenium of corpus callosum, and the DWI and ADC images demonstrated restricted diffusion in the same areas (Figure 2). Daily hemodialysis was performed for the next 3 days, and she was treated with dexamethasone. Over the next few days, symptoms gradually started to improve progressing to complete recovery. On day 5, her neurological symptoms resolved completely. She was discharged home well. One month after discharge follow-up, brain MRI did not show any residual lesion, which correlates with the complete recovery (Figure 3).

3. Discussion

CIE is rare, but with the growing use of endovascular interventions as a diagnostic and a therapeutic means, this complication is likely to become more common. The initial diagnosis is challenging mostly due to its close resemblance to acute stroke. One should have a high index of suspicion in every patient with new-onset neurological deficit who underwent angiographic procedure, especially in patients with hypertension and renal failure [9]. Imaging in the form of CT or MRI scanning is important at the early stage of CIE. It is essential to exclude embolic or hemorrhagic complications, to avoid the administration of potentially harmful treatment such as thrombolysis and to initiate treatment at an early stage [5]. There is no consensus on the treatment of CIE, but the general advice, according to some authors, is the use of aggressive intravenous hydration and daily hemodialysis with a short course of corticosteroids [10, 11]. We emphasize the need for increased awareness of CIE to make a valid diagnosis and to start supportive therapy as soon as possible.

Consent

Consent was obtained from the patient.

Authors' Contributions

All the authors were involved in the clinical management of the patient.

References

[1] N. H. Horwitz and L. Wener, "Temporary cortical blindness following angiography," *Journal of Neurosurgery*, vol. 40, no. 5, pp. 583–586, 1974.

[2] S. M. Sylverman, P. S. Bergman, and M. B. Bender, "The dynamics of transient cerebral blindness. Report of nine episodes following vertebral angiography," *Archives of Neurology*, vol. 4, no. 3, pp. 333–348, 1961.

[3] H. J. Mentzel, J. Blume, A. Malich, C. Fitzek, J. R. Reichenbach, and W. A. Kaiser, "Cortical blindness after contrast-enhanced CT: complication in a patient with diabetes insipidus," *American Journal of Neuroradiology*, vol. 24, no. 6, pp. 1114–1116, 2003.

[4] M. P. Merchut and B. Richie, "Transient visuospatial disorder from angiographic contrast," *Archives of Neurology*, vol. 59, no. 5, pp. 851–854, 2002.

[5] M. Baguma, N. Younan, F. London, M. Ossemann, and Y. Vandermeeren, "Contrast-associated transient cortical blindness: three cases with MRI and electrophysiology findings," *Acta Neurologica Belgica*, vol. 117, no. 1, pp. 195–199, 2017.

[6] K. R. Thomson and D. K. Varma, "Safe use of radiographic contrast media," *Australian Prescriber*, vol. 33, no. 1, pp. 19–22, 2010.

[7] Y. Uchiyama, T. Abe, M. Hirohata et al., "Blood brain barrier disruption of nonionic iodinated contrast medium following coil embolization of a ruptured intracerebral aneurysm," *American Journal of Neuroradiology*, vol. 25, no. 10, pp. 1783–1786, 2004.

[8] L. Junck and W. H. Marshall, "Neurotoxicity of radiological contrast agents," *Annals of Neurology*, vol. 13, no. 5, pp. 469–484, 1983.

[9] N. Matsubara, T. Izumi, S. Miyachi, K. Ota, and T. Wakabayashi, "Contrast-induced encephalopathy following embolization of intracranial aneurysms in hemodialysis patients," *Neurologia Medico-Chirurgica*, vol. 57, no. 12, pp. 641–648, 2017.

[10] J. Shinoda, Y. Ajimi, M. Yamada, and S. Onozuka, "Cortical blindness during coil embolization of an unruptured intracranial aneurysm," *Neurologia Medico-Chirurgica*, vol. 44, no. 8, pp. 416–419, 2004.

[11] Y. Niimi, M. J. Kupersmith, S. Ahmad, J. Song, and A. Berenstein, "Cortical blindness, transient and otherwise, associated with detachable coil embolization of intracranial aneurysms," *American Journal of Neuroradiology*, vol. 29, no. 3, pp. 603–607, 2008.

29

Diabetic Striatopathy: Case Report and Possible New Actors

Chiara Mozzini,[1] **Raffaele Ghirardi**,[2] **and Mauro Pagani**[1]

[1]*Department of Medicine, ASST Mantova, C. Poma Hospital Strada Lago Paiolo, Mantova 104600, Italy*
[2]*Department of Medicine, ASST Mantova, Presidio di Pieve, Via Bugatte, Borgo Mantovano, Mantova 146036, Italy*

Correspondence should be addressed to Chiara Mozzini; chiara.mozzini@asst-mantova.it

Academic Editor: Peter Berlit

Diabetic striatopathy is a very rare neurological complication of diabetes. We report the case of an 86-year-old woman with poorly controlled type 2 diabetes admitted to the internal medicine ward for sudden onset of altered sensorium and severe bilateral choreiform and ballistic movements. The precise pathophysiology of this condition is not well understood. Our communication aims to remind clinicians to consider the possibility of diabetic striatopathy when poor-controlled diabetic patients have sudden-onset choreiform and ballistic movements. Moreover, this case suggests the possibility that oxidative and endoplasmic reticulum stress may be involved in this process.

1. Introduction

Diabetic striatopathy (DS) is a very rare neurological complication of diabetes. The classic clinical manifestation of DS includes the triad of acute or subacute hemichorea-hemiballismus, hyperglycemic state, and unique reversible abnormalities limited to the striatum on neuroimaging [1]. It was first described in 1960 by Bedwell [2].

This case report aims to remind clinicians to consider DS when poor-controlled diabetic patients have sudden-onset choreiform and ballistic movements. Moreover, authors suggest the possibility that oxidative and endoplasmic reticulum stress may be involved in the pathogenesis of DS.

2. Case Presentation

2.1. Clinical Presentation. We report the case of an 86-year-old woman with poorly controlled type 2 diabetes admitted to the internal medicine ward for the sudden onset of altered sensorium and severe bilateral choreiform and ballistic movements. She had previously been admitted to the emergency department.

The patient had a history of hypertension, chronic coronary artery disease, and chronic atrial fibrillation. The diabetes was home-treated with repaglinide.

2.2. Laboratory Results. Laboratory results showed leukocytosis elevated *C*-reactive protein, hyperglycemia, and a positive urine test for infection. No faecal occult bloods was not detected nor were there any visible gastroenterological losses but iron, folic acid, and B12 vitamin deficiencies were detected (the main laboratory tests at admission and at discharge are depicted in Table 1). Ferritin values were in the normal range, likely due to the current infection.

2.3. Imaging and Instrumental Examinations. A noncontrast brain computed tomography revealed hyperdensity of the right basal nuclei, as depicted in Figure 1.

Afterwards, the patient underwent magnetic resonance that revealed hyperintensity on *T*1 in both the basal ganglia associated with areas of decreased signal intensity on *T*2 with pigments deposition (see Figure 2).

An electroencephalogram was also performed: it demonstrated nonspecific slow waves without spikes.

2.4. Therapeutic Approach. The patient received fluids, insulin, and symptomatic treatment to control choreiform and ballistic movements (clonazepam). *Staphylococcus aureus* was detected in the urine. Piperacillin-tazobactam therapy was administered.

TABLE 1: Main blood laboratory data at admission and discharge.

Blood laboratory data	Admission (Day 1)	Discharge (Day 14)
Haemoglobin (g/dL)	9.5	9.8
Hematocrit (%)	30	30.6
MCV (fL)	71	86
WBC ($10^3/mm^3$)	6220	8610
PLT per (mm^3)	429	322
Glucose (mg/dL)	356	90
Glycated Haemoglobin (%)	10	9.8
C-peptide (ng/mL)	4	4
Creatinine (mg/dL)	0.6	0.7
Sodium (mEq/L)	138	136
Potassium (mEq/L)	3.8	3.4
Calcium (mg/dL)	10	10
Magnesium (mEq/L)	1.48	1.48
C-reactive protein (mg/L)	64	4
Ammonium (μg/dL)	20	20
Iron (mcg/dL)	40	Not tested
Ferritin (mcg/L)	400	Not tested
Folates (ng/mL)	2	Not tested
B12 vitamin (pg/ml)	100	Not tested
Thyroid-stimulating hormone (mU/L)	2	Not tested
Urine culture	Positive: *Staphylococcus aureus*	Negative
Blood culture	Negative	Negative

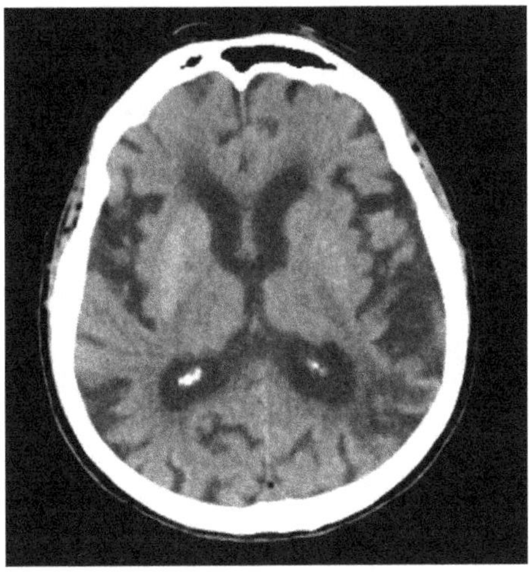

FIGURE 1: Patient's noncontrast brain computed tomography.

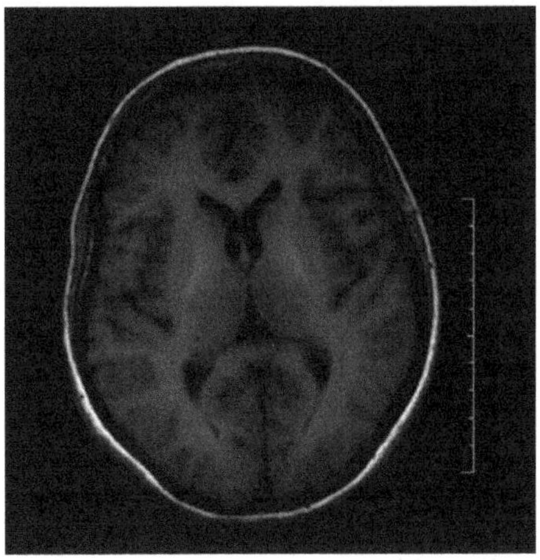

FIGURE 2: Patient's noncontrast brain magnetic resonance (on *T1* weighted).

Supplements with iron, folic acid, and B12 vitamins were administered due to deficiencies.

After two weeks, symptoms improved as well as the glucose control, and then she was discharged.

Oral antidiabetic dosage was improved, without insulin therapy because of sufficient insulin reserves. A close diabetes follow-up was organised. Nevertheless, the patients did not come to the following appointments.

3. Discussion

This case report of diabetic striatopathy (DS) is similar to others described [1, 3]. Now the challenge is the understanding of the pathogenic mechanisms of this condition.

Chorea is a hyperkinetic dyskinesia characterized as being involuntary, irregular, unpredictable, and small-amplitude. Ballismus is featured as being large-amplitude, arrhythmic, and more proximal. Chorea-ballismus can appear in the large majority of patients with DS [1].

Chorea-ballismus can also be observed in some ketotic diabetic patients, adolescents with newly diagnosed diabetes, and even children. In the elderly, other causes that could induce acute/subacute-onset choreiform movement must be considered: ischemic/hemorrhagic stroke, rheumatologic diseases, vascular malformations, electrolyte imbalance (hyponatremia/hypernatremia, hypercalcemia, and hypomagnesemia), autoimmune neurologic syndromes/paraneoplastic syndromes, tumors, carbon monoxide intoxication, hyperthyroidism, and hypoparathyroidism/hyperparathyroidism, demyelinating disease, psychostimulants (cocaine and amphetamines), infections (viral encephalitis, cryptococcal granuloma, mycoplasma, tuberculoma, neurosyphilis,

HIV encephalitis, and prion diseases), and drugs (neuroleptics, lithium, antiepileptic drugs, oral contraceptives, estrogen replacement therapy, steroids, methotrexate, cyclosporine and fluoroquinolones) [1, 2].

For our patient, the interaction of multiple mechanisms might explain the case: a hyperglycemic state due to an incipient infection together with vascular insufficiency in a poor-controlled diabetic patient.

The precise pathophysiology of DS is not well understood. Biopsy studies suggest that the lesion is a vasculopathy with gliosis restricted to the striatum. Postmortem findings have been somewhat inconsistent but include reactive astrocytosis, patchy ischemic necrosis, petechial hemorrhage, vascular proliferation, and arteriolar changes similar to the diabetic proliferative retinopathy.

Our communication aims to remind clinicians to consider the possibility of diabetic striatopathy when poor-controlled diabetic patients have sudden-onset choreiform and ballistic movements. Moreover, this case suggests the possibility that oxidative and endoplasmic reticulum (ER) stress may be involved in this process. This is only speculative because we have not examined the molecules involved in these pathways and no in vitro-tests have been performed.

However, this is the very first time that these mechanisms have been mentioned as possible mediators in DS.

In fact, these actors (oxidative and ER stress) are very prominent in neurological disorders, in both ischemic and hemorrhagic stroke, and in diabetes itself. Chronic hyperglycemia-associated oxidative stress and low-grade inflammation are considered to play critical roles in the progression of diabetic complications [4, 5].

After intracerebral hemorrage, both oxidative and ER stress levels are upregulated and alleviating either ER or oxidative stress limits secondary neuronal damage. Using nicotinamide adenine dinucleotide phosphate oxidase inhibitors and nonspecific reactive oxygen species scavengers, oxidative stress is reduced, cerebral vascular function improves, and cerebral amyloid angiopathy-related microhemorrhages are reduced. Reactive astrogliosis and apoptosis have been shown to be reduced using antioxidant compounds [6].

DS is a very uncommon disease, but its knowledge should be mandatory for physicians, and its mechanisms have to be better investigated. This case report adds same knowledge about this rare condition together with previous works [1, 3].

To conclude, in the future, the detection of circulating markers of oxidative and ER stress should be given serious consideration in patients with DS, in order to eventually propose antioxidant therapy and compounds ameliorating the ER stress, as is in the case of diabetes [7].

Postmortem studies in the brain tissues of DS patients should be focused on the detection of oxidative and ER stress markers. The results will strengthen or discard our hypothesis.

Authors' Contributions

CM, RG, and MP designed the manuscript and treated the patient, CM wrote the paper.

References

[1] C. B. Chua, C. K. Sun, C. W. Hsu, Y. C. Tai, C. Y. Liang, and I. T. Tsai, "Diabetic striatopathy: clinical presentations, controversy, pathogenesis, treatments, and outcomes," *Scientific Reports*, vol. 10, no. 1, p. 1594, 2020.

[2] S. F. Bedwell, "Some observations on hemiballismus," *Neurology*, vol. 10, no. 6, pp. 619–622, 1960.

[3] E. B. Lucassen, W. T. Delfyett, and M. C. Stahl, "Persistent hemichorea and caudate atrophy in untreated diabetic striatopathy: a case report," *Case Rep Neurol*, vol. 9, no. 3, pp. 299–303, 2017.

[4] S. I. Mohammed Thangameeran, S. T. Tsai, H. Y. Hung et al., "A role for endoplasmic Reticulum stress in intracerebral hemorrhage," *Cells*, vol. 9, no. 3, p. 750, 2020.

[5] C. Mozzini, L. Cominacini, U. Garbin, and A. M. Fratta Pasini, "Endoplasmic Reticulum stress, NRF2 signalling and cardiovascular diseases in a nutshell," *Current Atherosclerosis Reports*, vol. 19, no. 8, p. 33, 2017.

[6] A. Daverey and S. K. Agrawal, "Curcumin alleviates oxidative stress and mitochondrial dysfunction in astrocytes," *Neuroscience*, vol. 333, pp. 92–103, 2016.

[7] U. Ozcan, E. Yilmaz, L. Ozcan et al., "Chemical chaperones reduce ER stress and restore glucose homeostasis in a mouse model of Type 2 diabetes," *Science*, vol. 313, no. 5790, pp. 1137–1140, 2006.

30

Central Pain Mimicking Trigeminal Neuralgia as a Result of Lateral Medullary Ischemic Stroke

Abinayaa Ravichandran,[1] Kareem S. Elsayed,[2] and Hussam A. Yacoub [1]

[1]*Lehigh Valley Physician Group – Neurology, Lehigh Valley Health Network, Allentown, PA, USA*
[2]*Morsani College of Medicine, University of South Florida, Tampa, FL, USA*

Correspondence should be addressed to Hussam A. Yacoub; hyacoub123@yahoo.com

Academic Editor: Peter Berlit

Background. Central pain mimicking trigeminal neuralgia (TN) as a result of lateral medullary infarction or Wallenberg syndrome has been rarely reported. *Case Report.* We discuss a patient who presented with a lateral medullary infarct and shortly after developed facial pain mimicking TN. We also elaborate on the anatomical pathway of the trigeminal nerve explaining facial pain as a result of a lateral medullary lesion. *Discussion.* Clinicians should be aware of this typical complication of lateral medullary infarct in order to attain proper management and work-up.

1. Introduction

Trigeminal neuralgia is a common form of facial pain that is characterized by paroxysmal and excruciating pain along the distribution of the trigeminal nerve. Although this condition encompasses diverse etiologies, the International headache society has separated classical (or idiopathic) TN from the symptomatic form depending upon the presence of a structural lesion [1]. Increased utilization of magnetic resonance imaging (MRI) offers extensive evidence that most classical cases of TN are found to be associated with compression of the dorsal nerve root by tortuous or aberrant vessels (IHS) [1]. Space-occupying lesions including tumor, multiple sclerosis, and stroke account for 15% of all cases of TN [2]. Facial pain as a result of lateral medullary infarct can mimic TN with a wide reported incidence of 9% (Sacco et al.) [3] to 83% (Merritt and Finland) [4].

In this manuscript, we discuss a case of a patient who developed classic symptoms of central pain mimicking TN shortly after a lateral medullary infarct was diagnosed.

2. Case Report

A right-handed 81-year-old man with a past medical history of ischemic stroke, hypertension, hyperlipidemia, type-II diabetes mellitus, and paroxysmal atrial fibrillation presented to the hospital with symptoms of unsteadiness, mild dysphagia, and sharp stabbing right-sided facial pain. Neurological examination revealed decreased pin-prick sensation on the right side of the face. The patient had normal strength bilaterally. Coordination examination showed finger-to-nose dysmetria bilaterally, but more pronounced on the right. Ataxia with swaying to the right was observed on gait examination.

MRI of the brain revealed an area of restricted diffusion within the right posterior lateral medulla consistent with an acute or subacute infarction (Figure 1). Coagulation studies revealed an international normalized ratio of 2 while on warfarin; the patient endorsed some noncompliance with the recommended regimen.

The patient noted the concomitant onset of right "sharp-stabbing" intermittent pain merely hours after the onset of unsteadiness. The pain occurred in the ophthalmic and maxillary distribution of the trigeminal nerve and was acutely worsened by cold temperature. He was diagnosed with central facial pain secondary to lateral medullary infarct. The pain initially improved with the administration of carbamazepine, which was discontinued after hospital discharge due to adverse reactions. He was subsequently started on gabapentin 100 mg by mouth three times a day with some relief, but stopped the medication secondary to an adverse reaction of dizziness. The patient still experienced recurrent episodes of

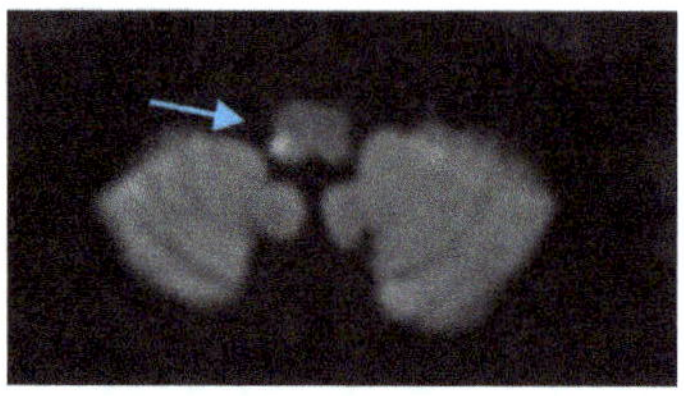

FIGURE 1: Diffusion weighted MRI demonstrating an area of restricted diffusion in the right posterior lateral medulla (arrow), consistent with an acute infarct.

right-sided facial pain. Several months after the initial event, he was evaluated in the office and was found to have a nonfocal examination. He continues to complain of brief episodes of right-sided lancinating pain in the forehead, cheek, nose, and periorbital region occurring on average three times a day. Symptoms were aggravated by cold temperature. The patient denied any associated symptoms of lacrimation or sweating.

3. Discussion

Central pain, by definition, is caused by lesions of the brain and spinal cord. Central pain caused by a brain stem infarct is well known and has been described since 1997, but published cases in literature are sparse [5].

Figure 2 illustrates the anatomy of the trigeminal sensory system. Cell bodies of the sensory nerves lie within the Gasserian ganglion. The central axons form the dorsal sensory root which extends into the brainstem and divides into the short ascending and long descending fibers. The former carries tactile, light pressure, and proprioceptive afferents, while the latter carries pain and temperature afferents and extends to the upper cervical segments, which is supported by the evidence of facial pain with medullary trigeminal tracheotomy [6]. From both the principal sensory and spinal trigeminal nuclei, second order fibers form the trigemino-thalamic tract which crosses to the contralateral thalamus. The peripheral fibers of the Gasserian ganglion form the three sensory divisions of the trigeminal nerve. The motor division of the trigeminal nerve arises at the motor nucleus in the mid pons and joins the mandibular division, but does not traverse through the ganglion. This explains motor function sparing with dorsal root compression. As reported by Fisher, pain is caused by a lesion affecting the cell bodies of the ganglion, whereas pressure on the axon typically causes isolated paresthesia [7].

In addition to ischemia, demyelination of the central trigeminal pathways may result in development of aberrant electrical impulses and alternatively irritation of the trigeminal structures creating an area with abnormal excitability [8].

Fitzek et al. evaluated the development and pathophysiology of facial pain following dorsolateral medullary infarct [9]. Eight of the 12 patients developed post-stroke pain within 12 days to 24 months following stroke. The findings on MRI supported the correlation of facial pain with lower medullary lesions, including infarcts affecting the spinal trigeminal tract and/or nucleus.

Ordás et al. reported a case of facial pain in the region supplied by the second division of the trigeminal nerve in a patient with right lateral medullary infarction secondary to dissection of the right vertebral artery [10]. A case of TN resulting from an infarction of the root entry zone of the trigeminal nerve was related by Golby et al. [8]. John et al. reported a case of a 73-year-old woman who developed brief paroxysms of pain on the left lower half of the face—described as sharp, electric shock like—4 days after an ipsilateral lateral medullary infarct [11].

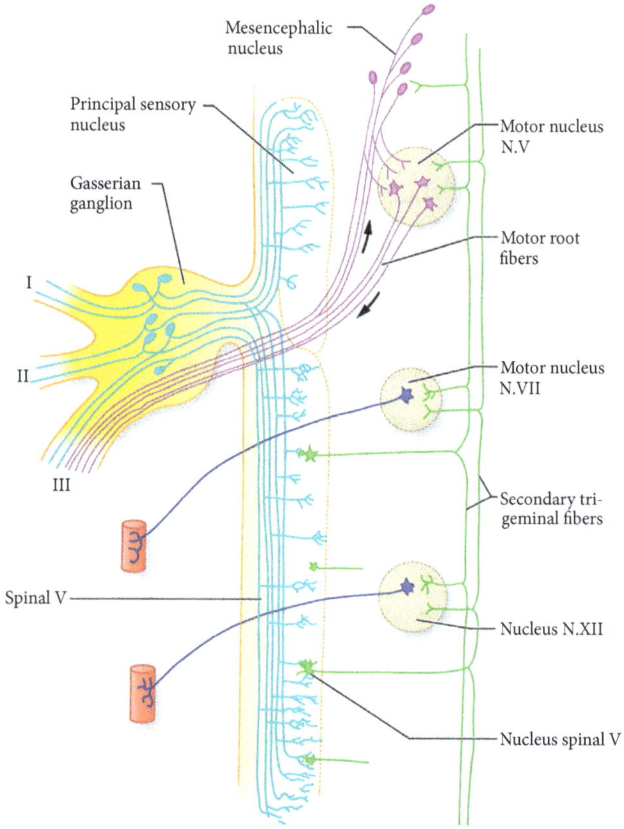

FIGURE 2: Anatomy of the trigeminal sensory system (adapted from Adams and Victor's Principals of neurology, 10th edition).

Cases of central pain mimicking TN as a result of pontine ischemia have also been reported since the 1990s [5]. Peker et al. reported sudden onset of facial pain symptoms similar to the classic pain experienced with TN in a patient with a chronic infarct in the left lateral pons [12]. Therefore, the timing between the infarct and development of central pain can vary. There are other cases reported with onset of symptoms several months to years after the infarction [9]. Central facial pain following pontine ischemia can be explained by the anatomical pathway of the trigeminal nerve as described above. We advise clinicians to be aware of this typical complication of lateral medullary infarct in order to avoid needless imaging and advanced work-up.

Acknowledgments

Jennifer Macfarlan, MPH; Debra Goldberg, MAMC; Network Office of Research and Innovation, Lehigh Valley Health Network, Allentown, PA.

References

[1] Headache Classification Committee of the International Headache Society (IHS), "The international classification of headache disorders, 3rd edition (beta version)," *Cephalalgia*, vol. 33, no. 9, pp. 629–808, 2013.

[2] G. Cruccu, G. Gronseth, J. Alksne et al., "AAN-EFNS guidelines on trigeminal neuralgia management," *European Journal of Neurology*, vol. 15, no. 10, pp. 1013–1028, 2008.

[3] R. L. Sacco, L. Freddo, J. A. Bello, J. G. Odel, S. T. Onesti, and J. P. Mohr, "Wallenberg lateral medullary syndrome clinical-magnetic resonance imaging correlations," *Archives of Neurology and Neuro Disorders*, vol. 50, no. 6, pp. 609–614, 1993.

[4] H. Merritt and M. Finland, "Vascular lesions of the hind-brain. (lateral medullary syndrome)," *Brain*, vol. 53, no. 3, pp. 290–305, 1930.

[5] M. Balestrino and M. Leandri, "Trigeminal neuralgia in pontine ischemia," *Journal of Neurology, Neurosurgery & Psychiatry*, vol. 62, no. 3, pp. 297–298, 1997.

[6] O. Sjöqvist, "Studies on pain conduction in the trigeminal nerve," *Brain*, vol. 62, no. 1, p. 125, 1939.

[7] C. M. Fisher, "Is pressure on nerves and roots a common cause of pain?" *Transactions of the American Neurological Association*, vol. 97, pp. 282–283, 1972.

[8] A. J. Golby, A. Norbash, and G. D. Silverberg, "Trigeminal neuralgia resulting from infarction of the root entry zone of the trigeminal nerve: case report," *Neurosurgery*, vol. 43, no. 3, pp. 620–623, 1998.

[9] S. Fitzek, U. Baumgärtner, C. Fitzek et al., "Mechanisms and predictors of chronic facial pain in lateral medullary infarction," *Annals of Neurology*, vol. 49, no. 4, pp. 493–500, 2001.

[10] C. M. Ordás, M. L. Cuadrado, P. Simal et al., "Wallenberg's syndrome and symptomatic trigeminal neuralgia," *The Journal of Headache and Pain*, vol. 12, no. 3, pp. 377–380, 2011.

[11] A. A. John, M. M. Abbas, M. Javali, R. Mahale, A. Mehta, and R. Srinivasa, "A rare presentation of trigeminal neuralgia in lateral medullary syndrome," *Neurology India*, vol. 65, no. 3, pp. 638–640, 2017.

[12] S. Peker, G. Akansel, I. Sun, and N. Pamir, "Trigeminal neuralgia due to pontine infarction," *Headache: The Journal of Head and Face Pain*, vol. 44, no. 10, pp. 1043–1045, 2004.

Multiple Cranial Nerve Palsies in a Pediatric Case of Lemierre's Syndrome due to *Streptococcus viridans*

Samantha Novotny,[1] **Kenneth Serrano,**[1] **Danielle Bazer,**[2] **and Louis Manganas**[2]

[1]*Renaissance School of Medicine at Stony Brook University, 101 Nicolls Road, Stony Brook, New York 11794, USA*
[2]*Department of Neurology at Stony Brook University Hospital, 101 Nicolls Road Stony Brook, New York 11794, USA*

Correspondence should be addressed to Samantha Novotny; samantha.novotny@stonybrookmedicine.edu

Academic Editor: Dominic B. Fee

Background. Lemierre's syndrome is a rare condition of internal jugular vein thrombosis following oropharyngeal infection. While it usually results from *Fusobacterium necrophorum* infection, atypical cases associated with other pathogens have been reported. *Objective.* To describe a unique case of pediatric Lemierre's syndrome with *Streptococcus viridans* infection resulting in cavernous sinus thrombosis and oculomotor, trochlear, and abducens nerve palsies. *Case Report.* A 14-year-old female initially presented after six days of fever, myalgias, and sore throat and was admitted for hyperbilirubinemia and acute kidney injury. She developed a fixed, dilated pupil with complete ophthalmoplegia, ptosis, and severe pain. Imaging revealed retromandibular space abscess, external and internal jugular vein thrombosis, cavernous sinus thrombosis, internal carotid artery stenosis, pulmonary embolism, and bilateral pneumonia. She was diagnosed with Lemierre's syndrome with cultures positive for *Streptococcus viridans* and treated with a combination of antibiotics and anticoagulation. *Conclusion and Relevance.* Both antibiotics and anticoagulation were effective management for this Lemierre's syndrome patient with cavernous sinus thrombosis. Early diagnosis and treatment of Lemierre's syndrome is essential. A multidisciplinary treatment team is beneficial for managing the sequelae of this condition.

1. Introduction

Lemierre's syndrome is a rare sequela of oropharyngeal infection in previously healthy young adults resulting in thrombosis of the internal jugular vein and septic embolism [1]. The most common offending organism is *Fusobacterium necrophorum* [2], although other organisms have been reported including *Staphylococcus aureus* and several strains of *Streptococcus* [3–9]. We describe a unique case of pediatric Lemierre's syndrome caused by *Streptococcus viridans* with multiorgan involvement and progression to cavernous sinus thrombosis with cranial nerves III, IV, and VI palsies. While Lemierre's syndrome associated with *Streptococcus viridans* infection has previously been described, our patient with development of complete ophthalmoplegia demonstrates an underreported sequela of this condition.

2. Case Presentation

A 14-year-old female with no medical history presented to the emergency department with a six-day history of fever, myalgias, pharyngitis, throbbing headache, and left eye ptosis. Her symptoms were associated with diplopia, blurred vision, photophobia, and phonophobia. Her neurological exam was significant for visual acuity of 20/200 in the left eye with an afferent pupillary defect. There were also cranial nerve III, IV, and VI palsies.

Throat swab cultures grew *Candida dubliniensis* and viridans group alpha hemolytic *Streptococcus.* Her hospital course was complicated by left retromandibular space abscess, left external jugular vein thrombosis, partial left internal jugular vein thrombosis, bilateral lower lobe pneumonia, and multiple pulmonary consolidations with wedge-shaped defects in the right upper lobe consistent with

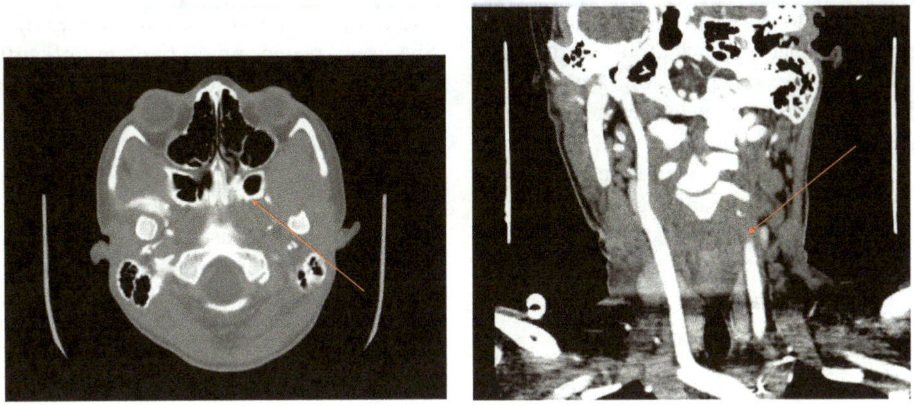

(a) (b)

FIGURE 1: CT angiography. (a) CT angiography venous phase of the head, demonstrating left CST. (b) CT angiography head demonstrating left ICA occlusion.

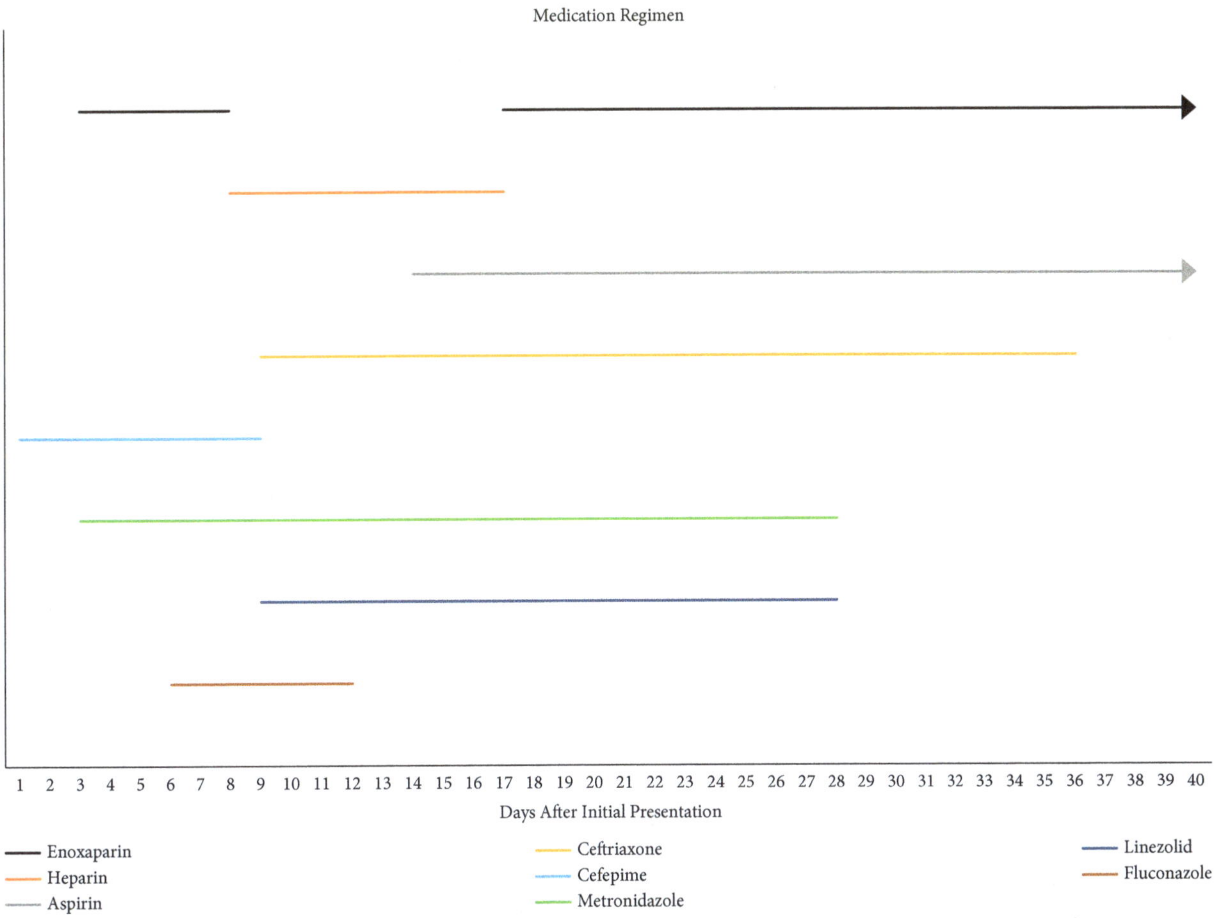

FIGURE 2: Timeline of the patient's medication regimen.

embolism. Additionally, compute tomography (CT) angiography head, magnetic resonance imaging (MRI) brain, magnetic resonance angiography (MRA) head and neck, and magnetic resonance venography (MRV) head and neck revealed left cavernous sinus thrombosis (CST) with adjacent pachymeningitis, possible cavernous sinus abscess, severe stenosis of the left distal petrous and cavernous internal carotid artery (ICA), focus of severe stenosis in the ICA terminus, and dural thickening and enhancement (Figure 1). The patient underwent two cerebral angiograms; the initial showed left ICA dissecting aneurysm with stenosis with posterior communicating artery collateral flow. The second angiogram four days later showed a complete, left ICA thrombosis.

The patient was managed with a medication regimen including both antibiotics and anticoagulation with age and weight-appropriate dosing. Her medication timeline is summarized in Figure 2. She was managed by various specialties including neurology, neurosurgery, ophthalmology, infectious disease, and hematology. The neurosurgery team determined that medical management without surgical intervention was sufficient. She remained on aspirin and enoxaparin after discharge. Unfortunately, her neurological deficits were persistent upon discharge home with outpatient follow-up. Repeat imaging 28 days after initial presentation revealed worsened left ICA occlusion and significant partial resolution of the cavernous sinus thrombosis.

3. Discussion

We describe a young female with cavernous sinus thrombosis and multiple cranial nerve palsies resulting from Lemierre's syndrome associated with *Streptococcus viridans*. Lemierre's syndrome is uncommon, particularly with organisms other than Fusobacteria [10]. A review by Riordan [10] suggests merely 8% of Lemierre's syndrome cases are due to other pathogens [10]. However, among patients with ophthalmic symptoms, 25% had *Streptococcus* infections [5]. Reports of Lemierre's syndrome with various strains of *Streptococcus* have described complications including CST and isolated cranial nerve palsies, as well as other findings including postseptal cellulitis, pulmonary embolism, pleural effusion, and bibasilar pneumonia [5–9]. While some of these case reports noted isolated trochlear or abducens nerve palsies, they did not report any instances of multiple cranial nerve palsies.

Lemierre's syndrome and its complications can be life-threatening [10, 11]. Thus, prompt diagnosis and treatment of the condition are essential. However, there is no clear consensus on treatment for Lemierre's syndrome. Management is typically focused on treating the infection via antibiotics and drainage as necessary [12]. Anticoagulative therapy is controversial. Riordan [10] suggested around 23% of patients receive anticoagulation [10], while a more current review by Johannesen and Bodtger [13] found up to 64% are treated with anticoagulation [13]. A systematic review by Adedeji et al. [14] studied 14 patients and found anticoagulation to be a safe therapeutic strategy in Lemierre's syndrome [14]. However, Gore [11] performed a meta-analysis that found anticoagulation did not significantly impact recanalization of thrombosed vessels or mortality rates [11]. Despite this, it has been suggested that decision to anticoagulate may be patient-specific. A review by Kristensen and Prag [15] recommended anticoagulation should only be given in patients at risk of thrombosis extension to the cavernous sinus [15]. Similarly, another review by Moore et al. [16] of 41 patients found 26.8% of patients improved with addition of anticoagulation and proposed use of anticoagulation in patients with extensive thrombosis [16]. For our patient, anticoagulation was initiated during hospitalization and continued after discharge.

4. Conclusion

We describe a pediatric case of Lemierre's syndrome caused by an unusual pathogen, *Streptococcus viridans*. Our patient developed extensive thrombosis, multiorgan involvement, and unique sequelae of cranial nerves III, IV, and VI palsies. She was treated on a regimen of antibiotics and anticoagulation. This case highlights the importance of a multidisciplinary, team-based approach to patient care. Rapid diagnosis of this rare syndrome is crucial for proper therapeutic management. It is beneficial for neurologists to be aware of Lemierre's syndrome, as there are potentially neurologically devastating sequelae of the syndrome. Moreover, future research and randomized controlled trials are warranted to develop consensus guidelines for anticoagulation and treatment of Lemierre's disease.

References

[1] S. P. Dasari and P. Jha, "A systematic review of Lemierre's syndrome with a focus on ophthalmologic complications," *Cureus*, vol. 12, no. 7, Article ID e9326, 2020.

[2] K. Kuppalli, D. Livorsi, N. J. Talati, and M. Osborn, "Lemierre's syndrome due to fusobacterium necrophorum," *The Lancet Infectious Diseases*, vol. 12, no. 10, pp. 808–815, 2012.

[3] R. K. Shah, M. M. Wofford, T. G. West, and A. K. Shetty, "Lemierre syndrome associated with group a streptococcal infection," *The American Journal of Emergency Medicine*, vol. 28, no. 5, pp. e643–e645, 2010.

[4] S. S. Gunatilake, L. G. Yapa, M. Gallala, R. Gamlath, C. Rodrigo, and H. Wimalaratna, "Lemierre's syndrome secondary to community-acquired methicillin-resistant *Staphylococcus aureus* infection presenting with cardiac tamponade, a rare disease with a life-threatening presentation: a case report," *International Journal of Emergency Medicine*, vol. 7, no. 39, p. 39, 2014.

[5] Y.-H. Wang, P.-Y. Chen, P.-J. Ting, and F.-L. Huang, "A review of eight cases of cavernous sinus thrombosis secondary to sphenoid sinusitis, including a12-year-old girl at the present department," *Infectious Diseases*, vol. 49, no. 9, pp. 641–646, 2017.

[6] J. Camacho-Cruz, H. Preciado, N. Beltrán, L. Fierro, and J. Carrillo, "Lemierre's syndrome caused by *Streptococcus anginosus* presenting as postseptal cellulitis in a pediatric patient," *ORL Journal for Otorhinolaryngology and its Related Specialties*, vol. 81, no. 4, pp. 234–239, 2019.

[7] M. A. Frizzola and J. H. Hertzog, "Lemierre syndrome in a 22-month-old due to Streptococcus pyogenes," *Pediatric Emergency Care*, vol. 27, no. 11, pp. 1078–1080, 2011.

[8] L. J. Rohowetz, S. M. Gratton, D. Dansdill, C. J. Miller, and S. Dubin, "Cavernous sinus thrombosis caused by Streptococcus constellatus-associated Lemierre syndrome presenting as an isolated abducens nerve palsy," *American Journal of Ophthalmology Case Reports*, vol. 18, Article ID 100592, 2020.

[9] S. Lee, T. Rutar, F. G. Velez, and A. L. Rosenbaum, "Lemierre's syndrome with fourth nerve palsy," *Journal of American Association for Pediatric Ophthalmology and Strabismus*, vol. 13, no. 1, pp. 107-108, 2009.

[10] T. Riordan, "Human infection with fusobacterium necrophorum (*Necrobacillosis*), with a focus on Lemierre's syndrome," *Clinical Microbiology Reviews*, vol. 20, no. 4, pp. 622–659, 2007.

[11] M. R. Gore, "Lemierre syndrome: a meta-analysis," *International Archives of Otorhinolaryngology*, vol. 24, no. 3, pp. e379–e385, 2020.

[12] J. Osowicki, S. Kapur, L. K. Phuong, and S. Dobson, "The long

shadow of Lemierre's syndrome," *Journal of Infection*, vol. 74, pp. S47–S53, 2017.

[13] K. Johannesen and U. Bodtger, "Lemierre's syndrome: current perspectives on diagnosis and management," *Infection and Drug Resistance*, vol. 9, pp. 221–227, 2016.

[14] A. Adedeji, O. Chukwura, T. Obafemi, S. B. McNulty, and J. P. Reinert, "Anticoagulation strategies in the management of Lemierre syndrome: a systematic review of the literature," *The Annals of Pharmacotherapy*, vol. 55, no. 5, pp. 658–665, 2021.

[15] L. H. Kristensen and J. Prag, "Human necrobacillosis, with emphasis on lemierre's syndrome," *Clinical Infectious Diseases*, vol. 31, no. 2, pp. 524–532, 2000.

[16] B. A. Moore, C. Dekle, and J. Werkhaven, "Bilateral Lemierre's syndrome: a case report and literature review," *Ear, Nose, & Throat Journal*, vol. 81, no. 4, pp. 234–252, 2002.

32

Medically Refractory Multiple Sclerosis is Successfully Treated with Plasmapheresis in a Super Morbidly Obese Pregnant Patient

Lindsey Dalka,[1] Antoine Harb,[2] Kael Mikesell,[3] and Gillian Gordon Perue[4]

[1]*Eastern Maine Medical Center, Department of Family Medicine, Bangor, USA*
[2]*Eastern Maine Medical Center, Department of Hematology and Oncology, Bangor, USA*
[3]*Eastern Maine Medical Center, Department of Patient Blood Management, Bangor, USA*
[4]*Eastern Maine Medical Center, Department of Neurology, Bangor, USA*

Correspondence should be addressed to Gillian Gordon Perue; ggordonperue@emhs.org

Academic Editor: Samuel T. Gontkovsky

Multiple sclerosis (MS) is a relapse remitting immune-mediated demyelinating neurological disorder that primarily affects women of childbearing age. In most patients, the hormonal changes during pregnancy are protective against MS relapses. When relapses do occur, treatment options are limited to use of intravenous steroids and plasmapheresis rescue therapy. We present a case of steroid refractory MS-transverse myelitis with quadriplegia in a 25-year-old pregnant super morbidly obese woman. Our clinical case is unique because the severity of her relapse early in pregnancy, which was intractable and resistant to steroids. This may have been a rebound demyelination due to the discontinuation of fingolimod; a newly recognized entity by the FDA. Our case report therefore seeks to raise awareness about a potential complication of discontinuing MS disease modifying therapies, highlighting that these rebound relapses can be steroid resistant and occur despite the usual protective hormonal influence of early pregnancy and that plasma exchange is a valid treatment option. Finally, we discuss the challenges of determining exchange volumes for plasmapheresis in the super morbid obese population to secure good maternal and fetal outcomes.

1. Introduction

Multiple sclerosis (MS) is an immune-mediated demyelinating neurological disorder that primarily affects women of childbearing age. Prior to the 1998 PRIMS study [1, 2], pregnancy in patients with MS was discouraged, fearing acute exacerbations, and poor maternal/fetal outcomes. With disease modifying treatments available and reassuring registry data, pregnancy in patients with MS is now common.

The hormonal changes of pregnancy are usually protective against exacerbations in MS. When exacerbations occur, they tend to be infrequent, mild, short lived, and responsive to intravenous methylprednisolone. Plasmapheresis is reserved for rescue therapy [3, 4]. However, rescue plasmapheresis is not well studied in pregnancy, and there are no studies on plasmapheresis in pregnancy with super morbid obesity as a comorbidity. We therefore present a case of a 25-year-old with severe disabling MS exacerbation, super morbid obesity in pregnancy successfully treated with plasma exchange.

2. Case Description

A 25-year-old G2 P0010 Caucasian female with past medical history of super morbid obesity (BMI 55.2), depression, and multiple sclerosis presented to us with bilateral lower extremity weakness and right-sided flank pain. At the time of presentation, she was at 18 weeks' gestation.

She was diagnosed with multiple sclerosis at age 17 after she developed right optic neuritis. Over a 3-year period, she tried multiple modifying agents including interferon beta 1-b which was associated with ovarian cyst formation requiring surgery and interferon beta 1-a, which had intolerable side effects and glatimer acetate. While on glatimer acetate, she had 2 relapses in 6 months. She was eventually transitioned to fingolimod with a single relapse shortly after initiation of therapy and treated with a 5-day course of solumedrol. Fingolimod was used successfully for 5 years and was discontinued 4 weeks prior to conception. Her pregnancy was complicated by a threatened abortion and persistent vaginal bleeding. She was placed on bed rest. During bed rest, she developed fever, flank pain, and severe paraparesis requiring hospitalization. She was diagnosed with an acute MS flare in the setting of pyelonephritis.

Antibiotics and intravenous methylprednisolone 1,000 mg daily were initiated. A noncontrast MRI of the brain and cervical spine revealed a new extensive demyelinating lesion from C1 to C4. After the completion of 6 days of intravenous (IV) methylprednisolone, her lower extremity function had moderately improved, and she was able to ambulate with a walker and was discharged to an acute inpatient rehabilitation center.

Three weeks later, she re-presented to the hospital with right-sided flank pain, generalized weakness resulting in a fall, and a tingling sensation in her extremities. Given the early recurrence, neurology was consulted. In the neurological exam, mental state was normal, pupils were normal symmetrical, and reactive to light. There was no facial asymmetry and the other cranial nerves were normal. Muscle tone was increased in her left upper extremity and bilateral lower extremities. In the motor exam, there was an asymmetrical moderate/severe tetraparesis mainly in the lower limbs and more pronounced distally. There was generalized hyperreflexia with bilateral clonus and bilateral Babinski. Sensation was impaired with decreased sensation to light touch, pinprick, and vibration without a clear sensory level.

Urinalysis was consistent with a urinary tract infection and a urine culture grew out pan-sensitive *Escherichia coli*. A new MRI of the head (Figure 1) showed progression T2 hyperintense signal abnormality in the craniocervical cord. To exclude other differentials, her vitamin B12 and ACE levels were checked and were within normal limits. To rule out a possible diagnosis of neuromyelitis optica, an aquaporin 4 AQR4 antibody was tested and was negative.

The patient was started on antibiotics for suspected pyelonephritis, which was eventually changed to oral amoxicillin after urine culture sensitivities resulted.

The patient was started on IV methylprednisolone 250 mg every 6 hours. After five days of steroid treatment, she showed minimal motor improvement. At this time, rescue plasmapheresis (TPE) was initiated. Five treatments of TPE were performed every other day, alternating treatment days with IV methylprednisolone. The patient tolerated her therapy well and had progressive improvement in her neurologic symptoms with near complete resolution of her tetraparesis and mild residual sensory loss in her left arm. She was discharged to the acute rehabilitation service.

For the reminder of her pregnancy, she was treated with methylprednisolone 1000 mg as a single infusion every 3 weeks. She presented to the hospital at 36 weeks' gestation with contractions, vaginal spotting, hypertension, headache, and lower extremity edema. She was taken to the operating room for a cesarean section due to concerns of severe preeclampsia and preterm labor. She delivered a 2495 g male with APGARs of 8 and 9. After delivery, fingolimod was reinitiated in the outpatient setting.

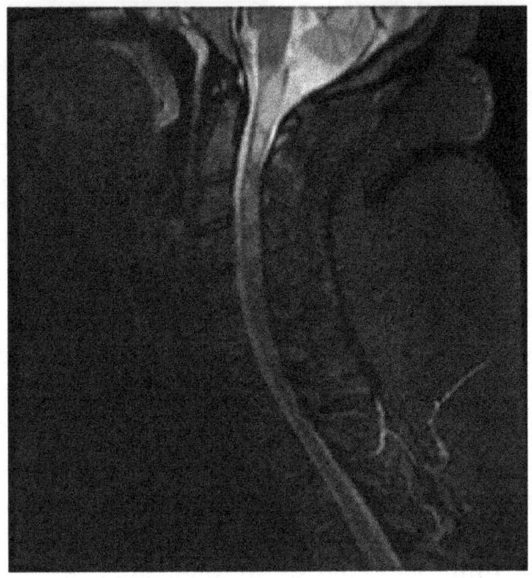

FIGURE 1: T2 sagittal flair image demonstrating an acute multiple sclerosis flare with longitudinally extensive transverse myelitis extending from the medulla to the upper cervical cord C3.

3. Discussion

Our case report therefore seeks to raise awareness about the potential complication of rebound demyelination due to the discontinuation of fingolimod, a newly recognized entity by the FDA [5], highlighting that these rebound relapses can be steroid resistant and occur despite the usual protective hormonal influence of early pregnancy and that plasma exchange is a valid treatment option. In the case of fingolimod cessation for pregnancy, scheduled IV methylprednisolone for maintenance may be considered.

Treatment with TPE rescue provided unique challenges. While TPE has been used to successfully treat pregnant patients with other diseases [6–8], to the best of our knowledge, our case is only the third report of TPE for acute MS exacerbation in pregnancy [9, 10]. In the previous two case reports, the Nadler formula was used to determine the patient's blood volume (BV) and plasma volume (PV). Once the PV was determined, a plasma exchange of 1.5 PV was used to account for the 45–55% increase in PV that occurs starting in the second trimester of pregnancy [11, 12].

A unique feature of our case report is the size of our patient, as she weighed 152.2 kg when plasmapheresis was initiated. Using the Nadler formula and her hematocrit of 29.8, her PV calculated to 4841 mL. If a 1.5 PV exchange was performed (accounting for pregnancy), this would have resulted in a 7262 mL exchange. An exchange of this volume would have put the patient and fetus at increased risk for complications and may be unnecessary. While PV increases with weight, it does not do so in a linear fashion [13]. A morbidly obese patient has more adipose tissue which requires less blood supply. As a result, the Nadler formula may give an erroneously elevated BV in the morbidly obesity.

One solution to overcome this miscalculation would be to use an adjusted body weight with the Nadler formula and then perform a 1.5 PV exchange based on the result. Alternatively, one could use a 1 PV exchange using the patient's actual body weight for the Nadler formula. Using the latter for our case led to 5000 mL exchange. TPE was successfully completed and improved the patient's symptoms appropriately. During TPE, the patient was positioned on the left lateral decubitus position to prevent inferior vena cava pressure and maximize venous return [9]. In addition, CMP and fibrinogen were monitored prior to each treatment to ensure that proper coagulation and calcium level was achieved. This method is safe and effective with good outcomes for both mother and child.

This case demonstrates that in patients with treatment refractory multiple sclerosis in pregnancy or fingolimod rebound demyelination therapeutic plasma exchange is safe and successful and that super morbid obesity should not be a contraindication. We hope that this will encourage future practitioners who face this dilemma to consider plasma exchange.

Consent

Informed consent was obtained from the patient.

Authors' Contributions

All authors have contributed substantially to the concept of this article as well as the drafting of the manuscript and critical revision for important intellectual content. All authors have given final approval of the version to be published. All authors agree to be accountable for all aspects of the work in ensuring that questions related to the accuracy or integrity of any part of the work are appropriately investigated and resolved.

Acknowledgments

The authors would like to thank the patient and her family for agreeing to participate and our team at EMMC who make care of these complex patients possible.

References

[1] G. C. Ebers, "Randomised double-blind placebo-controlled study of interferon beta-1a in relapsing/remitting multiple sclerosis. PRISMS (prevention of relapses and disability by interferon beta-1a subcutaneously in multiple sclerosis) study group," *The Lancet*, vol. 352, no. 9153, pp. 1498–1504, 1998.

[2] P. Cavalla and W. Gilmore, "Pregnancy in multiple sclerosis," *Neurology*, vol. 91, no. 17, pp. 771–773, 2018.

[3] I. Cortese, V. Chaudhry, Y. T. So, F. Cantor, D. R. Cornblath, and A. Rae-Grant, "Evidence-based guideline update: plasmapheresis in neurologic disorders: report of the therapeutics and technology assessment subcommittee of the American academy of neurology," *Neurology*, vol. 76, no. 3, pp. 294–300, 2011.

[4] J. E. Meca-Lallana, R. Hernández-Clares, A. León-Hernández, A. Genovés Aleixandre, M. Cacho Pérez, and J. J. Martín-Fernández, "Plasma exchange for steroid-refractory relapses in multiple sclerosis: an observational, MRI pilot study," *Clinical Therapeutics*, vol. 35, no. 4, pp. 474–485, 2013.

[5] FDA warns about severe worsening of multiple sclerosis after stopping the medicine gilenya (fingolimod) https://www.fda.gov/Drugs/DrugSafety/ucm626095.htm.

[6] W. J. Watson, V. L. Katz, and W. A. Bowes Jr., "Plasmapheresis during pregnancy," *Obstetrics & Gynecology*, vol. 76, no. 3, pp. 451–457, 1990.

[7] J. R. Tabares and P. F. A. Gonzalez, "Plasma exchange therapy for a severe relapse of devic's disease in a pregnant woman: a case report and concise review," *Clinical Neurology and Neurosurgery*, vol. 148, pp. 88–90, 2016.

[8] R. Basar, A. K. Uzum, B. Canbaz et al., "Therapeutic apheresis for severe hypertriglyceridemia in pregnancy," *Archives of Gynecology and Obstetrics*, vol. 287, no. 5, pp. 839–843, 2013.

[9] B. O. Khatri, O. D'Cruz, G. Priesler et al., "Plasmapheresis in a pregnant patient with multiple sclerosis," *Archives of Neurology*, vol. 47, no. 4, pp. 11-12, 1990.

[10] J. L. Cox, S. A. Koepsell, and S. M. Shunkwiler, "Therapeutic plasma exchange and pregnancy: a case report and guidelines for performing plasma exchange in a pregnant patient," *Journal of Clinical Apheresis*, vol. 32, no. 3, pp. 191–195, 2017.

[11] F. Hytten, "Blood volume changes in normal pregnancy," *Clinics in Haematology*, vol. 14, no. 3, pp. 601–12, 1985.

[12] B. C. McLeod, *Apheresis Principles and Practice*, AABB Press, Bethesda, MD, USA, 2010.

[13] H. Lemmens, D. Bernstein, and J. Brodsky, "Estimating blood volume in obese and morbidly obese patients," *Obesity Surgery*, vol. 16, no. 6, pp. 773–776, 2006.

33

A Co-Occurrence of Serologically Proven Myasthenia Gravis and Pharyngeal-Cervical-Brachial Variant of Guillain-Barré Syndrome

Stacey Ho and Antonio Liu

Ross University School of Medicine, Department of Neurology, California Hospital Medical Center, Los Angeles, California, USA

Correspondence should be addressed to Stacey Ho; staceyho62087@gmail.com

Academic Editor: Norman S. Litofsky

We report on a co-occurrence case of ocular myasthenia gravis with exacerbation leading to myasthenic crisis in addition to pharyngeal-cervical-brachial variant of Guillain–Barré syndrome in a patient with severe oropharyngeal dysphagia and acute respiratory failure.

1. Introduction

Myasthenia gravis (MG) is an autoimmune disease of the neuromuscular junction with a prevalence of approximately 20 per 100,000 in the US and between 15 and 179 per million worldwide [1, 2]. In patients less than 40 years of age, female to male ratio is 3:1. Patients between 40 and 50 years show an equal ratio between female and male. However, males over the age of 50 are more likely to have MG than their female counterpart [2]. MG causes fluctuating weakness that worsens with exertion and progresses throughout the day [1]. Approximately two-thirds of the patients with MG initially have extrinsic ocular muscles (EOMs) involvement that progresses to involve other bulbar muscles and limb musculature with the eventual presentation of generalized myasthenia gravis (gMG) [2]. In approximately 10% of MG patients, symptoms are limited to only EOMs causing the condition to be known as ocular MG (oMG) [2].

Guillain-Barré syndrome (GBS) is a fulminant polyradiculoneuropathy that is characterized by acute ascending weakness that is usually severe, and autoimmune-related leading to generalized paralysis [3]. The worldwide incidence of GBS is approximately 0.6–2.4 cases per 100,000 annually, with increased incidence with age and slightly more predominance in males [3, 4]. The etiology of GBS is believed to be autoimmune, in which the majority of cases (70%) showed upper respiratory infections that led to the stimulation of anti-ganglioside antibodies production [3]. Patients usually show signs and symptoms 1–3 weeks after acute infectious process, usually respiratory or gastrointestinal, that include the follow organisms: *Campylobacter jejuni*, *Mycoplasma pneumonia*, *Haemophilus influenzae*, cytomegalovirus, Epstein-Barr virus, and influenza [3, 4].

Although both MG and GBS present with weaknesses, the concurrent development of MG and GBS is rare [5]. A recent study found 13 cases of concurrent MG and GBS between 1982 and 2016 [6]. It has been suggested that concurrent development is due to molecular mimicry between infectious agents and self-antigens [5]. These antibodies may have shown cross-reactions against both myelin proteins of peripheral nerves and acetylcholine receptors of neuromuscular junctions; and thymoma-associated multiorgan autoimmunity may also play a factor in initiating autoimmune process [5].

2. Objective

We report on a co-occurrence case of ocular myasthenia gravis with exacerbation leading to myasthenic crisis in addition to pharyngeal-cervical-brachial variant of Guillain–Barré syndrome in a patient with severe oropharyngeal dysphagia and acute respiratory failure.

3. Case Report

An 83-year-old Hispanic male with an extensive past medical history including chronic hepatitis C, coccidioidomycosis, ocular myasthenia gravis, and interstitial lung disease presented to the Emergency Department (ED) with a complaint of chronic cough, shortness of breath, upper extremities weakness with diplopia, and dysphagia. The patient reported a daily cough with sputum production since Thanksgiving 2017 and became more severe in the past 3 days. He denied any weakness in his lower extremities and reported that he was able to garden up until 3 months ago when he started having upper extremities weakness. In the ED, the patient's SPO2 was 94%, initial chest X-ray showed no acute pathology, and CT of the chest showed no signs of thymoma or any other lung pathologies. He was admitted to telemetry with a BiPAP for further evaluation. The patient's Video Swallow Study showed severe oropharyngeal dysphagia. We were consulted as the patient had severe dysphagia and a history of ocular myasthenia gravis. However, the patient developed acute respiratory failure and was intubated before an assessment and evaluation can be performed.

Upon review of the patient's medical record, it showed that he was diagnosed with myasthenia gravis in 2017 when he was found to have AChR binding antibodies of 40.70 nmol/L, AChR blocking antibodies of 56%, and AChR modulating antibodies of 54%. He was prescribed pyridostigmine 60mg 1 tablet three times daily as treatment; however, his adherent to treatment regime was questionable; and he has had recurring follow-ups with his primary care physician for ocular myasthenia gravis. The patient's lab result in the ED showed AChR binding antibodies of 276 nmol/L, AChR blocking antibodies of 75%, and AChR modulating antibodies of 91%, all of which displayed a major increase in antibodies compared to his results at time of diagnosis. Due to the patient's history of ocular myasthenia gravis, his current state of severe dysphagia, and acute respiratory failure, we ordered a serum anti-GBS antibody work-up for our patient when he showed signs of improvement from diplopia but his respiratory status remained the same. The results revealed that the patient had GM1 antibodies of 81 units and GD1b antibodies of 52 units, which are serology markers seen in GBS. The patient was started on IVIG and methylprednisolone while continuing with pyridostigmine. Several days later, the patient exhibited significant improvement in respiratory status and clinical signs of improved swallow function, and his diplopia has been resolved.

4. Discussion

Myasthenia gravis is an autoimmune disease of the neuromuscular junction that presents with fluctuating pronounced exertional voluntary muscle weakness [7]. While Guillain-Barré syndrome and its variants are a group of autoimmune disease of the proximal peripheral nerves and nerve roots mediated by lymphocytic mononuclear cell infiltration and macrophage-associated segmental demyelination that is associated with limb weakness and areflexia [8].

Diagnosing MG is based on clinical history and neurologic examination and is confirmed by electrodiagnostic testing and the presence of serum autoantibodies directed against proteins—acetylcholine receptor (AChR) and muscle-specific tyrosine kinase (MuSK)—at the neuromuscular junction [1]. MG can be further divided into subtypes that includes (1) early-onset MG with age of onset <50 years, usually females, and has thymic hyperplasia, (2) late-onset MG with age of onset >50 years, usually males, and has thymic atrophy, (3) thymoma-associated MG, (4) MG with the presence of anti-MuSK antibodies, (5) oMG, and (6) MG with no detectable AChR and MuSK antibodies [2]. However, patients may present with overlapping of subtypes. The majority of patients with gMG (85%) and oMG (50%) will have anti-AChR antibodies, with an additional 8%-10% of those with gMG having anti-MuSK antibodies [1]. MG with evidence of thymoma is almost always detected to have anti-AChR antibodies; and it may also have additional paraneoplasia-associated antibodies, such as antivoltage-gated K^+ and Ca^{++} channels, anti-Hu, antidihydropyrimidinase-related protein 5, and antiglutamic acid decarboxylase antibodies [2]. In 40% of patients with no detectable anti-AChR antibodies, anti-MuSK and another postsynaptic neuromuscular junction (NMJ) protein are detected [2]. These patients have atypical clinical presentations, such as selective facial, bulbar, neck, or respiratory muscle weakness with occasional marked muscle atrophy and relative sparing of the ocular muscles [2]. Other MG patients can present with seronegative MG that lacks both anti-AChR and anti-MuSK antibodies.

Although our patient presented with an increase in AChR titers during myasthenic crisis, studies have shown that the level of AChR antibodies does not relate with the clinical severity of MG. A study done by Aurangzeb et al. showed that out of the 71 seropositive MG patients in their study, 57.7% of the patients had low titers and 42.2% had high titers [9]. And while the majority of those patients exhibited Osserman's stage III (acute severe generalized disease with respiratory failure), there was no correlation between AChR antibodies titers and Osserman's classification [9].

Treatment for MG is immunosuppressive therapies, such as prednisone, azathioprine, cyclosporine, and mycophenolate mofetil [1]. Cholinesterase inhibiting agents typically only provide temporary relief from symptoms without altering the course of MG [1]. Thymectomy is usually beneficial in those with evidence of thymoma on chest CT [1]. Plasmapheresis and IV immunoglobulin (IVIG) are usually reserved for patients who encounter a myasthenic crisis [1].

The presentation of GBS include areflexia and limb weakness and rarely sensory loss proceeding to neuromuscular paralysis involving bulbar, facial, and respiratory function with maximum severity of symptoms in 2–4 weeks [3]. Patients typically presents initially with lower and upper extremities weakness (32%) or selective proximal and distal lower extremities weakness (56%) that often spreads to the arm while some have onset of weakness in the upper extremities (12%) [8]. Lower extremities are usually affected more often than upper extremities, and facial diparesis occurs in 50% of patients [3]. The weakness exhibited in GBS is typically seen in a pyramidal distribution with ankle dorsiflexion and knee and hip flexion often severely affected, while weakness in the arms is usually more severe in shoulder abduction and elbow extension [4]. Lumbar pain is also common and may represent inflammation in the nerve roots and breakdown in the nerve CSF barrier that leads to protein leaking into the CSF [4]. Respiratory involvement may be acute with vital capacity falling steadily, and intubation and ventilation are required at level of approximately 1 liter [4]. Studies have shown that mortality in GBS is between 5% and 10%, and 60% of patients who recover are able to walk unaided by 12 months [4].

Patients with GBS may present with clinical variants based on the types of nerve fibers involved (motor, sensory, and cranial or autonomic), predominant mode of fiber injury (demyelinating versus axonal), and the presence of alteration of consciousness [8]. In a study done by Koga et al., IgG anti-GT1a and anti-GM1b were particularly valuable in diagnosing GBS and its variants in which early appearance of bulbar involvement was observed [10]. The major gangliosides GM1 and GD1a and the minor ones GM1b, GalNAc-GD1a, and GT1a are target molecules for autoantibodies found in GBS and its variants [10].

Pharyngeal-cervical-brachial (PCB) variant of Guillain-Barré syndrome presents in 3% of cases and causes rapidly progressive oropharyngeal and cervicobrachial weakness associated with areflexia in the upper extremities without ophthalmoplegia or lower extremities weakness [11]. Motor and strength of lower extremities are typically preserved, thus making PCB a localized subtype of GBS that is a form of acute motor axonal neuropathy (AMAN) [11]. Autoantibodies that are associated with PCB include IgG anti-GM1, anti-GD1a, anti-GD1b, and anti-GT1a [11]. Our patient had serum antibodies showing GM1 antibodies of 81 units and GD1b antibodies of 52 units and presented with clinical symptoms of a pure motor bulbar palsy typically seen in PCB. Although anti-GD1b is commonly seen in cases of GBS with ataxia and is usually associated with sensory neuropathy [12], both ataxia and sensory neuropathy presentation were not observed in our patient.

Treatment of GBS includes admission to intensive care with respiratory support when required and early recognition of respiratory failure [13]. Patients with severe dysphagia may require nasogastric and feeding tubes, while intubation should be considered for patients who cannot tolerate their secretions or who have an ineffective cough [8]. Treatment with pain modulating drugs such as antidepressants, gabapentin, pregabalin, carbamazepine, tramadol, and mexiletine in patient with marked radicular back pain or neuropathic pain refractory to acetaminophen or NSAIDs [13]. Patients with weakness impairing function or any respiratory involvement should be treated with plasmapheresis or IVIG [13].

In summary, the diagnosis of PCB can be challenging due to its overlapping features with other variants of GBS. A history of prior respiratory tract infection (as seen in our patient) or diarrheal illness is common in GBS and can be often overlooked. The rate of disease progression can also provide clues and is typically acute with steady progression [11]. Particularly, PCB should be differentiated from MG patients who display early or prominent ocular-bulbar weakness, which may be associated with anti-MuSK in the absence of anti-AChR antibodies. In our case, the patient was already diagnosed with MG and presented with myasthenic crisis. Furthermore, our patient showed signs of severe bulbar palsy that required further investigation. Thus, a good history and neurological findings can help differentiate PCB from other causes of orpopharyngeal and cervicobrachial weakness [11].

References

[1] J. M. Statland and E. Ciafaloni, "Myasthenia gravis: five new things," *Neurology: Clinical Practice*, vol. 3, no. 2, pp. 126–133, 2013.

[2] A. Jayam Trouth, A. Dabi, N. Solieman, M. Kurukumbi, and J. Kalyanam, "Myasthenia gravis: a review," *Autoimmune Diseases*, vol. 2012, Article ID 874680, 2012 (Basque).

[3] S. R. Sudulagunta, M. B. Sodalagunta, M. Sepehrar et al., "Guillain-barré syndrome: clinical profile and management," *GMS German Medical Science*, vol. 13, no. Doc16, 2015.

[4] J. B. Winer, "An update in guillain-barré syndrome," *Autoimmune Diseases*, vol. 2014, Article ID 793024, 2014.

[5] S.-L. Kung, J.-M. Su, S.-J. Tsai, T.-M. Lu, and C.-M. Chen, "Concurrent Guillain-Barré syndrome and myasthenia gravis: the first case in Taiwan," *Acta Neurologica Taiwanica*, vol. 18, no. 3, pp. 193–197, 2009.

[6] J. Yuan, J. Zhang, B. Zhang, and W. Hu, "The clinical features of patients concurrent with guillain-barré syndrome and myasthenia gravis," *Neurosciences*, vol. 23, no. 1, pp. 66–70, 2018.

[7] J. P. Sieb, "Myasthenia gravis: an update for the clinician," *Clinical & Experimental Immunology*, vol. 175, no. 3, pp. 408–418, 2014.

[8] M. M. Dimachkie and R. J. Barohn, "Guillain-Barré syndrome and variants," *Neurologic Clinics*, vol. 31, no. 2, pp. 491–510, 2013.

[9] S. Aurangzeb, M. Tariq, M. Irshad, M. Badshah, and R. S. Khan, "Relationship between anti-acetylcholine receptor antibody titres and severity of myasthenia gravis," *Journal of Pakistan Medical Association*, vol. 59, no. 5, pp. 289–292, 2009.

[10] M. Koga, N. Yuki, and K. Hirata, "Antiganglioside antibody in patients with Guillain-Barré syndrome who show bulbar palsy as an initial symptom," *Journal of Neurology, Neurosurgery & Psychiatry*, vol. 66, no. 4, pp. 513–516, 1999.

[11] B. R. Wakerley and N. Yuki, "Pharyngeal-cervical-brachial variant of Guillain-Barré syndrome," *Journal of Neurology, Neurosurgery & Psychiatry*, vol. 85, no. 3, pp. 339–344, 2014.

[12] M. Uysalol, B. Tath, N. Uzel, A. Çitak, E. Aygün, and S. Kayaoğlu, "A rare form of Guillan Barre syndrome: a child diagnosed with Anti-GD1a and Anti-GD1b positive pharyngeal-cervical-brachial variant," *Balkan Medical Journal*, vol. 30, no. 3, pp. 337–341, 2013.

[13] J. B. Winer, "Guillain Barré syndrome," *Journal of Clinical Pathology: Molecular Pathology*, vol. 54, no. 6, pp. 381–385, 2001.

Transient Global Amnesia as the Sole Presentation of an Acute Stroke in the Left Cingulate Gyrus

Lawrence Chau and Antonio Liu

Department of Neurology, Adventist Health White Memorial, USA

Correspondence should be addressed to Antonio Liu; liuak@ah.org

Academic Editor: Isabella Laura Simone

We discuss a patient who presented to our hospital with signs, symptoms, and clinical course consistent with transient global amnesia (TGA). Her hospital work-up was overall unremarkable except for the presence of a diffusion weighted imaging (DWI) abnormality on MRI suggestive of acute infarction in the left cingulate gyrus. Symptoms quickly resolved, and she was discharged home in stable condition. While the etiology of TGA remains controversial, in discussing this case and the current literature we hope to provide further data supporting the possibility of an underlying ischemic process, as well as help better illustrate the neurologic structures involved.

1. Introduction

Transient global amnesia is a clinical phenomenon described as the sudden onset of acute amnesia (mostly anterograde, but retrograde is also frequently observed) with neither altered consciousness nor cognitive impairment. It subsequently resolves within 24 hours, and there are no known long-term sequelae aside from a mild amnestic period in some patients. In the decades since it was first observed, its characteristics have been defined clearly, yet the cause remains elusive. Vascular processes, epilepsies, and migraines have been postulated as possible etiologies, yet the lack of prevalence of these disorders in cases of TGA as noted in prior studies suggests against them as causes [1]. Another hypothesis is that TGA may be associated with ischemia, and while the evidence is sparse, multiple case reports have been written to explore this theory. The hippocampus has typically been sited as the affected structure [2, 3], as review of MRIs in retrospective cases of TGA has shown a predominance of DWI hyperintensities in that region [4, 5]. Here, we report a case of TGA in downtown Los Angeles with findings in the left cingulate gyrus as seen on DWI, a much rarer occurrence. In doing so, we hope to provide more data to the medical community regarding both incidence and areas of involvement in ischemic TGA to better our understanding of this condition.

2. Case

A 60-year-old woman was initially brought to the emergency room by concerned family members. Her only past medical history is obesity, hyperlipidemia, and hyperthyroidism, for which she takes levothyroxine 75mcg and simvastatin 40mg. She also takes a daily aspirin 325mg. Family described that the patient had a sudden change in her behavior just prior to admission. There was no reported loss of consciousness or altered level of consciousness, just noting that she was acting "strange." She was cooking at the time and suddenly left the food unattended on the stove. She appeared lost and seemed to have forgotten what she was doing. She remained generally oriented with no focal complaints, and there was no headache or pain. She could walk, and she had no weakness of any kind. There was no precipitating seizure and no incontinence. However, she was not following conversations and did not recognize her own sister who dropped by for dinner. En route to the hospital as well as in the emergency room, she kept asking the very same question, "where am I?" and "how did I get here?" Someone will offer the answer only to be met with the same questions minutes later. During her ER stay, she had a completely normal and non-focal neurologic examination. NIHSS score was zero. She scored 3/3 on registration but was unable to recall objects after a while. She had no idea

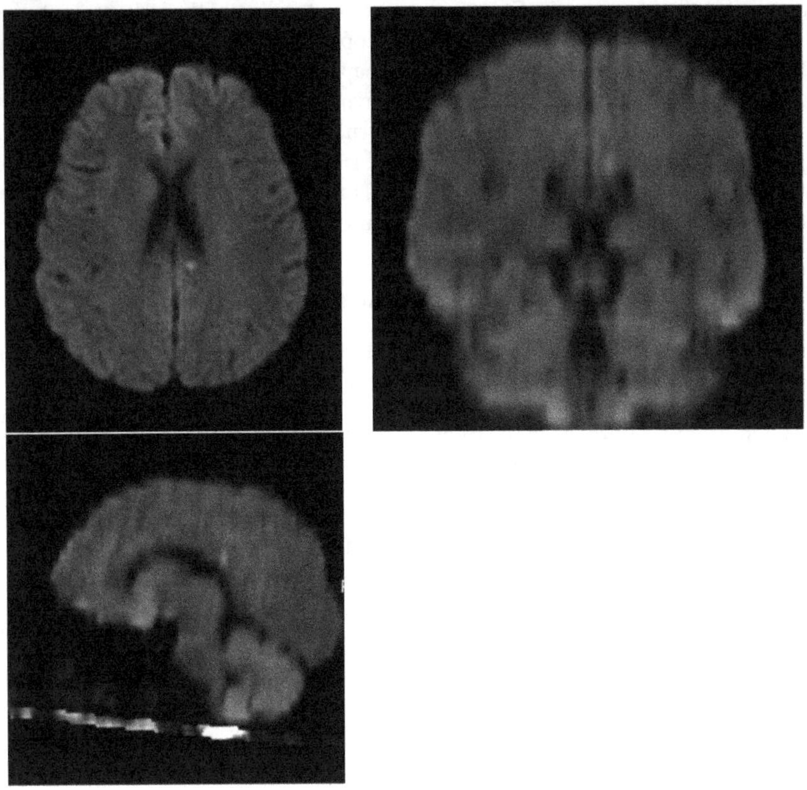

Figure 1: DWI in axial, coronal, and sagittal views (Siemens Aera 1.5T) (ST 5mm, TE 16ms, TR 5230ms) showing a single diffusion abnormality in left cingulate gyrus.

how she got to the emergency room, but she is oriented to person and time. Her toxicology screen was negative. Blood pressure was 117/71 and patient was afebrile throughout her hospital course. Further work-up for altered mental status was unremarkable, chemistry and CBC were negative, GFR 113, and random sugar was 97. TSH was 5.96. There was no evidence of acute infection. Initial CT of the head was negative. She was admitted to the hospital for overnight observation. The next morning, patient was back to her baseline but still had no idea how she got to the hospital. The last event she recalled from the day prior was leaving the bathroom and walking towards her living room, apparently before she started cooking. She knew she had a complete lapse of memory and was concerned about developing dementia like her father. Her registration and recall returned to normal. Family at bedside also confirmed that she appeared to be at her baseline. Her repeat neurological examination that morning remained non-focal. MRI of the brain, however, showed a small DWI signal abnormality at the left cingulate gyrus (see Figures 1 and 2). No other lesions were noted. Stroke workup eventually showed no other abnormality and she was sent home on Plavix and Lipitor 80mg daily.

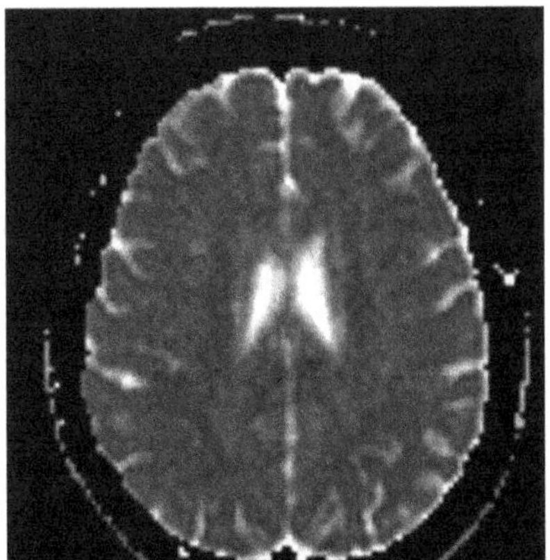

Figure 2: ADC view (same values).

3. Discussion

Currently, cases of transient global amnesia with DWI findings has typically implicated the hippocampus. Naldi et al. reported a clear case of TGA in 2016 with findings of DWI hyperintensity in the right hippocampus on MRI and stenosis of the right posterior cerebral artery on CT angiography. Even then, they further cited multiple prior cases with similar hippocampal involvement [2], albeit small variations in clinical presentation, such as in Carota et al. where the patient had additional findings of anomic aphasia (coined a “TGA plus” syndrome) [3]. In a retrospective study of 86 patients with TGA, Enzinger et al. found that, of the 10 patients with significant DWI findings, there was a predominance of lesions in the hippocampus [5]. Forster et al. in Germany looked at 386 patients diagnosed with TGA at their hospital, and, of the 27 patients who received MRI evaluation, all 12 with DWI lesions were in the hippocampus [4]. Furthermore, it was noted that the properties of these lesions compared to those of pure hippocampal strokes were indistinguishable in terms of DWI and apparent diffusion coefficient (ADC) [6], which seems to suggest that these are true infarctions.

TGA with findings solely in the cingulate gyrus, as was seen with our patient, is a significantly rare occurrence. To our understanding, only one other case has been reported. Gallardo-Tur et al. In 2014 described a patient who presented with classical TGA symptoms with no recurrence of symptoms noted on a one-year follow-up. MRI findings at the time 3 days after presentation is significant for findings in the right cingulate gyrus. In our patient, clinical presentation was similar, with the exception that imaging findings were noted on the left. Other case reports of TGA with DWI hyperintensities include involvement of the corpus callosum [7, 8], putamen [9], uncinate gyrus [10], and the fornix [11]. Thus, while the affected neurologic structures that have been reported in TGA are all in some manner associated with memory or mental development, the fact that a similar clinical presentation arises from various affected structures only highlights how the current literature is lacking in data to establish a comprehensive relationship between ischemia and transient amnesia.

Also, it should be reiterated that despite the numerous cases of TGA with DWI lesions reported, the overall incidence remains low. As noted by Enzinger et al. and Forster et al., only 11% and 3% of all TGA cases seen at their institutions, respectively, were positive for significant MRI findings. This is likely in part because TGA remains a clinical diagnosis, and decision to obtain further work-up with MRI and work-up for ischemia is to the discretion of the provider. Thus, the true incidence of ischemic events in TGA may be underreported. Detection methods and timing of MRI studies may also be limiting factors, as Scheel et al. in a retrospective study of 198 TGA cases showed a significant increase in detection of lesions when slice thickness of 3 mm is utilized and when MRI studies are performed 2 days after the amnestic event [12]. Furthermore, in the retrospective study by Enzinger et al., the hyperintensity findings drastically differed amongst patients with similar presentations, as 9 lesions were found in the left hemisphere, 5 were in the right, and 2 were found bilaterally. Lesion sizes varied between 3 and 6 mm. Comparatively, patients with pure hippocampal strokes could have no memory involvement whatsoever [6]. Thus, the fact that neither the presence, nor the location, nor the size of DWI hyperintensities can consistently correlate with the severity of TGA findings only highlights how lacking the current literature is in understanding the significance of these ischemic-like lesions in the pathogenesis of TGA. An ischemic event may only be a factor in a cascade of neurologic processes that lead to an amnestic event, possibly alongside concurrent metabolic or vascular processes that have also been implicated as possible causes [1] and as such requires further study. Thus, while this is not the first documented case of TGA with ischemic findings in the cingulate gyrus, it takes a step forward in expanding the literature's currently limited understanding of the involvement of ischemic events in TGA. Hopefully, this will help us as the scientific community better map the structures other than the hippocampus that are involved. Doing so may provide a better correlation between structural involvement and disease, furthering the possibility of ischemia or other etiology of cerebrovascular involvement as the culprit of this clinical condition and aid in refining the diagnostic criteria.

Acknowledgments

The authors thank their colleagues, Dr. Jedediah Dixon, M.D. and Dr. Arman Yaghoubian, M.D. at the Adventist Health White Memorial Department of Radiology who helped with interpretation of the images, providing insight and expertise that greatly assisted the writing of this article.

References

[1] D. Owen, B. Paranandi, R. Sivakumar, and M. Seevaratnam, "Classical diseases revisited: transient global amnesia," *Postgraduate Medical Journal*, vol. 83, no. 978, pp. 236–239, 2007.

[2] F. Naldi, S. Baiardi, M. Guarino, L. Spinardi, F. Cirignotta, and A. Stracciari, "Posterior hippocampal stroke presenting with transient global amnesia," *Neurocase*, vol. 23, no. 1, pp. 22–25, 2016.

[3] A. Carota, A. P. Lysandropoulos, and P. Calabrese, "Pure left hippocampal stroke: a transient global amnesia-plus syndrome," *Journal of Neurology*, vol. 259, no. 5, pp. 989–992, 2012.

[4] A. Förster, M. Al-Zghloul, H. Wenz, J. Böhme, C. Groden, and E. Neumaier-Probst, "Isolated punctuate hippocampal infarction and transient global amnesia are indistinguishable by means of MRI," *International Journal of Stroke*, vol. 12, no. 3, pp. 292–296, 2017.

[5] C. Enzinger, F. Thimary, P. Kapeller et al., "Transient global amnesia," *Stroke*, vol. 39, no. 8, pp. 2219–2225, 2008.

[6] A. Gallardo-Tur, J. Romero-Godoy, C. D. L. C. Cosme, and A. Arboix, "Transient global amnesia associated with an acute infarction at the cingulate gyrus," *Case Reports in Neurological Medicine*, vol. 2014, Article ID 418180, 4 pages, 2014.

[7] R. Beyrouti, M. Mansour, A. Kacem, J. Zaouali, and R. Mrissa, "Transient global amnesia like syndrome associated with acute infarction of the corpus callosum: a case report," *Acta Neurologica Belgica*, vol. 116, no. 3, pp. 375–377, 2016.

[8] K. Saito, K. Kimura, K. Minematsu, A. Shiraishi, and M. Nakajima, "Transient global amnesia associated with an acute infarction in the retrosplenium of the corpus callosum," *Journal of the Neurological Sciences*, vol. 210, no. 1-2, pp. 95–97, 2003.

[9] K. Yoshida, "A case of transient global amnesia with small left putamen infarction," *Journal of Stroke and Cerebrovascular Diseases*, vol. 26, no. 1, pp. e27–e28, 2017.

[10] D. M. Greer, P. W. Schaefer, and L. H. Schwamm, "Unilateral temporal lobe stroke causing ischemic transient global amnesia: Role for diffusion-weighted imaging in the initial evaluation," *Journal of Neurogenetics*, vol. 11, no. 3, pp. 317–319, 2001.

[11] M. Gupta, M. A. Kantor, C. E. Tung, N. Zhang, and G. W. Albers, "Transient global amnesia associated with a unilateral infarction of the fornix: Case report and review of the literature," *Frontiers in Neurology*, vol. 5, 2015.

35

A Patient with Combined CADASIL and MTHFR Homozygosity

Sidonie Ibrikji, Tarek El Halabi, and Bassem Yamout

American University of Beirut Medical Center, Department of Neurology, Beirut, Lebanon

Correspondence should be addressed to Bassem Yamout; yamoutba@gmail.com

Academic Editor: Tapas Kumar Banerjee

Cerebral Autosomal Dominant Arteriopathy with Subcortical Infarcts and Leukoencephalopathy (CADASIL) is an inherited disorder caused by a mutation in the NOTCH 3 gene, characterized by early onset of subcortical lacunar infarcts in the absence of vascular risk factors and cerebral microbleeds. Homozygosity for the factor Methylenetetrahydrofolate Reductase (MTHFR) is also associated with lacunar stroke risk and cerebral small-vessel disease regardless of the homocysteine level. The coexistence of MTHFR C677T homozygosity and NOTCH 3 mutation has never been reported in the literature previously, and that brings up the challenge of antithrombotic treatment in the presence of cerebral microbleeds.

1. Introduction

This is the case of a 49-year-old man presenting for stepwise speech impairment and progressive mental slowing of 14 years duration. In his early 30s, he developed recurrent attacks of migraine, preceded by visual aura, for which he was symptomatically treated. At the age of 35, he had a left posterior frontal subcortical ischemic infarct resulting in heavy speech that progressively improved with time. At the age of 37, another subcortical ischemic infarct occurred in his right centrum semioval, leading to left-sided hemiparesis with partial recovery. Three years prior to his presentation, a second left frontotemporal stroke led to severe dysarthria with only minimal recovery. All through this period, he reported mild forgetfulness and mental slowing in retrieving ideas. He had no vascular risk factors except for heavy smoking (more than a 100-pack-year). His family history was significant for a 30-year-old daughter with migraines without aura, and a 25-year-old son with unclear seizure disorder.

On neurological exam, he had moderate flaccid dysarthria and left-sided hemiparesis. His MMSE (Mini-Mental Status Exam) score was 26/30; showing intact attention, orientation, and registration, while losing points on memory (2 out 3 objects recalled at 5 minutes), visuospatial capacities, repetition, and writing.

Cerebrospinal fluid studies (CSF) taken from a lumbar puncture were unremarkable. Magnetic Resonance Imaging (MRI) of the brain showed high T2W lesions involving the external capsules and anterior temporal poles bilaterally, multiple old subcortical infarcts involving predominately the frontal lobes, and bilateral low signal lesions on Susceptibility Weighted Imaging (SWI), in the basal ganglia and thalami suggesting microhemorrhages (Figure 1). Magnetic Resonance Angiography (MRA) of the cervical and cerebral vessels was normal.

A hypercoagulable panel and Cerebral Autosomal Dominant Arteriopathy with Subcortical Infarcts and Leukoencephalopathy (CADASIL) genetic testing were ordered and revealed a homozygous Methylenetetrahydrofolate Reductase (MTHFR) C677T mutation with a normal homocysteine level (10 μmol/L) and a NOTCH3 gene mutation (Heterozygous for c.3691CT p.Arg1231Cys). The patient was on folate, vitamin B12, and vitamin B6 supplements, with normal serum folate and vitamin B12 levels.

Given the presence of microbleeds on MRI and the high risk they confer for bleeding, the patient was not put on antithrombotic treatment. A follow-up 6 months later revealed no new strokes, and the patient was physically and cognitively unchanged.

2. Discussion

CADASIL is a rare, adult-onset inherited disorder, with a mean age at onset of 36.7 years. The earliest clinical

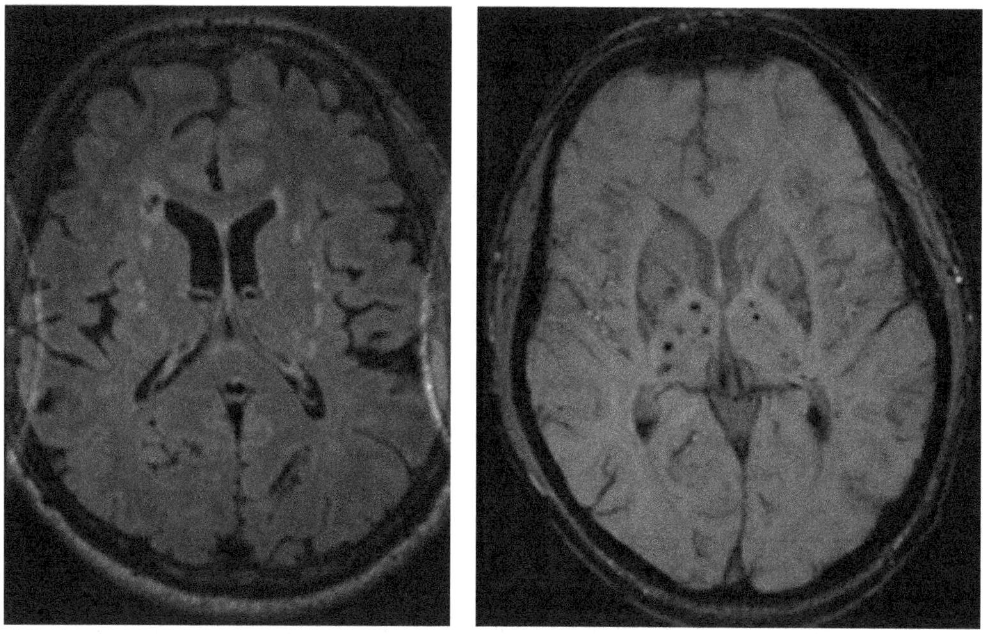

(a) (b)

Figure 1: MRI brain showing abnormal FLAIR signal (a) along the bilateral external capsules, with abnormal hypo intensities in bilateral basal ganglia on T2 FFE (b).

manifestation is migraine with aura, followed by subcortical lacunar ischemic events, considered as the most common manifestation, occurring in 60 to 85% of cases, in the absence of conventional vascular risk factors [1]. Cognitive decline is the second most frequent symptom, and consists of impairment in attention and memory, alteration in executive function, and later on affecting language, reasoning, and verbal and visual memory. Apathy is less common, occurring in 40% of cases. Abnormalities on brain MRI are present in virtually all individuals carrying the mutation after the age of 35 years and consist of high-FLAIR signals indicating leukoencephalopathy, predominating in the periventricular areas, centrum semioval, anterior temporal poles, and external capsules. The 2 latter MRI abnormalities have the highest diagnostic sensitivity, nearing 90%. Cerebral microbleeds are also commonly seen in cortical and subcortical areas, white matter, brainstem, and thalamus [2]. Treatment focuses on primary and secondary prevention by controlling vascular risk factors and smoking avoidance. The benefit of aspirin alone or in combination with clopidogrel in secondary stroke prevention in CADASIL is still questionable. In the presence of cerebral microbleeds, the risk of aspirin-associated intracranial bleed increases, but is still much lower than the rate of ischemic attacks [3].

Pathophysiologically, CADASIL is caused by a mutation in the NOTCH3 gene on chromosome 19. NOTCH3 contributes to arterial development through a cell-surface protein expressed on vascular smooth muscle cells, playing a major role in the stability of those cells' phenotype [4]. The patient can be homozygous or heterozygous for the mutation, homozygosity predicting a slightly more severe course whether clinically or radiologically [5].

Furthermore, MTHFR polymorphism increases the risk of lacunar stroke risk and cerebral small-vessel disease, especially in association with hypertension, but can occur in the absence of other vascular risk factors [6]. The MTHFR mutation reduces the activity of the enzyme responsible for the remethylation of homocysteine to methionine, elevating the plasma concentrations of homocysteine, an independent risk factor for small-vessel ischemic disease through endothelial dysfunction [4]. Our patient had normal homocysteine levels, probably secondary to supplementation with folic acid, vitamin B12, and vitamin B6. Lowering homocysteine levels did not demonstrate a significant effect in decreasing the risk of stroke [7].

The coexistence of MTHFR C677T homozygosity and NOTCH 3 mutation has never been reported in the literature previously and increases the risk of small-vessel ischemic strokes and silent brain lesions, secondary to a combination of endothelial dysfunction on top of microangiopathic changes.

Authors' Contributions

Sidonie Ibrikji and Tarek El Halabi were responsible for literature review, data collection, and writing the case. Bassem Yamout was responsible for literature review, case supervision, and clinical follow-up.

References

[1] H. Chabriat, A. Joutel, M. Dichgans, E. Tournier-Lasserve, and

M.-G. Bousser, "CADASIL," *The Lancet Neurology*, vol. 8, no. 7, pp. 643–653, 2009.

[2] D. Mandellos, G. Limbitaki, A. Papadimitriou, and D. Anastasopoulos, "Cerebral autosomal dominant arteriopathy with subcortical infarcts and leukoencephalopathy (CADASIL) in a Greek family," *Neurological Sciences*, vol. 26, no. 4, pp. 278–281, 2005.

[3] A. Bersano, G. Bedini, J. Oskam et al., "CADASIL: treatment and management options," *Current Treatment Options in Neurology*, vol. 19, no. 9, pp. 1–15, 2017.

[4] J. Liu, K. Sun, Y. Bai et al., "Association of three-gene interaction among MTHFR, ALOX5AP and NOTCH3 with thrombotic stroke: a multicenter case-control study," *Human Genetics*, vol. 125, no. 5-6, pp. 649–656, 2009.

[5] H. Abou Al-Shaar, N. Qadi, M. H. Al-Hamed, B. F. Meyer, and S. Bohlega, "Phenotypic comparison of individuals with homozygous or heterozygous mutation of NOTCH3 in a large CADASIL family," *Journal of the Neurological Sciences*, vol. 367, pp. 239–243, 2016.

[6] V. K. Gadiyaram, M. A. Khan, T. Hogan et al., "Significance of MTHFR gene mutation with normal homocysteine level in vascular events," *Journal of Clinical Oncology*, vol. 27, no. 15, 2016.

[7] M. Lee, K.-S. Hong, S.-C. Chang, and J. L. Saver, "Efficacy of homocysteine-lowering therapy with folic acid in stroke prevention," *Stroke*, vol. 41, no. 6, pp. 1205–1212, 2010.

"At-Home" Photobiomodulation: A New Approach for Bell's Palsy Treatment

Carlo Fornaini[1,2,3] **Zhao Meng,**[3] **Elisabetta Merigo**[1] **and Jean-Paul Rocca**[1,3]

[1]*Micoralis Laboratory EA7354, Faculty of Dentistry, University of Nice Sophia Antipolis, 24 Avenue des Diables Bleus, Nice 06357, France*
[2]*Group of Applied ElectroMagnetics, Department of Engineering and Architecture, University of Parma, Viale G. P. Usberti 181/A, Parma 43124, Italy*
[3]*Department of Stomatology, 2nd Hospital, Gonguong Road 425, Shijiazhuang, Hebei, China*

Correspondence should be addressed to Carlo Fornaini; carlo@fornainident.it

Academic Editor: Dominic B. Fee

Objective. This report is the first one to describe the possibility to use "self-administered" photobiomodulation (PBM) for Bell's palsy (BP) treatment. *Background.* BP is a peripheral disorder of the facial nerve causing sudden paralysis of unilateral facial muscles, and PBM has been successfully suggested for its treatment without any side effect. This is the first case report where a laser device was successfully used at home by the patient herself to treat BP opening new perspectives on the therapy of this disease. *Methods.* This report describes the "at-home PBM" treatment performed on a 15-year-old girl who presented BP consisting of acute pain on the right side of her face, difficulty in biting and dripping saliva from the right side of her lips. The treatment was performed twice a day by cutaneous applications, each of 15 minutes (total fluence 48 J/cm^2) in an area corresponding to the parotid gland by a device emitting at 808 nm at 250 mW output power. *Results.* Two weeks after PBM treatment, performed at home twice a day by the patient herself without any kind of pharmacological therapy, the complete disappearing of the disease was noticed with no side effects. *Conclusion.* With the limitations due to a single case report and with the need of further clinical trials to confirm it, "at-home PBM" seems to represent a good and safe approach to the treatment of BP.

1. Introduction

Bell's palsy (BP) was first described by Sir Charles Bell (1774–1842) as an idiopathic disorder of the peripheral facial nerve causing sudden paralysis of monolateral facial muscles [1].

The incidence of BP is around 20–30 cases per 100,000 persons yearly, regardless of age and gender [2], and even if a relight of herpes simplex infection has been largely hypothesized as the main cause, this has never been demonstrated [3].

Although several patients with BP totally recover in some months, 30% of them exhibit an incomplete healing, sometimes related to social, aesthetic, or psychological problems [4].

Therefore, an immediate diagnosis and a prompt therapeutic intervention seem to be vital for achieving an optimal result [5].

Two main pharmacological kinds of drugs, steroids, and antivirals have been proposed for improving the recovery from BP, chosen on the basis of the hypothesis of its etiopathogenesis, consisting on inflammation and viral infection [6], and also for the reason that, in the saliva and facial nerve endoneural fluid of BP patients, the presence of herpes simplex virus was observed [7].

Recently, also photobiomodulation (PBM) has been suggested for the treatment of BP [8] demonstrating an immediate pain decrease as well as an antiinflammatory effect [9].

In PBM treatment, a photochemical laser-tissue interaction is involved; the energy emitted by the device is given to the mitochondria and absorbed by chromophores (endogenous porphyrins and respiratory chain components such as cytochrome c oxidase); finally, laser energy is converted into metabolic energy by the respiratory chain with the production of adenosine triphosphate (ATP); thanks to the use of parameters characterized by low-energy density, PBM can be considered free of possible side effects [10].

Its mechanism of action in BP derives both by a direct effect on nerves and by an anti-inflammatory action.

The first consists on functional activity of the injured peripheral nerve increasing, degeneration in corresponding motor neurons of the spinal cord decreasing, and axonal growth and myelinization improving [11].

The second may be provoked by levels of proinflammatory cytokines, such as interleukin-1 alpha (IL-1α) and IL-1 beta (IL-1β), reduction, and levels of anti-inflammatory growth factors and cytokines, such as basic fibroblast growth factor (bFGF), platelet-derived growth factor (PDGF), and transforming growth factor-beta (TGF-β), increasing [12].

Several clinical trials and case reports have demonstrated that PBM administered with adequate protocols by trained professionals may represent a good option for accelerating the recovery process in both adults and children [13–17].

Javaherian and co-authors, in a systematic review, concluded that the PBM with 830 nm and 100 mW power for a period of 6 weeks might be beneficial on recovery for the patients with subacute Bell's palsy, reporting no adverse effects during treatment and/or follow-up sessions [18].

Aghamohamdi and co-authors, in a clinical study on 30 diabetic patients with Bell's palsy, demonstrated that PBM is a safe, reliable, and proper alternative approach for the treatment of facial nerve palsy, especially in the presence of underlying conditions such as diabetes mellitus [19].

Unfortunately, the main practical problem related to PBM is the necessity for short sessions for two or three times a week and sometimes even daily [20]. To permit the patients to perform their treatment without reaching the therapist, a new laser family has recently appeared on the market; due to these devices belonging to class II of the American National Standard Institute (ANSI), they may be used directly by the patients themselves in a very simple way, thanks to the preset parameters; moreover, the use of protective goggles is not necessary, cost and size are reduced, as well as the risk of side effects and contraindications are absent; nevertheless, patients evaluation by a specialist before its use remains mandatory [21].

This case report is the first to describe the effectiveness of "at-home PBM" in the treatment of BP disease and to evidence the advantages of this technique when related to classic PBM.

2. Materials and Methods

2.1. Clinical Case. R B, a 15-year-old girl, came to our unit for evaluating facial paralysis on the right side. As reported by her mother, the anamnesis was totally negative not describing any important diseases, and drugs assumption and family occurrence of this condition as well as previous episodes of facial paralysis were also excluded.

The patient reported that the symptoms appeared the day before the medical examination and consisted in acute pain on the right side of the face, difficulty in biting, dripping saliva from the mouth right corner, and impossibility to obtain a complete closure of the left eye. The clinical observation revealed a facial asymmetry with edema in the right jaw, difficulty of facial movements on the right side when smiling, and asymmetry of the eyes. Due to these aspects, the diagnosis was established as an idiopathic facial paralysis, and according to the House Brackmann scale, it was classified as IV degree (moderate severe dysfunction) (Figure 1).

It was decided to treat the disease with an "self-administered PBM," and the patient received the device as well as the instructions to correctly use it. The same day, the patient started the treatment applying the laser device (B-Cure Laser Pro, Good Energies Ltd., Haifa, Israel) on her own; this device is a class II laser according to ANSI classification, emitting in the near IR portion of the spectrum (808 nm) with a green LED aiming beam for indicating the irradiated zone of 4.5 cm^2; its output power of 250 mW is emitted in micropulses with a frequency of 15 kHz (energy per minute of 14.4 J and fluence per minute of 3,2 J/cm^2).

Treatment was performed twice a day by cutaneous applications, each 15 minutes (total fluence: 48 J/cm^2) by putting the device in contact with the skin of the right side in the area corresponding to the parotid gland, as reported in other different case reports [9].

3. Results

One week after the first session, the facial observation revealed an important improvement of the clinical condition and the patient described a great relief of the pain; the eyes asymmetry had disappeared as well as the incapacity to close the left eye, while the asymmetry of the mouth, even if diminished, was still present (II degree of House Brackmann scale = moderate dysfunction) (Figure 2).

Two weeks later, the complete disappearing of the disease was noticed, with the normal facial functions in all areas (grade I of House Brackmann scale = normal) (Figure 3).

The patient had an important change also in her psychological sphere; she was a young girl temporarily disfigured and also worried about the prognosis of her disease which suddenly appeared compromising also her aesthetical aspect, and the rapid resolution of these signs improved her quality of life.

4. Discussion

Even if several cases of BP spontaneously recover some months after the initial insult, its management is focused on minimizing the risk of incomplete resolution and reducing the possibility of morbid sequelae such as facial tissues contracture, synkinesis, autonomic dysfunction, and moderate to severe facial weakness [22].

Current pharmacological approach of BP is based, as described above, on the combination of steroids and antiviral agents [23].

Recently, as PBM has shown beneficial outcome in the regeneration of peripheral nerves [24], it was proposed also in the treatment of BP to minimize the side effects of the drugs assumption [15].

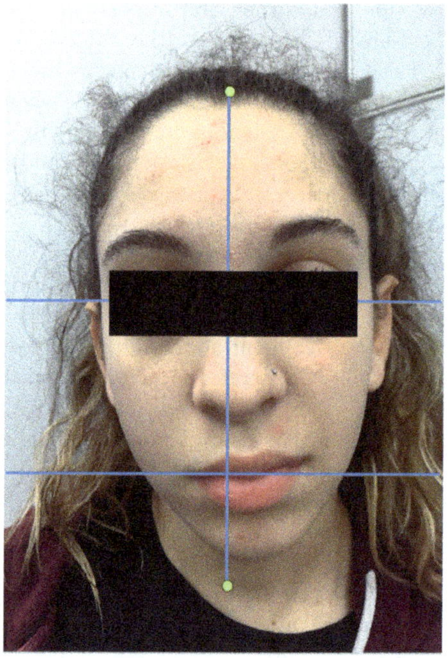

Figure 1: Facial observation before treatment.

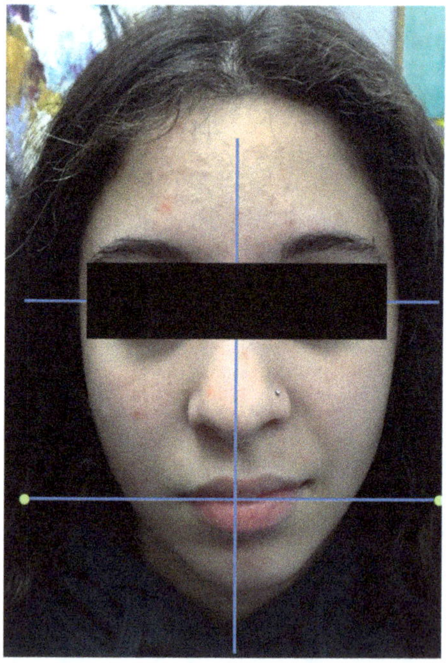

Figure 2: One week treatment follow-up.

PBM therapy is a noninvasive therapy defined by Anders et al. as "a form of light therapy that utilizes nonionizing forms of light;" it is a photothermal reaction which involves endogenous chromophores resulting in beneficial therapeutic phenomena, the most important being promotion of wound healing, tissue regeneration, pain and inflammation reduction, and immunomodulation [25]. The only negative aspect of PBM is represented by the need for the patient to go to the clinics two or three times weekly for performing very short sessions (five/ten minutes), which sometimes limits the compliance during the treatment.

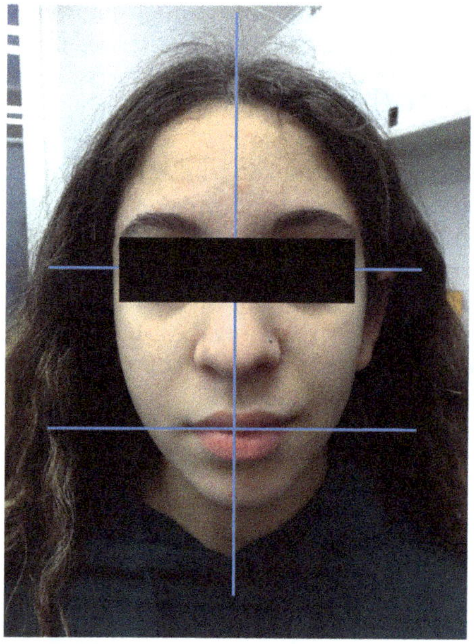

Figure 3: Two weeks treatment follow-up.

The "at-home PBM" devices, recently introduced on the market, are very small, certified as class II lasers according to the ANSI classification and with fixed parameters; for these reasons, their utilization at home by the patients themselves is very easy and with minimal risk of overtreatment.

The energy delivered by this kind of laser devices is in the range of these suggested by the other different studies where conventional PBM was employed and, in every case, it did not exceed the fluence of 10 J, condition for avoiding the possibility to obtain an opposite effect, as established by the Arndt–Schulz rule [26].

The particularity of the "at-home PBM," as shown in this case report, is the short time for completing the treatment and achieve the clinical result; it might be explained by the opportunity, due to the possibility to perform the treatment at home, to give the irradiation daily or twice a day, so accelerating the healing process.

5. Conclusion

This short case report wants to contribute to enlarge the range of "at-home PBM" clinical applications by the demonstration of the advantages of this technique: easiness of use, possibility to perform more daily sessions, no need to go to clinics for treatment, and no overtreatment risk.

With the limitations due to it is a single case report and with the necessity to confirm these results by clinical trials, "at-home PBM" seems to be a good and safe approach to the treatment of Bell's palsy.

Authors' Contributions

CF and EM were responsible for the clinical diagnosis and performed the treatment and follow-up. MG and J-PR were involved in drafting the manuscript and revised it critically for important intellectual content. All authors read and approved the final manuscript.

References

[1] A. Greco, A. Gallo, M. Fusconi, C. Marinelli, G. F. Macri, and M. de Vincentiis, "Bell's palsy and autoimmunity," *Autoimmunity Reviews*, vol. 12, no. 2, pp. 323–328, 2012.

[2] J. D. Tiemstra and N. Khatkhate, "Bell's palsy: diagnosis and management," *American Family Physician*, vol. 76, no. 7, pp. 997–1002, 2007.

[3] A. Zandian, S. Osiro, R. Hudson et al., "The neurologist's dilemma: a comprehensive clinical review of Bell's palsy, with emphasis on current management trends," *Medical Science Monitor: International Medical Journal of Experimental and Clinical Research*, vol. 20, pp. 83–90, 2014.

[4] F. M. Sullivan, I. R. Swan, P. T. Donnan et al., "Early treatment with prednisolone or acyclovir in Bell's palsy," *New England Journal of Medicine*, vol. 357, pp. 1598–1607, 2007.

[5] K. Mantsopoulos, G. Psillas, G. Psychogios, C. Brase, H. Iro, and J. Constantinidis, "Predicting the long-term outcome after idiopathic facial nerve paralysis," *Otology & Neurotology*, vol. 32, no. 5, pp. 848–851, 2011.

[6] E. C. Quant, S. S. Jeste, M. Gagyor et al., "Antiviral treatment for Bell's palsy (id- iopathic facial paralysis)," *Cochrane Database of Systematic Reviews*, vol. 5, Article ID CD001869, 2015.

[7] T. Uscategui, C. Doree, I. J. Chamberlain, and M. J. Burton, "Antiviral therapy for Ramsay Hunt syndrome (herpes zoster oticus with facial palsy) in adults," *The Cochrane Database of Systematic Reviews*, vol. 71, 2008.

[8] M. S. Alayat, A. M. Elsodany, and A. A. El Fiky, "Efficacy of high and low level laser therapy in the treatment of Bell's palsy: a randomized double blind placebo-controlled trial," *Lasers in Medical Science*, vol. 29, pp. 335–342, 2014.

[9] M. M. Poloni, N. P. Marques, N. V. Ribeiro Junior, F. F. Sperandio, J. A. C. Hanemann, and M. L. de Carli, "Bell's palsy treated with photobiomodulation in an adolescent: rare case report and review of the published literature," *International Journal of Paediatric Dentistry*, vol. 02, pp. 1–5, 2018.

[10] E. Merigo, J.-P. Rocca, A. L. B. Pinheiro, and C. Fornaini, "Photobiomodulation therapy in oral medicine: a guide for the practitioner with focus on new possible protocols," *Photobiomodulation, Photomedicine, and Laser Surgery*, vol. 37, no. 11, pp. 669–680, 2019.

[11] R. I. Barbosa, A. M. Marcolino, R. R. de Jesus Guirro, N. Mazzer, C. H. Barbieri, and M. de Cássia Registro Fonseca, "Comparative effects of wavelengths of low-power laser in regeneration of sciatic nerve in rats following crushing lesion," *Lasers in Medical Science*, vol. 25, no. 3, pp. 423–430, 2010.

[12] P. V. Peplow, T.-Y. Chung, and G. D. Baxter, "Application of low level laser technologies for pain relief and wound healing: overview of scientific bases," *Physical Therapy Reviews*, vol. 15, no. 4, pp. 253–285, 2010.

[13] B. Ordahan and A. Y. Karahan, "Role of low-level laser therapy added to facial expression exercises in patients with idiopathic facial (Bell's) palsy," *Lasers in Medical Science*, vol. 32, no. 4, pp. 931–936, 2017.

[14] T. F. Montero, M. S. H. Zayas, L. R. C. Andino, and V. C. Correoso, "Evaluación clínica y funcional de pacientes con parálisis de Bell tratados con láser," *Medisan*, vol. 19, no. 12, 2015.

[15] C. R. Fontana and V. S. Bagnato, "Low-Level laser therapy in pediatric Bell's palsy: case report in a three-year-old child," *Journal of Alternative & Complementary Medicine*, vol. 19, no. 4, pp. 376–382, 2013.

[16] T. A. Alfaya, P. N. Tannure, E. C. Dip, L. Uemoto, R. Barcelos, and C. V. D. Gouvêa, "Association of Bell's palsy and temporomandibular dysfunction: clinical management," *Revista da Faculdade de Odontologia- UPF*, vol. 17, no. 2, pp. 222–227, 2012.

[17] J. P. C. Tanganeli, S. S. I. de Oliveira, T. da Silva, K. P. S. Fernandes, L. J. Motta, and S. K. Bussadori, "Complete and fast recovery from idiopathic facial paralysis using laser-photobiomodulation," *Case Reports in Dentistry*, vol. 2020, Article ID 9867693, 4 pages, 2020.

[18] M. Javaherian, B. Attarbashi Moghaddam, S. Bashardoust Tajali, and N. Dabbaghipour, "Efficacy of low-level laser therapy on management of Bell's palsy: a systematic review," *Lasers in Medical Science*, vol. 35, no. 6, pp. 1245–1252, 2020.

[19] D. Aghamohamdi, S. Fakhari, M. Farhoudi, and H. Farzin, "The efficacy of low-level laser therapy in the treatment of Bell's palsy in diabetic patients," *Journal of Lasers in Medical Sciences*, vol. 11, no. 3, pp. 310–315, 2020.

[20] L. Gavish and N. N. Houreld, "Therapeutic efficacy of home-use photobiomodulation devices: a systematic literature review," *Photobiomodulation, Photomedicine, and Laser Surgery*, vol. 37, no. 1, pp. 4–16, 2019.

[21] M. L. Juhász, M. K. Levin, and E. S. Marmur, "A review of available laser and intense light source home devices: a dermatologist's perspective," *Journal of Cosmetic Dermatology*, vol. 16, no. 4, pp. 438–443, 2017.

[22] N. J. Holland and G. M. Weiner, "Recent developments in Bell's palsy," *BMJ*, vol. 329, pp. 553–7, 2004.

[23] K. K. Adour, J. M. Ruboyianes, P. G. VonDoersten, F. M. Byl, C. S. Trent, and C. P. Quesenberry Jr, "Bell's palsy treatment with acyclovir and prednisone compared with prednisone alone: a double-blind, randomized, controlled trial," *Annals of Otology, Rhinology & Laryngology*, vol. 105, pp. 371–378, 1996.

[24] S. Rochkind, V. Drory, M. Alon, M. Nissan, and G. E. Ouaknine, "Laser phototherapy (780 nm), a new modality in treatment of long-term incomplete peripheral nerve injury: a randomized double-blind placebo-controlled study," *Photomedicine and Laser Surgery*, vol. 25, no. 5, pp. 436–442, 2007.

[25] J. J. Anders, R. J. Lanzafame, and P. R. Arany, "Low-level light/laser therapy versus photobiomodulation therapy," *Photomedicine and Laser Surgery*, vol. 33, no. 4, pp. 183-184, 2015.

[26] R. Zein, S. Wayne, and M. R. Hamblin, "Review of light parameters and photobiomodulation efficacy: dive into complexity," *Journal of Biomedical Optics*, vol. 23, no. 12, Article ID 120901, 2018.

37

Treatment of a Woman with Inoperable Meningioma using Mifepristone for 26 Years

Maria das Dores Medina-Lopes[1] and Luiz Augusto Casulari[2]

[1]*The Secretariat of Health of the Federal District and the Ministry of Health, Brasília, DF, Brazil*
[2]*The University Hospital of Brasília and Clinic of Endocrinology and Neurology (CLINEN), Brasília, DF, Brazil*

Correspondence should be addressed to Luiz Augusto Casulari; lacasulari@unb.br

Academic Editor: Hidetoshi Ikeda

Meningioma treatment includes observation of its growth or surgery with or without associated radiotherapy. However, drug treatment can be used for tumors deemed inoperable because of their size and location. Due to the presence of progesterone receptors, the use of antiprogestin mifepristone is recommended. This study describes a case of inoperable meningioma treated with mifepristone for 26 years without interruption. The patient is a 45-year-old woman diagnosed with plaque meningioma, extending from the bottom of her right orbit, through the length of the small wing of the sphenoid, part of the large wing of the sphenoid, especially near the superior orbital fissure, and at the ceiling of the orbit. As this meningioma was considered inoperable, treatment with 200 mg oral mifepristone was administered uninterruptedly for 26 years. This treatment initially halted the growth of the meningioma and subsequently resulted in a small reduction of its volume; however, the meningioma has persisted until the last evaluation. After five years of mifepristone use, hydroxyurea was added for nine months but was discontinued due to anemia and leucopenia. In conclusion, mifepristone was useful for the survival of the patient for those 26 years. The drug interfered with the natural history of the meningioma, which generally evolves to death in such long follow-up durations without associated surgery or radiation therapy.

1. Introduction

Meningiomas are classified into types I, II, or III. Type I meningiomas have very slow growth; however, rare variants (clear cell, chordal, papillary, and rhabdoid), as well as invasive or atypical grade II and type III anaplastic, are much aggressive. The specific chromosomal changes of these histological types account for their variable evolution [1].

Typically, type I meningioma does not require treatment, but only observation, in cases of growth that may require surgical intervention [2–5]. However, type II and type III meningiomas usually grow and require treatment. The suggested treatment strategies of these two types include maximum removal of the tumor that can be performed safely, active observation when the entire tumor has not been removed, and radiotherapy after partial tumor removal [6].

Several medical treatments have been developed for cases in which tumor growth cannot be controlled. These developments have occurred due to increased knowledge of specific molecular changes and the immune environment. Advances in molecular biology and genomics have led to new therapeutic modalities with promising results. Generally, therapies directed to hormones, cytotoxic chemotherapy, and molecular therapies with genomic analysis have been used (review, [7]).

Following the discovery of progesterone receptors on meningiomas [8–10], mifepristone has been of interest for the treatment of inoperable tumors or in cases for which surgery had no effect [11–17].

Mifepristone has been studied for many years for its potential therapeutic use as a potent antagonist of progesterone and glucocorticoids [18]. It is the first antisteroid with activity greater than or equal to that of the naturally occurring hormone agonist used clinically. It binds weakly to androgen receptors and does not bind to mineralocorticoid and estrogen receptors. Its use in the treatment of endometriosis, breast cancer, interruption of pregnancy, and contraception has been described, due to its antiprogestin activity [18]. Recently, its potential use in the treatment of vestibular schwannoma has been suggested [19]. Regarding the antiglucocorticoid effect of mifepristone, its use in depression, immunological abnormalities, inoperable adrenal cancer [18], tumors producing ectopic adrenocorticotropic hormone (ACTH) [20], and Cushing's disease [21] has been evaluated.

This article examined the antiprogestin action of mifepristone in the treatment of meningioma in a woman treated for 26 years without surgery and/or radiotherapy. For nine months, she also received hydroxyurea. To our knowledge, this case has the longest follow-up described in the literature.

2. Case Presentation

A white woman, 41 years of age, started having frequent headaches accompanied by extreme fatigue, nauseas, vomiting, and diplopia. She had a history of migraines since childhood. After successive consultations with several ophthalmologists, nothing was identified except diplopia. Exercises to correct the diplopia were prescribed without success.

At age 43, proptosis developed in her right eye; again, ophthalmological evaluations did not detect any abnormality. Therefore, the condition was considered a variation from normality. Subsequently, she observed that her right eye was on a lower plane in relation to her left eye and had altered motility, as if there were a lesion in the third cranial nerve. At that time, a cranioencephalic tomography revealed a pronounced thickening of the ceiling of the orbit and the small and large wings of the sphenoid; the upper rectus muscle was also lowered and thickened, especially posteriorly, suggesting meningioma in plaque, extending from the bottom of the right orbit, by the small wing of the sphenoid, in practically all its extension, and in part of the large wing of the sphenoid, especially along the superior orbital fissure, and at the ceiling of the orbit.

Cranioencephalic magnetic resonance imaging (MRI) confirmed the diagnosis of meningioma (Figures 1–3) with the presence of a right parasellar lesion related to the cavernous sinus, previously involving superior orbital fissure impairment and later following the free edge of the tentorium. The lesion progressed to the suprasellar cistern, mainly to the right of the midline, apparently involving the pituitary infundibulum. These findings were highly suggestive of parasellar meningioma, with extension to the suprasellar cistern to the right of the midline and, later, to the free edge of the tentorium.

In her personal history, the patient had menarche at the age of 11, with later catamenias always regular; she was pregnant four times but had a spontaneous abortion in the first weeks of her second pregnancy. She had three children aged 23, 25, and 27 years from normal births. In the second full-term pregnancy, she had contractions from the seventh month of gestation and required rest until delivery.

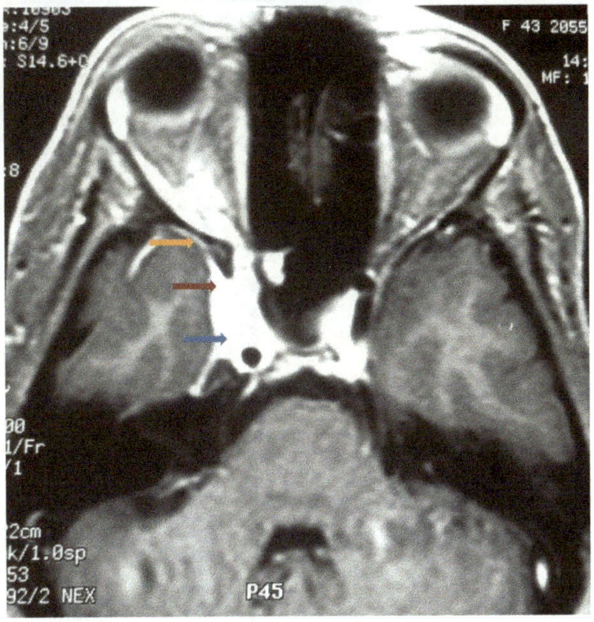

Figure 1: Axial sequence, after contrast, in T1, showing expansive, extra-axial, parasellar lesion, with intense enhancement after contrast infusion, involving the cavernous sinus and the carotid, without compromising their diameters (blue arrow); the lesion involves the apex of the orbit (red arrow), and there is thickening and enhancement of the dura mater (yellow arrow), suggestive of meningioma.

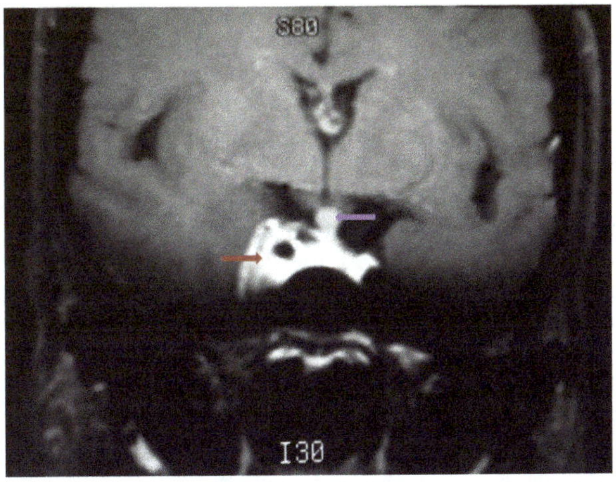

Figure 2: Coronal sequence, after contrast, in T1, showing expansive, extra-axial, parasellar lesion, with intense enhancement after contrast infusion, involving the right cavernous sinus and the carotid, without compromising their diameters (red arrow); thickening of the pituitary stem of an indeterminate nature (purple arrow).

In the family history, her parents were immigrants to Brazil from Graciosa Island, in the archipelago of the Azores, and were not consanguineous. She was the eldest of six children. Her father died at 78 years of age due to metastatic prostate cancer. He was also a carrier of ankylosing spondylitis. Her uncle, five years younger than her father, had a history of seizures since adolescence; at the age of 55 years, he underwent surgery to remove a meningoteliomatous

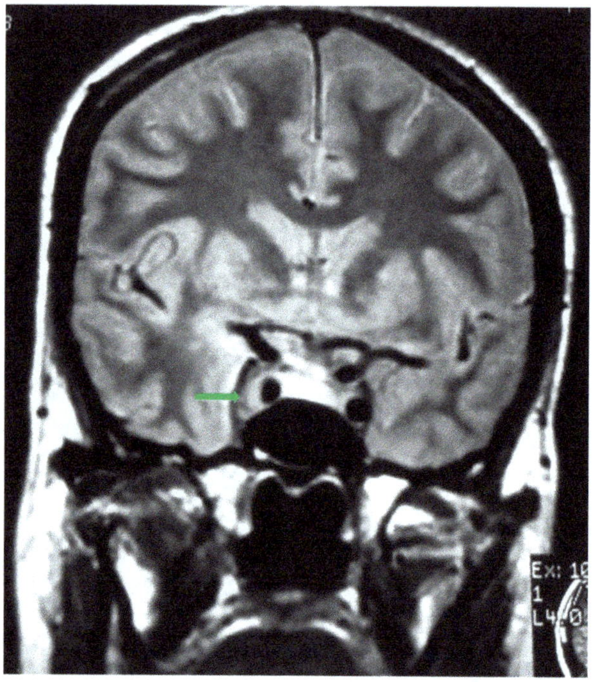

Figure 3: Coronal sequence, in T2, showing expansive, extra-axial, parasellar lesion, involving the right cavernous sinus and the carotid, without compromising their diameters (red arrow) with intermediate signal (green arrow).

meningioma, as shown in Figure 4. Meningioma was found in the mother when she was 80 years of age.

The unanimous opinion of several neurosurgeons was that the patient had a tumor with no possibility of surgery.

She was started on 200 mg mifepristone daily, at age 44, as part of a research process being carried out by the Exelgyn Laboratory in France. She has uninterruptedly maintained this treatment to this day, for 26 years.

In the month following the diagnosis of meningioma, and before using mifepristone, her diplopia became pronounced and episodes of transient amaurosis appeared. Table 1 shows the evolution of proptosis in the right eye and exotropia in the left eye before and during the 26 years of treatment. Significant worsening of both assessments was observed shortly after the tumor diagnosis was performed eight months before the start of mifepristone treatment. Relative stabilization of proptosis occurred after seven years. Exotropia, however, also worsened after diagnosis but with greater intensity than proptosis. She improved after four years of treatment and remained so until she was 66 years old. After 25 years of treatment, the motility of her eyeball was normal.

Other eye changes described were papilla edema observed during nine months of treatment with the drug, which disappeared after the fourth year.

The symptoms of headache, nausea, and vomiting were progressively decreased during the course of mifepristone treatment.

Five years after starting mifepristone treatment, oral hydroxyurea was initiated (500 mg three times daily). This treatment was continued for nine months and stopped due to major decreases in red and white blood cell counts. During the treatment, she had a 0.5 mm decrease in proptosis and wrinkles developed on the forehead. However, brain MRI showed no significant change in the tumor images.

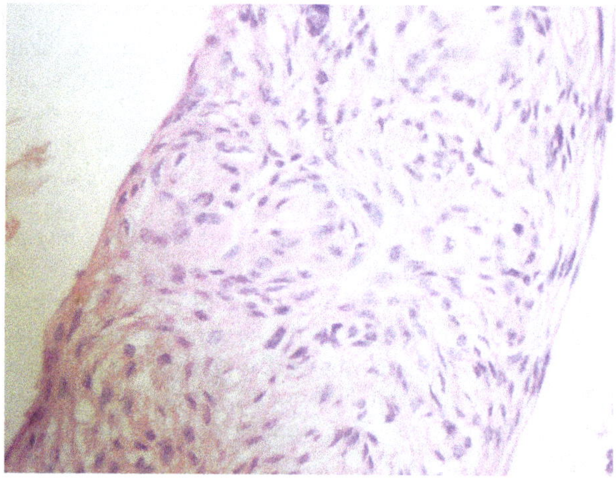

Figure 4: Neoplasia consisting of masses of elongated cells with imprecise limits, finely granular cytoplasm, and large rounded or oval nuclei; cytoplasmic invaginations configuring nuclear pseudoinclusions are visible at the top left, and the cells are arranged in lobes separated by fibrous tissue with some vorticilar aspects.

Serial MRI evaluations did not show significant changes in the images until 13 years of follow-up. However, a small decrease in tumor size was observed with 16 years of treatment (figures not shown). As shown in Figures 5(a) and 5(b), MRI at 23 years of treatment had a greater tumor decrease compared to the previous examination. The last MRI, after 26 years of treatment (figures not shown), showed no alteration in the tumor in relation to the evaluation at 23 years.

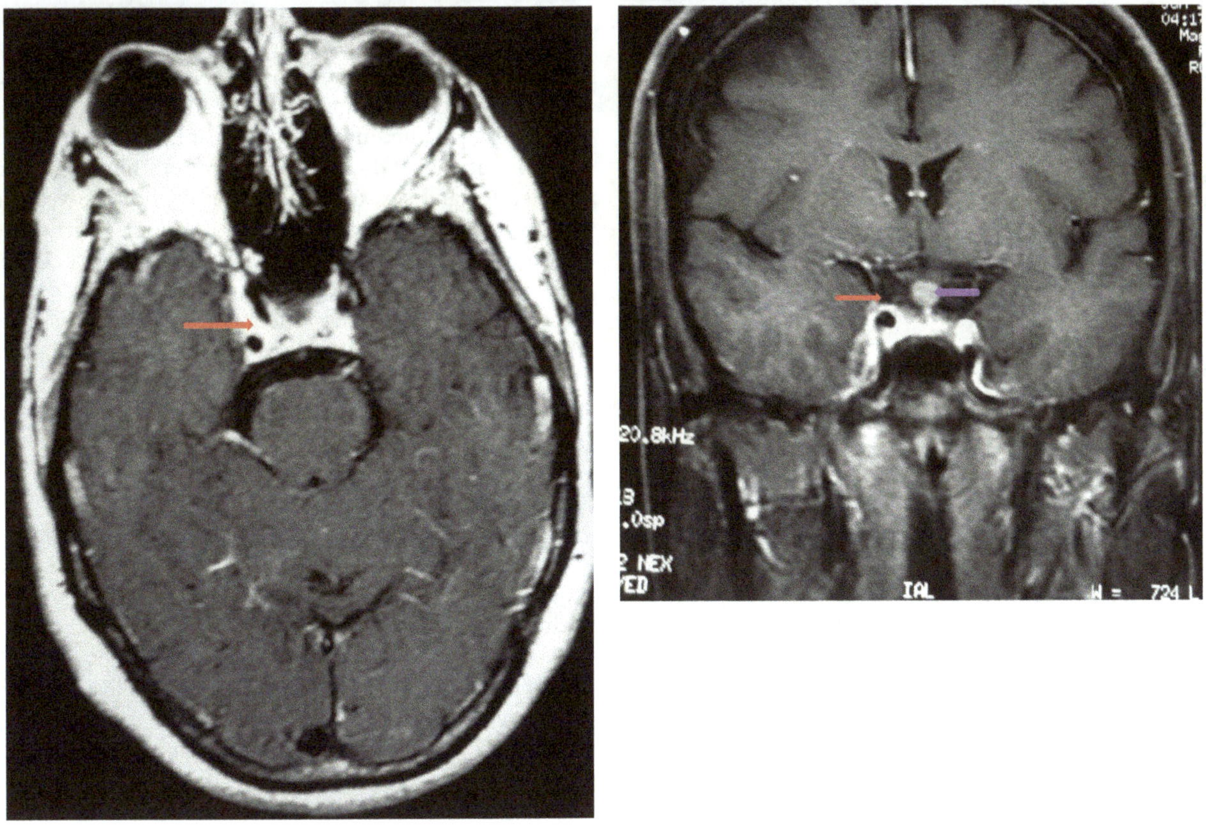

(a) (b)

Figure 5: Magnetic resonance imaging after 23 years of mifepristone treatment. (a) Axial and (b) coronal sequences, in T1, after contrast, show significant reduction of the parasellar and dura mater expansive lesion (red arrow), with persisting thickening of the pituitary stem (purple arrow).

Table 1: Evolution of right eye proptosis and left eye exotropia before and during treatment with mifepristone.

	Exophthalmometry (mm)	Exotropia (diopters)
Before mifepristone (month)		
8	3	8
4	5	12
After mifepristone (year)		
0.2	6	18
2	6.5	18
4	7	—
5	6	8
6	6.5	8
7	6.5	7
9	5.5	—
10	5.5	8
16	5.0	6
25	Normal	Normal

Table 2 shows the results of hormonal dosages before and during mifepristone use.

Four months before starting treatment with mifepristone, ACTH and cortisol concentrations were normal at 8-hour and 16-hour evaluations. However, after the start of the drug, both hormones increased above normal values and thus remained until the last evaluation after 26 years.

The patient's cycles were regular, and she should have menstruated four days after she started treatment with mifepristone, and also, the progesterone was 15 ng/mL; however, she never menstruated. Table 2 shows that the evaluations of gonadotropins (FSH and LH), estradiol, and progesterone were within the follicular phase of the menstrual cycle. After initiation of treatment with mifepristone, their FSH and LH levels remained above normal for the

TABLE 2: Hormonal dosages before and during mifepristone use.

Hormone*	Basal	After mifepristone	
Cortisol 8 h (NV 4.3–22.4 ng/mL)	6.0	239	
Cortisol 16 h (NV 2–15 ng/dL)	3.0	37	
ACTH 8 h (NV up to 160 pg/mL)	90	420	
ACTH 16 h (NV up to 50 pg/mL)	110	85	
FSH (NV follicular phase 2.5–10.2 mIU/mL)	9.4	0,1†	8.3‡
LH (NV follicular phase 2.5–12 mIU/ml)	6.75	0,8†	6.77‡
Estradiol (NV 19.5–144 pg/mL)	151	—	35.8‡
Progesterone (NV follicular phase < 1.4 ng/mL)	0.22	—	
TSH (NV 0.6–4.5 mcUI/mL)	6.8	<0.01$	
T4 total (NV 5.2–12,7 mcg/dL)	6.47	—	
T4 free (NV 0.72–1.72 ng/mL)	0.68	1.38$	
T3 total (NV 60–181 ng/dL)	92	—	
Prolactin (NV up to 26 ng/mL)	76.8	17.0	
IGF-1 (37–219 ng/mL)	90.6	91	

*ACTH = adrenocorticotropic hormone; FSH = follicle-stimulating hormone; LH = luteinizing hormone; TSH = thyroid-stimulating hormone; IGF-1 = insulin growth factor 1. †Use of 0.625 mg equine-conjugated estrogen; ‡after bilateral oophorectomy performed at age 57; $use of 100 mcg L-thyroxine.

follicular phase for three months and then remained within the normal range. However, she started using 0.627 mg of conjugated estrogen which she continued for 14 years, concomitantly with mifepristone. During this period, FSH and LH remained suppressed.

Serial gynecological control showed that the endometrium was thickened. She underwent endometrial biopsies twice, showing cystic hyperplasia. After 29 months of using mifepristone, at age 47, she underwent a total hysterectomy. Histopathological examination showed uterine body leiomyomas, adenosis, and cystic endometrial hyperplasia, without cytological atypia.

Ultrasound monitoring of the patient's ovaries showed bilateral growth, with cystic cavities with septations. Bilateral oophorectomy was performed at age 57, after 12 years of mifepristone use. The histopathological diagnosis was follicular cysts and albicans bodies and serous cyst on the right and left ovary, respectively. After this procedure, her hormone levels were never compatible with menopause, even after 24 years of starting mifepristone treatment.

As shown in Table 2, about four years after the onset of the signs and symptoms of meningioma and one month before starting mifepristone treatment, the patient had thyroid-stimulating hormone (TSH) slightly above normal (6.8 μUI/mL) and free T4 was below normal, but total T4 and total T3 had normal levels. Antithyroglobulin, antimicrosomal, and antiperoxidase antibodies were always undetectable. TSH levels increased four months after starting mifepristone (8.26 μUI/mL) and remained at similar concentrations for up to 20 months; some levels of total T4 and free T4 during this same period were below the normal limit; however, total T3 levels were always normal. Replacement was started with 100 μg L-thyroxine, and her TSH level remained below detectable concentrations. Her free T4 level was between 0.80 and 1.4 ng/mL until the last evaluation, 26 years after starting mifepristone therapy.

Before treatment, her prolactin levels were elevated, remained high (42.0 ng/mL) at two months, and normalized (17.0 ng/mL) at eight months after starting mifepristone. Until the last evaluation, 26 years after starting treatment, the levels remained normal (6.8 ng/mL).

The patient's IGF-1 level was always within normal limits for her age and sex, until the last evaluation, 26 years after the use of mifepristone. A growth hormone (GH) stimulus test to check for hormone deficiency was never performed.

Laboratory exams, such as complete blood count, lipidogram, liver and renal function tests, and levels of electrolytes, calcium, phosphorus, and parathyroid hormone (PTH), were within normal limits before the treatment was started and did not change during the 26 years of observation.

3. Discussion

We describe the case of a woman with inoperable meningioma treated using mifepristone without interruption for 26 years. The lack of tumor growth and its decrease may have been due to the chronic use of this drug; this possibility was evaluated by clinical improvements and radiological imaging.

Serial ophthalmological assessments suggested tumor growth within three years after diagnosis. The first ophthalmic signs of meningioma growth stabilization appeared after two years of mifepristone use. However, they were more remarkable after seven years, with improvement of proptosis and exotropia of the right eye. At 10 years of treatment, there was a marked improvement of these parameters in both eyes. At age 57, she underwent bilateral oophorectomy 12 years after starting mifepristone. After 16 years of mifepristone use and four years of surgical removal of the ovaries, there was an even greater improvement in ophthalmologic assessments.

Some characteristics of the patient were compared with those more commonly observed in patients with meningioma. For example, in a cohort of 12,384 patients diagnosed with meningioma, women (75%), white (79%), and married (53%) predominated [22]. An extensive case-control study [23] found that a family history of meningioma was associated with a higher frequency of this tumor. In the present case, the patient's paternal uncle and the mother had meningiomas.

Any comparison of the 26-year long-term survival with mifepristone with published results must consider the type of meningioma. This is because the survival of patients with type I meningioma is much greater than that of types II and III [2–5, 7]. As there was no histological study of the tumor, some of its characteristics in presentation led us to believe it to be a type II or atypical meningioma. The signs and symptoms included rapid tumor growth, which does not occur with type I, but with a much less intense evolution than those observed in type III. Type III has very rapid growth, with a 10-year survival rate of 14–34% [7]. In addition, the MRI images were suggestive of type II or atypical tumors.

In the follow-up of 244 untreated meningioma patients, 44% had growth during monitoring for 3.8 years. The factors associated with this evolution were age under 60 years, hyperintensity in MRI, absence of calcification, and a diameter greater than 26 mm [5]. All these factors were present in the current patient, which suggests that she would have had a worse prognosis if she had not been treated with mifepristone.

A mifepristone dose of 200 mg per day is most commonly used for the treatment of meningioma because it has significant antiprogesterone but less antiglucocorticoid activity [14]. The ingestion of doses greater than 100 mg results in constant serum concentrations. This is due to the saturation of alpha 1 acid glycoprotein, the serum protein to which mifepristone binds. This limits and regulates drug availability in tissues [24]. This is one of the justifications for not using dosages greater than 100 mg [24]. However, mifepristone exceeding that dose has been shown to be metabolized [25, 26] by demethylation and hydroxylation, resulting in monodemethylated, didemethylated, and hydroxylated metabolites [24, 27]. These metabolites retain considerable affinity for progesterone and glucocorticoid receptors [24, 27]. Serum concentrations of monodemethylated metabolite exceed those of mifepristone [25, 26]. When a dosage of 100 mg mifepristone is increased to 800 mg, serum concentrations remain the same, while concentrations of metabolites increase [27, 28]. Mifepristone has difficulty crossing the blood-brain barrier, but concentrations of demethylated metabolites were four times greater than those of mifepristone in the rat brain [27]. It is possible that the metabolites of mifepristone are more important for their antiprogestin and antiglucocorticoid effects than mifepristone [25, 26]. Thus, higher doses of mifepristone may be more useful in the successful treatment of intracranial tumors. However, this possibility needs to be demonstrated in further research.

Evaluation of the action of mifepristone on meningioma is difficult due to the low growth rate of these tumors. Thus, in addition to the imaging evaluation, cranial pair paralysis and ophthalmological evaluations for acuity and visual fields should also be objectively documented, along with neurological examinations [16]. To our knowledge, this is the first case in which these serial evaluations, along with imaging evaluations, were performed in the long term, with the use of mifepristone for the treatment of meningioma.

The first publication evaluating mifepristrone in the treatment of inoperable meningiomas at a dose of 200 mg per day, ranging from two to 31 months, observed objective improvements in tomography or resonance images of 5/14 treated patients [11]. In a subsequent publication with 28 patients, ranging from 2 to 157 months, they concluded that minor regression of meningioma that can result in significant clinical benefit is suggested in the male and premenopausal female subgroups of patients [14].

More recently, Touat et al. [15] treated three women with multiple meningiomas with mifepristone, with follow-up time duration ranging from five to nine years. Radiologically, they observed a decrease in two patients and stabilization in the third. Long-term treatment with mifepristone has been described for up to 13 years in one patient and 10 to 12 years in six patients [13]. The patient described here was followed for 26 years, a long time not yet described in the literature.

Although mifepristone is well-tolerated, a systematic literature review found no evidence to recommend its use in inoperable meningiomas [16].

The only randomized placebo study showed no significantly greater effect of mifepristone. The multicenter, prospective, randomized, placebo-controlled, phase III research study assessed 80 patients who received mifepristone and 84 who received a placebo. Twenty-four patients (30%) completed two years of mifepristone use without disease progression, adverse effects, or other reasons to discontinue treatment. The 28 (33%) patients administered that the placebo also completed the study. No statistical difference was observed between the two groups in relation to failure-free or overall survival [17]. The authors did not reach a conclusion because 88% of the meningiomas in the sample had progesterone receptors but did not respond to treatment with mifepristone. Nevertheless, they speculated that meningiomas without progesterone receptors have a higher likelihood of recidivism than those with such receptors [29]. Thus, the latter would be less responsive to mifepristone and would see meningioma progression and those with a good response would be progesterone receptor-positive. An interesting suggestion for the nonaction of mifepristone in progesterone receptor-positive meningiomas may be linked to the presence of an estrogen receptor. The anticancer action of progesterone in hormonally sensitive tumors usually occurs through the downregulation of the estrogen receptor, which is present in less than 5% of meningiomas [17].

Soon after beginning mifepristone treatment, the patient experienced amenorrhea, which persisted for the entire follow-up period. In the hormonal evaluations, FSH and LH levels increased in the first three months of mifepristone use but later remained within the range of the follicular phase of the cycle, which is the lowest during the menstrual cycle. These gonadotropin behaviors were also observed in treatment with mifepristone [12, 30]. Decreases in LH and FSH secretion in normal women during the menstrual cycle, with the use of mifepristone, have been described [31, 32]. This behavior of gonadotropins may be due to the negative feedback effect of increased testosterone, estradiol, and estrone caused by mifepristone [12]. In a randomized study, the 14 premenopausal patients who used mifepristone had menstrual cycle alteration [17].

Serial evaluations showed cystic endometrial hyperplasia. After two years, the patient underwent a total hysterectomy, following which the histopathological examination showed leiomyomas of the uterus body, adenosis, and cystic endometrial hyperplasia, without cytological atypia. Endometrial hyperplasia with the chronic use of mifepristone for the treatment of meningioma [13, 14, 17] and in Cushing's disease [21] has been described. Endometrial polyps due to the blockage of the contraregulatory action of estradiol progesterone have also been described [30]. In a case-control study [23], women with meningiomas were more likely to develop hormone-related diseases such as uterine leiomyoma, as observed in the present case.

Twelve years after starting mifepristone, at 57 years of age, she presented bilateral growths on her ovaries. She underwent bilateral oophorectomy, and serous cystadenoma was found in her left ovary. This association was also reported in one of the three patients treated with mifepristone for multiple meningioma [15].

The patient developed subclinical hypothyroidism soon after starting mifepristone, which has also been described previously [13]. The mechanism may be linked to mifepristone interference in the hypothalamic-pituitary-adrenal axis. Excess cortisol in Cushing's syndrome is associated with decreased TSH level; the action of mifepristone may block this effect on TSH [33]. In the randomized study, no hypothyroidism was observed in either the mifepristone or placebo group [17].

However, it is more likely that the patient developed hypothyroidism secondary to the presence of the meningioma in the region near the hypothalamus and hypophysis. Patients with lesions in this region may secrete TSH that is biologically inactive, although it is immunologically active and recognized by the antibody used in the assay of its dosage. In this case, the control of hormone replacement with L-thyroxine is with the dosage of free T4, kept above 1.0 ng/mL. Unlike primary hypothyroidism, in which TSH plays an important role in hypothyroidism secondary to hypothalamic injury, the levels may be normal or slightly elevated. With L-thyroxine replacement, its secretion is quickly suppressed [34, 35].

The patient was treated with hydroxyurea for nine months. There was a decrease in proptosis, and she began to develop wrinkles on her forehead. However, MRI assessment showed no alterations in the tumor. Due to anemia and leukopenia, we opted not to continue this treatment. A first publication that reported the use of hydroxyurea for the treatment of meningioma had very good results: three patients had tumor reductions of 74%, 60%, and 15%, respectively, and a fourth patient with type III meningioma had no tumor recurrence two years after surgery [36]. Retrospective and prospective studies showed that hydroxyurea had an initial beneficial effect, followed by disease progression (review, [7]). However, hydroxyurea in association with imatinib [37, 38] and verapamil [39] presented promising results.

In conclusion, ophthalmological serial evaluations showed that the tumor grew in the first three years, with progressive worsening of exotropia and ocular proptosis. If mifepristone had not been started, most probably, the patient would have developed a loss of vision and even died within a few years, as described for grade II meningiomas. Given the natural history of type II meningiomas, with or without treatment, it is unlikely that the patient would have survived for 26 years if she had not been receiving mifepristone.

Consent

Informed consent for this publication was obtained from the patient.

Acknowledgments

The authors thank Dr. Miguel Farage Filho, the neurosurgeon who followed the case since the time of diagnosis; Professor Dr. Anibal Faundes, for including the patient in the RU486 research program for inoperable meningioma at Exelgyn Laboratory, France; Dr. José Luiz Mendonça, for reviewing the MRIs; and Professor Albino Verçosa de Magalhães, for reviewing the histology of meningioma.

References

[1] C. Mawrin and A. Perry, "Pathological classification and molecular genetics of meningiomas," *Journal of Neuro-Oncology*, vol. 99, no. 3, pp. 379–391, 2010.

[2] W. C. Olivero, J. R. Lister, and P. W. Elwood, "The natural history and growth rate of asymptomatic meningiomas: a review of 60 patients," *Journal of Neurosurgery*, vol. 83, no. 2, pp. 222–224, 1995.

[3] M. Nakamura, F. Roser, J. Michel, C. Jacobs, and M. Samii, "The natural history of incidental meningiomas," *Neurosurgery*, vol. 53, no. 1, pp. 62–71, 2003.

[4] L. A. Zeidman, W. J. Ankenbrandt, H. Du, N. Paleologos, and N. A. Vick, "Growth rate of non-operated meningiomas," *Journal of Neurology*, vol. 255, no. 6, pp. 891–895, 2008.

[5] S. Oya, S. H. Kim, B. Sade, and J. H. Lee, "The natural history of intracranial meningiomas," *Journal of Neurosurgery*, vol. 114, no. 5, pp. 1260–1266, 2011.

[6] S. Q. Sun, A. H. Hawasli, J. Huang, M. R. Chicoine, and A. H. Kim, "An evidence-based treatment algorithm for the management of WHO Grade II and III meningiomas," *Neurosurgical Focus*, vol. 38, no. 3, p. E3, 2015.

[7] S. Gupta, W. L. Bi, and I. F. Dunn, "Medical management of meningioma in the era of precision medicine," *Neurosurgical Focus*, vol. 44, no. 4, p. E3, 2018.

[8] M. A. Blankenstein, J. W. van't Verlaat, R. J. M. Croughs et al., "Hormone dependency of meningiomas," *The Lancet*, vol. 333, no. 8651, pp. 1381-1382, 1989.

[9] M. A. Blankenstein, F. M. Verheiien, J. M. Jacobs, T. H. Donker, M. W. van Duijnhoven, and J. H. Thijssen, "Occurrence, regulation, and significance of progesterone receptors in human meningiomas," *Steroids*, vol. 65, no. 10-11, pp. 795–800, 2000.

[10] F. M. Verheijen, M. Sprong, H. M. Jacobs et al., "Progesterone receptor isoform expression in human meningiomas," *European Journal of Cancer*, vol. 37, no. 12, pp. 1488–1495, 2001.

[11] S. M. Grunberg, M. H. Weiss, I. M. Spitz et al., "Treatment of unresectable meningiomas with the antiprogesterone agent mifepristone," *Journal of Neurosurgery*, vol. 74, no. 6, pp. 861–866, 1991.

[12] O. Heikinheimo, S. Ranta, S. Grunberg, and I. M. Spitz, "Alterations in sex steroids and gonadotropins in postmenopausal women subsequent to long-term mifepristone administration," *Steroids*, vol. 65, no. 10-11, pp. 831–836, 2000.

[13] I. M. Spitz, S. M. Grunberg, N. Chabbert-Buffet, T. Lindenberg, H. Gelber, and R. Sitruk-Ware, "Management of patients receiving long-term treatment with mifepristone," *Fertility and Sterility*, vol. 84, no. 6, pp. 1719–1726, 2005.

[14] S. M. Grunberg, M. H. Weiss, C. A. Russell et al., "Long-term administration of mifepristone (RU486): clinical tolerance during extended treatment of meningioma," *Cancer Investigation*, vol. 24, no. 8, pp. 727–733, 2006.

[15] M. Touat, G. Lombardi, P. Farina, M. Kalamarides, and M. Sanson, "Successful treatment of multiple intracranial meningiomas with the antiprogesterone receptor agent mif-

epristone (RU486)," *Acta Neurochirurgica*, vol. 156, no. 10, pp. 1831–1835, 2014.
[16] G. Cossu, M. Levivier, R. T. Daniel, and M. Messerer, "The role of mifepristone in meningiomas management: a systematic review of the literature," *BioMed Research International*, vol. 2015, Article ID 267831, 11 pages, 2015.
[17] Y. Ji, C. Rankin, S. Grunberg et al., "Double-blind phase III randomized trial of the antiprogestin agent mifepristone in the treatment of unresectable meningioma: SWOG S9005," *Journal of Clinical Oncology*, vol. 33, no. 34, pp. 4093–4098, 2015.
[18] E.-E. Baulieu, "The steroid hormone antagonist RU486: mechanism at the cellular level and clinical applications," *Endocrinology and Metabolism Clinics of North America*, vol. 20, no. 4, pp. 873–891, 1991.
[19] J. E. Sagers, A. S. Brown, S. Vasilijic et al., "Computational repositioning and preclinical validation of mifepristone for human vestibular schwannoma," *Scientific Reports*, vol. 8, no. 1, p. 5437, 2018.
[20] T. Wannachalee, A. F. Turcu, and R. J. Auchus, "Mifepristone in the treatment of the ectopic adrenocorticotropic hormone syndrome," *Clinical Endocrinology*, vol. 89, no. 5, pp. 570–576, 2018.
[21] R. S. Newfield, I. M. Spitz, C. Isacson, and M. I. New, "Long-term mifepristone (RU486) therapy resulting in massive benign endometrial hyperplasia," *Clinical Endocrinology*, vol. 54, no. 3, pp. 399–404, 2001.
[22] K. S. Cahill and E. B. Clauss, "Treatment and survival of patients with nonmalignant intracranial meningioma: results from the surveillance, epidemiology, and end results program of the national cancer institute," *Journal of Neurosurgery*, vol. 115, no. 2, pp. 259–267, 2011.
[23] E. B. Claus, L. Calvocoressi, M. L. Bondy, J. M. Schildkraut, J. L. Wiemels, and M. Wrensch, "Family and personal medical history and risk of meningioma," *Journal of Neurosurgery*, vol. 115, no. 6, pp. 1072–1077, 2011.
[24] O. Heikinheimo, R. Kekkonen, and P. Lähteenmäki, "The pharmacokinetics of mifepristone in humans reveal insights into differential mechanisms of antiprogestin action," *Contraception*, vol. 68, no. 6, pp. 421–426, 2003.
[25] O. Heikinheimo, K. Kontula, H. Croxatto, I. Spitz, T. Luukkainen, and P. Lähteenmäki, "Plasma concentrations and receptor binding of RU 486 and its metabolites in humans," *Journal of Steroid Biochemistry*, vol. 26, no. 26, pp. 279–284, 1987.
[26] O. Heikinheimo, P. L. A. Laähteenmaäki, E. Koivunen et al., "Metabolism and serum binding of RU 486 in women after various single doses," *Human Reproduction*, vol. 2, no. 5, pp. 379–385, 1987.
[27] O. Heikinheimo and R. Kekkonen, "Dose-response relationships of RU 486," *Annals of Medicine*, vol. 25, no. 1, pp. 71–76, 1993.
[28] O. Heikinheimo, M. Haukkamaa, and P. Lähteenmäki, "Distribution of RU 486 and its demethylated metabolites in humans," *The Journal of Clinical Endocrinology & Metabolism*, vol. 68, no. 2, pp. 270–275, 1989.
[29] P. E. Fewings, R. D. E. Battersby, and W. R. Timperley, "Long-term follow up of progesterone receptor status in benign meningioma: a prognostic indicator of recurrence?" *Journal of Neurosurgery*, vol. 92, no. 3, pp. 401–405, 2000.
[30] P. A. Martineau and M. Levental, "Large endometrial polyp in a patient on long-term mifepristone therapy," *Journal of Ultrasound in Medicine*, vol. 19, no. 2, pp. 487–489, 2000.
[31] G. Schaison, M. George, N. Lestrat, A. Reinberg, and E. E. Baulieu, "Effects of the antiprogesterone steroid RU 486 during midluteal phase in normal women," *The Journal of Clinical Endocrinology & Metabolism*, vol. 61, no. 3, pp. 484–489, 1985.
[32] V. G. Garzo, J. Liu, A. Ulmann, E. Baulieu, and S. S. C. Yen, "Effects of an antiprogesterone (RU486) on the hypothalamic-hypophyseal-ovarian-endometrial Axis during the luteal phase of the menstrual cycle," *The Journal of Clinical Endocrinology & Metabolism*, vol. 66, no. 3, pp. 508–517, 1988.
[33] D. Rubello, N. Sonino, D. Casara, M. E. Girelli, B. Busnardo, and M. Boscaro, "Acute and chronic effects of high glucocorticoid levels on hypothalamic-pituitary-thyroid axis in man," *Journal of Endocrinological Investigation*, vol. 15, no. 6, pp. 437–441, 1992.
[34] J. Abuncham, T. C. A. Vieira, E. R. Barbosa, R. S. Ribeiro, and M. R. A. Martins, "Hormone replacement therapy in hypopituitarism," *Brazilian Archives of Endocrinology and Metabolism*, vol. 47, no. 4, pp. 492–508, 2003.
[35] S. Y. Kim, "Diagnosis and treatment of hypopituitarism," *Endocrinology and Metabolism*, vol. 30, no. 4, pp. 443–455, 2015.
[36] U. M. H. Schrell, M. G. Rittig, M. Anders et al., "Hydroxyurea for treatment of unresectable and recurrent meningiomas. II. Decrease in the size of meningiomas in patients treated with hydroxyurea," *Journal of Neurosurgery*, vol. 86, no. 5, pp. 840–844, 1997.
[37] D. A. Reardon, A. D. Norden, A. Desjardins et al., "Phase II study of Gleevec plus hydroxyurea (HU) in adults with progressive or recurrent meningioma," *Journal of Neuro-Oncology*, vol. 106, no. 2, pp. 409–415, 2012.
[38] E. Mazza, A. Brandes, S. Zanon et al., "Hydroxyurea with or without imatinib in the treatment of recurrent or progressive meningiomas: a randomized phase II trial by Gruppo Italiano Cooperativo di Neuro-Oncologia (GICNO)," *Cancer Chemotherapy and Pharmacology*, vol. 77, no. 1, pp. 115–120, 2016.
[39] M. Karsy, N. Hoang, T. Barth et al., "Combined hydroxyurea and verapamil in the clinical treatment of refractory meningioma: human and orthotopic xenograft studies," *World Neurosurgery*, vol. 86, no. 2, pp. 210–219, 2016.

38

Anti-NMDAR-Positive Small-Cell Lung Cancer Paraneoplastic Limbic Encephalitis: A Case Report and Literature Review

Raman Sohal,[1] Steven H. Adams,[2] Vishal Phogat,[1] Abha Harish,[1] Carlos Ynigo D. Lopez,[3] Michael P. A. Williams,[2] Kamal K. Khurana,[2] Basel Abuzuaiter,[1] Nia Jagroop,[1] and Bhavya Narapureddy[3]

[1]*Department of Medicine, SUNY Upstate Medical University Hospital, 750 E Adams St., Syracuse, NY 13210, USA*
[2]*Department of Pathology, SUNY Upstate Medical University Hospital, 750 E Adams St., Syracuse, NY 13210, USA*
[3]*Department of Neurology, SUNY Upstate Medical University Hospital, 750 E Adams St., Syracuse, NY 13210, USA*

Correspondence should be addressed to Raman Sohal; sohalr@upstate.edu

Academic Editor: Peter Berlit

Introduction. Paraneoplastic limbic encephalitis (PLE) is a rare disease that presents as rapid onset dementia characterized by short-term memory loss (STM), anxiety, and behavioral changes. Anti-NMDAR antibodies are unfrequently reported in PLE associated with small-cell lung cancer (SCLC). Given that PLE can precede the diagnosis of cancer, it is very important that once infectious, metabolic, nutritional, or structural disorders associated with short-term memory loss are ruled out that vigorous effort must be made to rule out underlying malignancy. *Case.* We report a rare case of PLE as the presenting symptom of SCLC. A 72-year-old male with history of COPD was brought to the ED by his wife after he was found to have short-term memory loss, including forgetfulness of his wedding anniversary the day before, and anxiety. Neurological exam showed impaired short-term recall on MOCA. CT head showed no evidence of infarct. Lumbar puncture was performed which showed lymphocytic pleocytosis, a nonspecific inflammatory change. CSF panel was negative for HSV, *Neisseria*, *Hemophilus*, *E. coli*, and HIV. Initial EEG was unremarkable, though a repeat EEG showed mild slowing of the posterior dominant rhythm consistent with mild encephalopathy. MRI showed equivocal increased FLAIR on T2-weighted images in the bilateral temporal lobes, left greater than right. CTA thorax showed bulky mediastinal and right hilar LAD. FNA of the R4 lymph node revealed SCLC. The NM bone scan showed no osteoblastic lesions. While the serum autoantibody panel was positive for anti-NMDAR, the CSF autoantibody panel returned entirely negative. Chemotherapy with etoposide and cisplatin was started on Day 4 of admission. The patient's neurological symptoms showed improvement following chemotherapy. *Conclusion.* This case highlights the importance of recognizing short-term memory loss as a feature of PLE.

1. Case

Our patient is a 72-year-old Caucasian right-handed male with a past medical history significant for hypertension, hypercholesterolemia, COPD, coronary artery disease, and status post a recent umbilical hernia repair, admitted for short-term memory loss that began acutely on a mid-September morning (Day 1). The patient arrived anxious, worried that he was losing his memory. As per the patient's wife, he was feeling well, driving, and behaving normally on the previous day. He had gone to sleep at approximately 21:00 in his normal state of health but awoke the following morning with inability to recall events, including their 50th wedding anniversary party, of the prior day. His wife denied any symptoms of behavioral or personality changes in her husband prior to that ominous morning. The patient had a 50-pack-year smoking history, quitting 2.5 years prior to presentation, but was without any illicit drug or significant alcohol history. The patient's review of systems was positive for cough, congestion, anxiety, confusion, dizziness, and light-headedness only, denying any chest pain, shortness of breath, abdominal pain, loss of consciousness, history of recent falls or injury, weakness, numbness, tingling, speech difficulty, slurred speech, vision changes, headache, vertigo, photophobia, neck pain, nausea, or vomiting.

His vitals were within normal limits, with the exception of his blood pressure which measured 153/78 mm Hg (supine). On neurological examination, the patient was alert and oriented to person, place, month, and year. He was able to follow complex commands crossing his body's midline. On memory span testing, he recalled all three words accurately and immediately with categorical prompts. On the digit span test, he was able to recall five digits forward and four in reverse. Abstraction was preserved. He was without aphasia. Serial 7's were intact, and he was able to spell "world" forward and backwards. He was able to name all his children's names and their spouses but had difficulty with some of his grandchildren's names. He had only 1/3 object recall at three minutes, prompting with these categories did not improve his recall. His cranial nerve, sensory, and motor exams, and cerebellar tests for coordination and gait, were unremarkable. The remainder of the physical exam was normal. His CBC, BMP, LFT, and ammonia values were within normal limits. Ethyl alcohol tested negative. Serum thyroglobulin (0.9 IU/mL) and thyroperoxidase antibody (0.4 IU/mL) counts were normal; however, serum thyroglobulin antibody was elevated at 24.5 IU/mL.

Routine EEG was within range of normal variation. Noncontrast CT head was insignificant for any acute ischemic or hemorrhagic event. MRI brain with and without gadolinium showed no evidence of edema, mass effect, or metastasis, although patchy areas of T2 prolongation in the subcortical and periventricular white matter were noted. These were initially attributed to moderate chronic microvascular white matter ischemic changes in light of the patient's chronological age. Because his chest X-rays showed a widened mediastinum with apparent mass effect and tracheal deviation to the left, a CTA thorax was obtained, which showed bulky mediastinal and right hilar lymphadenopathy concerning for malignancy. Fine-needle aspiration of the R4 lymph nodes was positive for small-cell carcinoma (Figure 1).

At this point, the patient's neurological symptoms were considered to be of possible paraneoplastic etiology. With this new consideration in mind, the MRI brain findings of bilateral (left more than right) medial temporal lobe hyperintensity compared with the rest of the temporal lobes were reassessed by the neurology service as possible manifestations of PLE. However, the neuroradiology service, upon reviewing the brain MRI, was not convinced that the findings represented limbic encephalitis (Figure 2).

Cerebrospinal fluid tests were ordered: protein was WNL at 34 mg/dl and glucose was WNL at 62. CSF was colorless and clear, with 14 RBCs and 6 total nucleated cells. Lymphocytic CSF pleocytosis was detected with 93% lymphocytes and 7% monocytes/macrophages. CSF culture and stain showed 3+ WBCs (WNL) with no organism growth. CSF pathogen panel PCR was negative for the 14 common pathogens responsible for community-acquired meningitis or encephalitis including viruses, bacteria, and yeast. CSF cytology showed no evidence of malignancy. Thus, both MRI and CSF cytology confirmed no metastasis to the brain.

On Day 3 of hospitalization, his MOCA score was 21/30 with deficits in delayed recall, visuospatial ability, and orientation. NM bone scan whole body imaging showed no evidence of osteoblastic metastatic bone disease.

On Day 4, chemotherapy was initiated and the patient received three rounds (a 3-day treatment regimen) of cisplatin/etoposide.

On Day 5, neurological improvement was noted on the second day of cycle 1 of chemotherapy, with the patient able to complete the visuospatial part of MOCA that he had missed previously, although he still had impaired delayed recall. The patient did receive 1 g of solumedrol before deciding with the neurology team to not continue with an IV steroid course because he was improving with chemotherapy. He was discharged after three days of cycle 1 of chemotherapy with encouraging signs of neurological improvement. Radiation oncology was also consulted to initiate radiation therapy as outpatient with a plan for radiation to begin with cycle 2 of chemotherapy.

On Day 13, 18F-FDG PET/CT imaging showed right upper lobe metabolically active lung mass compatible with a lung primary, and right hilar and mediastinal lymphadenopathy compatible with metastatic disease. Otherwise, no metastatic disease was detected. His SCLC was described as cT1cN2M0, stage IIIA. His forgetfulness showed slight improvement.

On Day 18, a serum encephalopathy autoantibody panel returned positive for NMDAR Ab (CBA). Anti-NMDAR antibody was detected when testing at 1 : 10 dilution by a cell-based assay only. Higher titers of antibody were not detected by reflex testing at 1:120 dilution by a tissue-based assay. Samples were sent to Mayo Clinic Laboratories, Rochester, for encephalopathy, autoimmune evaluation, and serum (Test ID: ENS2) which tests for AChR ganglionic neuronal Ab, S; AMPA-R Ab CBA, S; amphiphysin Ab, S; anti-glial nuclear Ab, type 1; anti-neuronal nuclear Ab, type 1; anti-neuronal nuclear Ab, type 2; anti-neuronal nuclear Ab, type 3; CASPR2-IgG CBA, S; CRMP-5-IgG, S; DPPX Ab IFA, S; GABA-B-R Ab CBA, S; GAD65 Ab assay, S; GFAP IFA, S; LGI1-IgG CBA, S; mGluR1 Ab IFA, S; NMDAR Ab CBA, S; N-type calcium channel Ab; P/Q-type calcium channel Ab; Purkinje cell cytoplasmic Ab type 1; Purkinje purkinje cell cytoplasmic Ab type 2; Purkinje cell cytoplasmic Ab type Tr.

On Day 26, on follow-up with the neurologist, the patient's wife reported that the patient's memory had significantly improved, although he intermittently would forget small details or events that happened one day back. No improvement was reported for the patient's anxiety.

On Day 32, a second routine EEG performed in the awake and asleep states showed during drowsiness an increased emergence of theta and delta rhythms and during sleep showed vertex sharp transients and K-complexes. The clinical interpretation of the EEG was that it showed abnormal results with mild slowing of the posterior dominant rhythm consistent with mild encephalopathy.

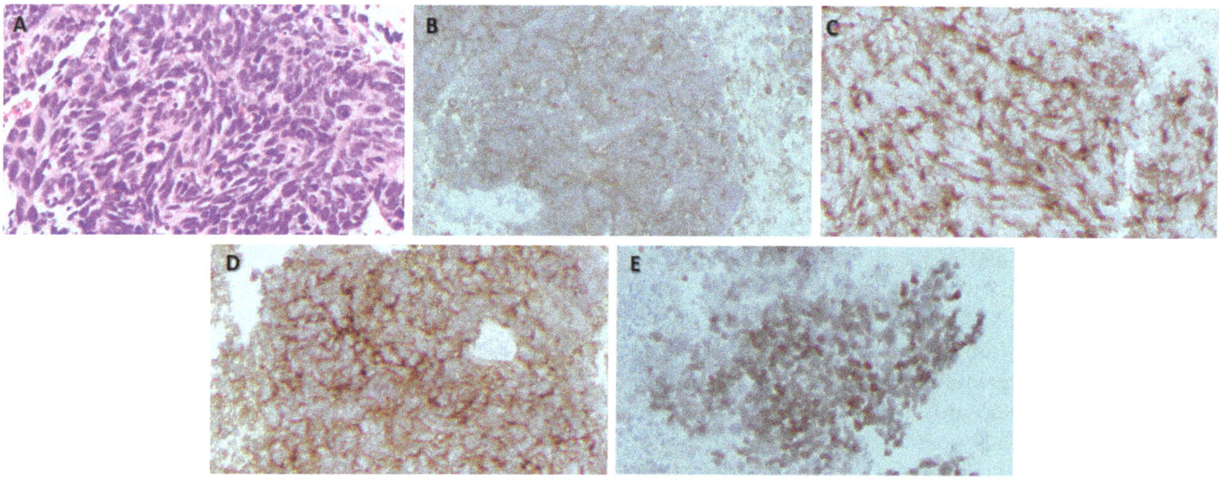

FIGURE 1: Microscopy (slides prepared for cell block analysis): (a) hematoxylin and eosin (H&E) slides consists of malignant cells, single and molding in groups with increased nuclear to cytoplasmic ratios, irregular nuclear contours, and hyperchromatic (200x magnification). ((b)–(e)) Immunohistochemistry (IHC) stains of synaptophysin (b), chromogranin (c), CD56 (d), and TTF-1 (e) are positive in the malignant cells (200x magnification). P63 IHC stain is negative (not shown).

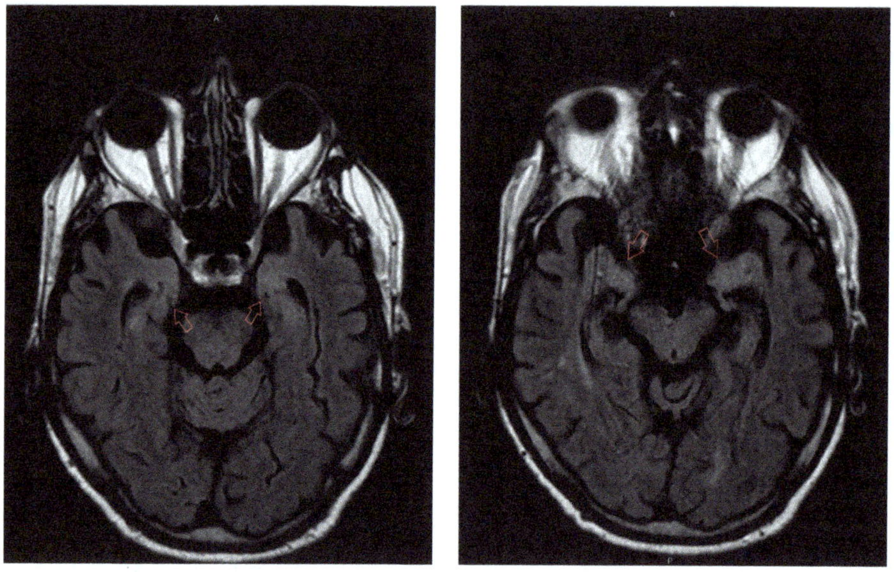

(a) (b)

FIGURE 2: ((a) and (b)) Axial FLAIR MRI showing slight increased signal in bilateral temporal lobes.

On Day 33, paraneoplastic and autoimmune CSF antibody panels returned negative for all antibodies. Specifically, the patient's spinal fluid was sent to Mayo Clinic Laboratories, Rochester, for the encephalopathy, autoimmune evaluation, and spinal fluid (Test ID: ENC2) which tests for AMPA-R Ab CBA, CSF; amphiphysin Ab, CSF; anti-glial nuclear Ab, type 1; anti-neuronal nuclear Ab, type 1; anti-neuronal nuclear Ab, type 2; anti-neuronal nuclear Ab, type 3; CASPR2-IgG CBA, CSF; CRMP-5-IgG, CSF; DPPX Ab IFA, CSF; GABA-B-R Ab CBA, CSF; GAD65 Ab assay, CSF; GFAP IFA, CSF; LGI1-IgG CBA, CSF; mGluR1 Ab IFA, CSF; NMDAR Ab CBA, CSF; Purkinje cell cytoplasmic Ab type Tr; Purkinje cell cytoplasmic Ab type 1; Purkinje cell cytoplasmic Ab type 2.

On Day 46, the patient completed carboplatin/etoposide (cisplatin was discontinued due to kidney disfunction) concurrent with 45 Gy in 1.5 Gy fractions BID radiation.

On Day 96, repeat Brain MRI showed no bitemporal hyperintensities or other acute intracranial processes.

On Day 131, repeat serum encephalopathy autoantibody panel returned entirely negative for any autoantibodies.

On Day 133, complete neurological and cognitive exams showed no deficits. As per the family, he is significantly better, although he still forgets some important dates but can recall them properly when reminded.

On Day 151, the patient completed prophylactic cranial irradiation with 25 Gy/10fx.

On Day 178, the patient continued to remain fully functional and stable.

2. Discussion

Limbic encephalitis (LE) is a rare disorder characterized by rapidly progressive memory loss, acute onset dementia, and personality change. LE may be autoimmune, inflammatory, i.e., paraneoplastic or infectious in etiology. It typically involves components of the limbic system including the anteromedial temporal cortex, hippocampus, and amygdala.

There are multiple causes of rapidly progressive dementia including infectious and metabolic etiologies. The patient should be evaluated for common infectious causes of altered mentation including HSV, HIV, and Creutzfeldt-Jakob disease. Once other metabolic or nutritional deficiencies (e.g., TSH, niacin, thiamine, celiac disease, and alcohol abuse) have been excluded, one must consider the possibility of a paraneoplastic presentation of encephalopathy [1].

Although the etiology of LE is not well understood, the current hypothesis suggests that the body reacts against particular antigens expressed on tumor cells, resulting in antibodies that then cross-react with similar antigens expressed on cells in the limbic system. Anti-Hu Ab, also known as anti-ANNA1, is most closely associated with paraneoplastic LE in SCLC [2], while anti-NMDAR Ab is associated with teratomas [3].

The definition and diagnostic criteria of autoimmune limbic encephalitis are steadily evolving in recent decades as data accumulates. In 2000, Gultekin presented the original diagnostic criteria, which include all four of the following:

(a) Symptoms of short-term memory loss, seizures, or psychiatric symptoms
(b) <4 year between the onset of neurological symptoms and the cancer diagnosis
(c) Exclusion of metastasis, infection, metabolic and vitamin deficits, and stroke etiologies
(d) ≥1 of the following:
    (i) CSF with inflammatory abnormalities (pleocytosis, increased protein concentration)
    (ii) Hyperintensities on MRI FLAIR or T2 in the uni or bilateral temporal lobes
    (iii) EEG with epileptic or slow activity involving the temporal lobes focally [4]

Our patient meets each of the abovementioned criteria: (a) he presented with STM loss, (b) with only two days between the onset of neurological symptoms and the cancer diagnosis. (c) CT and MRI showed no evidence of stroke or metastasis. The patient was afebrile, without leukocytosis, and without focal neurological deficits beyond his STM loss. The CSF pathogen panel returned negative. EEG showed no evidence of CJD. (d) (i) CSF showed lymphocytic pleocytosis, (ii) bilateral medial temporal lobe hyperintensities were present (left more than right) on Axial FLAIR. However, the latter finding had some degree of ambiguity and disagreement on interpretation. (iii) Notably, a repeat EEG showed mild slowing of the posterior dominant rhythm. Some experts opine that slowing of any kind on EEG, taken together with other clinical and imaging findings, is supportive of limbic encephalitis [5].

In 2005, Graus and Saiz suggested a revised set of criteria which included laboratory detection of a paraneoplastic antibody. More recently, there is a growing consensus that antibody status should not be included in the mandatory diagnostic criteria of autoimmune or paraneoplastic limbic encephalitis. This is because several weeks may pass before antibody tests' results return and, importantly, absence of antibodies does not necessarily exclude an autoimmune origin (see discussion below). Rather, the diagnosis should be driven by clinical presentation, imaging studies, and exclusion of infectious etiologies through more rapid serum and CSF laboratory tests [5, 6].

In 2016, several experts suggested a revised set of diagnostic criteria for definitive autoimmune limbic encephalitis, which includes all four of the following:

(1) Subacute onset (less than 3 months) of working memory deficits, seizures, or psychiatric symptoms
(2) Bilateral MRI brain abnormalities on medial temporal lobes
(3) At least one of the following: (a) CSF pleocytosis and (b) EEG with epileptic or slow wave activity in the temporal lobes
(4) Reasonable exclusion of alternative causes

If one of the first three criteria is not met, a diagnosis of definite LE can be made only by the detection of antibodies against cell-surface, synaptic, or onconeural proteins [6].

These criteria were intended for an umbrella diagnosis of limbic encephalitis. However, studies by Dalmau et al. in 2007-2008 of anti-NMDA-receptor-positive LE suggest that this particular form of LE should be treated as a new subcategory with its own diagnostic criteria. Of 92 anti-NMDAR-Ab-positive patients with EEG monitoring, 77% showed slow delta or theta activity, generalized or in frontotemporal regions. Only 22 of 100 anti-NMDAR-positive patients showed increased signal in the medial temporal lobes [7]. These findings of Dalmau et al. suggest that unlike the diagnostic criteria for the umbrella LE disease entity in anti-NMDAR encephalitis, MRI abnormalities on medial temporal lobe abnormalities should be unnecessary for diagnosis.

Of note, anti-NMDAR Ab alone is not specific to limbic encephalitis as it also can be found in multiple sclerosis and neuromyelitis optica [8].

It is significant that unlike our elderly male patient positive for serum anti-NMDAR Abs with SCLC, anti-NMDAR Abs have been more frequently described in younger women presenting with ovarian teratomas and in young men with testicular germ cell tumors [9]. Furthermore, in the literature, PLE SCLC is closely linked to anti-Hu Abs, not anti-NMDAR Abs of our patient [2].

Ironically, in our patient with neurological symptoms, the CSF was negative for autoimmune antibodies, while serum was found to be positive for anti-NMDAR Abs. The reason for such findings is unclear. However, in general, approximately half of autoimmune encephalitis cases are found to be antibody negative. Reasons for these frequent negative findings may include insensitivity of current clinical antibody testing, false-negative results caused by an insufficient quantity of antibody, and other technical issues such as antigen denaturation during tissue fixation. Furthermore, as in recent years, many new CNS autoantibodies have been discovered (e.g., anti-NMDAR, anti-LGI1, anti-Caspr2, and anti-GABAB receptor), and it is plausible that CNS inflammation in LE in some cases is caused by unknown or newly discovered autoantibodies that are not yet available for laboratory testing. In addition, there is a possibility that the temporal lobe inflammation is not antibody mediated [5, 8].

The goal of PLE therapy is to decrease the presentation of the antigen-expressing tumor cells, thereby limiting the number of cross-reactive antibodies. This goal is accomplished by tumor resection, radiation, chemotherapy, and immunosuppressive therapies [10]. In the study of Dalmau et al., at median 17-month follow-up, 47% attained full recovery, 46% remained with neuropsychiatric deficits, and 7% died from the disease—with treatments including tumor resection, intravenous immunoglobulin, plasma exchange, corticosteroids, rituximab, cyclophosphamide, and azathioprine [7] Patients typically do not have good response to first-line therapy. Our patient received only a single dose of one gram of solumedrol prior to decision to discontinue due to significant improvement with initiation of chemotherapy (cisplatin and etoposide). Not only did the patient have a remarkably good response without the need for immunotherapy but also improvement was noted almost immediately following the administration of chemotherapy. Such a response is not typically anticipated and noteworthy in this case for 3 reasons. Firstly, drastic improvement was seen despite this patient not being of the typical age group (young, female). Secondly, the presenting malignancy was atypical to the corresponding autoantibody (small-cell lung cancer which is more tightly associated with anti-Hu antibodies and present in elderly men). Thirdly, there was no CSF detection of the NMDAR antibody which is unusual but possible in the proper clinical context, and it was the likely diagnosis in this case as patient had significant response to a decrease in antigen burden once chemotherapy was initiated. Our patient with SCLC showed significant improvement in neurological status after chemotherapy and radiation. He remained stable at 6-month follow-up.

3. Conclusion

Our case brings attention to anti-NMDAR SCLC PLE, an uncommon disease entity. It is clear that the understanding of PLE, its subcategories, and accurate diagnostic criteria are continuously evolving as more data are reported and studied.

References

[1] I. W. Altabakhi, H. M. Babiker, Paraneoplastic limbic encephalitis-StatPearls-NCBI bookshelf, https://www.ncbi.nlm.nih.gov/books/NBK519523/.

[2] H. Senties-Madrid and F. Vega-Boada, "Paraneoplastic syndromes associated with anti-Hu antibodies," *The Israel Medical Association Journal : IMAJ*, vol. 3, no. 2, pp. 94–103, 2001.

[3] J. A. Braverman, C. Marcus, and R. Garg, "Anti-NMDA-receptor encephalitis: a neuropsychiatric syndrome associated with ovarian teratoma," *Gynecologic Oncology Reports*, vol. 14, pp. 1–3, 2015.

[4] S. H. Gultekin et al., "Paraneoplastic limbic encephalitis: neurological symptoms, immunological findings and tumour association in 50 patients," *Brain*, vol. 123, no. 7, pp. 1481–1494, 2000.

[5] A. Ganesh and S. F. Wesley, "Practice Current: when do you suspect autoimmune encephalitis and what is the role of antibody testing?" *Neurology: Clinical Practice*, vol. 8, no. 1, pp. 67–73, 2018.

[6] F. Graus, M. J. Titulaer, R. Balu et al., "A clinical approach to diagnosis of autoimmune encephalitis," *The Lancet Neurology*, vol. 15, no. 4, pp. 391–404, 2016.

[7] J. Dalmau, A. J. Gleichman, E. G. Hughes et al., "Anti-NMDA-receptor encephalitis: case series and analysis of the effects of antibodies," *The Lancet Neurology*, vol. 7, no. 12, pp. 1091–1098, 2008.

[8] S. K. Lee and S.-T. Lee, "The laboratory diagnosis of autoimmune encephalitis," *Journal of Epilepsy Research*, vol. 6, no. 2, pp. 45–50, 2016.

[9] S. Boangher, P. Mespouille, C.-M. Filip, and S. Goffette, "Small-cell lung cancer with positive anti-NMDAR and anti-AMPAR antibodies paraneoplastic limbic encephalitis," *Case Reports in Neurological Medicine*, vol. 2016, Article ID 3263718, 3 pages, 2016.

[10] K. Shen, Y. Xu, H. Guan et al., "Paraneoplastic limbic encephalitis associated with lung cancer," *Scientific Reports*, vol. 8, no. 1, 2018.

39

Thunderclap Headache: A Primary Symptom of a Steroid-Responsive Encephalopathy with Autoimmune Thyroiditis

Naman Zala[1] **Lena Wirth,**[1] **Berit Jordan,**[1] **Hagen Meredig,**[2] **and Timolaos Rizos**[1]

[1]*Department of Neurology, Heidelberg University Hospital, Im Neuenheimer Feld 400, Heidelberg 69120, Germany*
[2]*Department of Neuroradiology, Heidelberg University Hospital, Im Neuenheimer Feld 400, Heidelberg 69120, Germany*

Correspondence should be addressed to Naman Zala; namanz@gmail.com

Academic Editor: Ritsuo Hashimoto

Thunderclap headache is frequently associated with serious intracranial vascular disorders and a usual reason for emergency department admissions. Association of thunderclap headaches with autoimmune disorders, such as steroid-responsive encephalopathy with autoimmune thyroiditis (SREAT), is highly unusual. Here, we report a patient who presented with high-intensity headache of abrupt onset. Cerebrospinal fluid (CSF) analysis revealed moderate lymphocytic pleocytosis without evidence of infectious, neoplastic, or metabolic causes. Brain magnetic resonance imaging showed no specific pathologies, and examinations for neuronal antibodies in serum and CSF were negative. The medical history revealed that seven years before, an episode of an aseptic meningoencephalitis with remarkable response to steroids was present. Finally, increased levels of serum anti-TPO antibodies were identified, and against the background of a previous steroid-responsive aseptic meningoencephalitis, diagnosis of SREAT was highly probable. Methylprednisolone therapy was initiated, and the patient recovered completely. In particular, because most SREAT patients respond very well to steroids, this case underlines the importance of taking SREAT into consideration during the assessment of a high-intensity headache of abrupt onset.

1. Introduction

A high-intensity headache of abrupt onset (thunderclap headache) is a very common reason for seeking urgent medical advice [1]. By definition, thunderclap headache is of abrupt onset, reaching maximum intensity in less than 1 minute and lasting for at least 5 minutes or more [2]. Thunderclap headache is frequently associated with serious intracranial vascular disorders, including all types of intracranial hemorrhage (epidural, subdural, subarachnoid, or intracerebral hemorrhage), cerebral venous thrombosis, unruptured or thrombosed vascular malformation (mostly aneurysm), arterial dissection (intra- and extracranial), reversible cerebral vasoconstriction syndrome (RCVS), and pituitary apoplexy [3]. Other causes of thunderclap headache are meningitis, colloid cysts, spontaneous intracranial hypotension, and acute sinusitis (particularly with barotrauma) [2, 3]. A randomized population-based prospective study estimated an annual incidence of 43 cases per 100,000 adults [4].

In contrast to thunderclap headache, steroid-responsive encephalopathy with autoimmune thyroiditis (SREAT) is a rare disease, affecting only approximately 2.1 in 100.000 people [5]. SREAT is an autoimmune disorder presenting with neurological and neuropsychiatric symptoms and elevated titers of antithyroid antibodies. By definition, SREAT is associated with subacute onset of encephalopathy, presence of thyroid antibodies (antithyroid peroxidase antibodies and antithyroglobulin antibodies), and proven neurological improvement after immunotherapy, in the absence of other neural autoantibodies [6]. It is recognized as a rare disease with diagnosis based on a rigorous clinical assessment and comprehensive testing for well-characterized neuronal antibodies to exclude other potential causes of encephalopathy [7]. The clinical presentation of patients with SREAT is highly variable, encompassing a broad spectrum of complaints and symptoms [8]. Particularly due to the broad variety of clinical manifestations and subtlety of symptoms, which may be acute or chronic [9], diagnosing SREAT remains a major challenge.

Although headache and, in particular, migraine-like headaches are reported in SREAT patients, sudden and severe headache (i.e., thunderclap headache) as the first symptom has not yet been documented. Thus, we here report a case with thunderclap headache being the initial symptom of a relapsing SREAT.

2. Case Report

A 79-year-old Caucasian female with known history of hypertension, diabetes mellitus type 2, hypothyroidism, and mild renal impairment was admitted to our emergency department (ED) because of a sudden onset of severe bifrontal headache. The headache was rated by the patient as 8/10 on the numeric rating scale for pain. Along with that, she complained of difficulties in concentration. There were no preceding trauma and no history of migraine or other intermittent headaches. The initial neurological examination was normal. Cranial computer tomography showed minor microangiopathic and major macroangiopathic changes and strio-pallido-dentate calcifications but no other pathologies. Standard laboratory results revealed a mild microcytic hypochrome anaemia (Hb: 9,9 g/dl, MCV: 77fl, and MCH: 25pg) and a mild impaired renal function (glomerular filtration rate: 48 ml/min). Metamizole (2 g/d) was administered, which led to significant improvement and discharge.

Within 24 hours of being discharged, the patient experienced difficulty in speaking, and she was referred again to our ED. The neurological examination at admission still remained normal, especially with no signs of aphasia or dysarthria. Within hours, the patient became delirious with partially aggressive behavior accompanied by optic hallucinations. Brain magnetic resonance imaging (MRI) showed minor microangiopathic changes along with small left temporoparietal postischemic defects. Moreover, bilateral strio-pallido-dentate calcifications and minor artifacts in the left occipital region related to calcification of the tentorium were noticed. A cerebrospinal fluid (CSF) analysis showed moderate lymphocytic pleocytosis (48 cells/μl; total protein: 0.695 g/l; glucose: 78.0 mg/dl; lactate: 1.8 mmol/l). Under the suspicion of an infectious meningoencephalitis, broad-spectrum antimicrobial and antiviral therapy with ceftriaxone and acyclovir was initiated. The microbiological analysis of CSF showed no evidence of any bacterial or fungal pathogen. The polymerase chain reaction tests for herpes simplex 1&2 DNA, varicella zoster DNA, cytomegalovirus DNA, Ebstein–Barr virus DNA, enterovirus RNA, as well as specific anti-Borrelia burgdorferi antibodies (IgG & IgM) were negative. We then considered an ictal phenomenon as a possible differential diagnosis for the presenting symptoms and started antiepileptic therapy with valproic acid (900 mg/d). Nevertheless, the electroencephalography (EEG) showed no signs of epileptiform discharges or any abnormal background EEG frequencies. Even after an intravenous antimicrobial therapy for seven days, the patient's clinical state remained to a large extent unchanged. The neuropsychological screening (Montreal Cognitive Assessment: 13/30 points) showed a considerable cognitive deterioration. We decided to perform a follow-up CSF analysis to rule out the presence of paraneoplastic neuronal antibodies as a probable cause of the meningoencephalitis. Again, a moderate lymphocytic pleocytosis was observed (34 cells/μl; total protein: 0.609 g/l; glucose: 59.0 mg/dl; lactate: 1.7 mmol/l), and a serological and CSF analysis provided no signs of any pathogens. Antineuronal antibody analysis revealed normal results for anti-Hu, Ri, ANNA-3, Yo, Tr/DNER, Ma/Ta, GAD65, amphiphysin, aquaporin-4, MOG, glutamate receptors (Type NMDA and AMPA), GABA A/B receptors, LGI1, CASPR2, IgLON5, ZIC4, DPPX, anti-myelin, glycin receptors, mGluR1, mGluR5, Rho-GTPase activating protein 26, ITPR1, Homer 3, recoverin, neurochondrin, GluRD2, and flotillin ½. In conjunction to this, the CSF biomarkers for dementia showed elevated levels of tau protein (478 pg/ml, norm: <450 pg/ml) and phospho-tau protein (90 pg/ml, norm: <61 pg/ml) as well as a reduced Aß ratio (0.38, norm: >0.5). On the 10th day after hospitalization, the symptoms remained mostly unchanged, and follow-up brain MRI was conducted. Compared to the first MRI, progressive leptomeningeal and sulcal T2/fluid-attenuated inversion recovery (FLAIR) hyperintensities parieto-occipital on both sides and temporoparietal on the left side were seen. Moreover, increasing unspecific subcortical and periventricular T2-FLAIR hyperintensities were observed (Figure 1). Careful reevaluation of the medical history revealed a preceding episode of aseptic meningoencephalitis seven years before with comparable clinical findings. Although an extensive diagnostic analysis at that occasion showed no conclusive cause of the meningoencephalitis, there were remarkable effects of the steroid therapy. Based on this, we recommended a probatoric treatment with steroids. However, because the medication with steroids initially caused severe worsening of neuropsychiatric symptoms seven years ago, the patient's legal representatives rejected this recommendation and urged to discharge the patient which was then done.

Five days later, our patient was again referred to our ED because of the worsening of the neuropsychiatric symptoms, in particular, the visual and the auditory hallucinations. We again conducted a CSF analysis which showed no relevant changes (lymphocytic pleocytosis: 43 cells/μl; protein: 0.457 g/l; glucose: 59 mg/dl; and lactate 1.8 mmol/l; and no evidence of intrathecal IgG or IgM synthesis). Although the patient had a known history of hypothyroidism, autoimmunological laboratory diagnostic regarding thyroid antibodies was never conducted. Taking the aforementioned medical history into consideration, we augmented previous laboratory tests with autoimmune thyroid antibodies which was not done seven years ago. Here, antithyroid peroxidase antibodies (anti-TPO antibodies) were markedly increased (344 IU/l, norm: <60IU/l). Nevertheless, the thyroid-stimulating hormone (TSH), thyroxine (T4), and the triiodothyronine (T3) were within normal ranges. The ultrasound

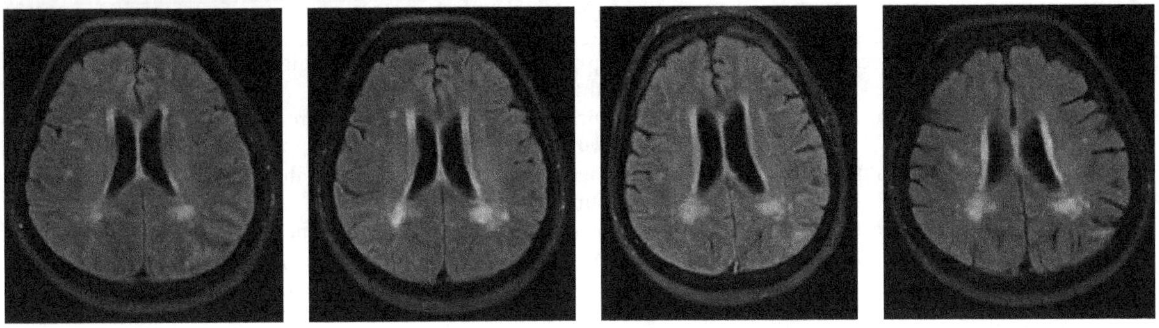

(a) (b) (c) (d)

FIGURE 1: FLAIR images (a–d) showing progressive diffuse signal abnormality involving the white matter of both cerebral hemispheres over 7-year period (a–c) with gradual resolving after steroid treatment (d). (a) June 2012. (b) October 2012. (c) July 2019. (d) February 2020.

of the thyroid gland revealed no clear evidence of thyroiditis, and the patient was clinically in an euthyroid state.

Together with the history of steroid-responsive aseptic meningoencephalitis in 2012, diagnosis of SREAT was highly probable, and a high-dose immunosuppressive therapy with intravenous methylprednisolone (1000 mg i.v. for 3 days, with tapering oral dose at a rate of 10 mg/week thereafter and eventual maintenance dose of 10 mg/day) was commenced. Under this treatment regime, neuropsychiatric symptoms showed clear and fast improvements. Visual and auditory hallucinations resolved completely after 3 days. Also, the neuropsychological screening (Montreal Cognitive Assessment: 19/30 points) showed improvement. Three months later, the patient was seen in our outpatient department. The CSF analysis at that time was completely normal (3 cells/μl; protein: 0.52 g/l; glucose: 72.0 mg/dl; lactate: 1.88 mmol/l). In addition to this, the neuropsychological deficits had improved remarkably. A follow-up brain MRI showed clear signs of improvement. Maintenance dose of oral steroids was further reduced to 5 mg/day and continued to prevent a further relapse of SREAT.

3. Discussion and Conclusion

Steroid-responsive encephalopathy with autoimmune thyroiditis is a rare but very serious illness. Importantly, no SREAT-specific clinical, laboratory, or radiological findings are existent, and the disease is often missed, underdiagnosed, or diagnosed with a substantial time delay. Hence, it can be assumed that, because of low overall awareness and due to limited diagnostic workup in patients with otherwise unexplained encephalopathy, the incidence of SREAT is underestimated.

Clinically, both sudden onset of focal neurological symptoms and gradually increasing neurological complaints are described. A Chinese study identified cognitive impairment and psychiatric symptoms as the most common presentation [10]. However, in a review by Ferracci and colleagues, seizures and myoclonus were among the most frequently reported events [5]. Two types of SREAT have been suggested. The first being relapsing/remitting, also referred to as vasculitic type, which manifests with encephalopathy and stroke-like episodes [9]. The other is a diffuse progressive type, which has an insidious onset and a progressive course with occasional fluctuations, and manifests with psychiatric symptoms (including confusion and hallucinations), dementia, and impairment of the sleep-wake cycle [9]. Either type may also present with tremor, myoclonus, seizures, stupor, or coma [9]. Importantly, the presence of thyroid autoantibodies and steroid responsiveness of symptoms is deemed mandatory for the final diagnosis (Table 1). Nevertheless, titers of anti-TPO antibodies do not clearly correlate with the severity of the disease or improvement of clinical symptoms [11].

Thunderclap headache in a patient without a history of migraine or other intermittent headaches being the primary symptom of a steroid-responsive encephalopathy with autoimmune thyroiditis represents a peculiarity of our case. In SREAT, headache may occur in up to 80% of the patients, but it is normally mild or periodic, not a presenting sign, and is usually attributed to previous migraine and hypothyroidism. The pathogenesis of SREAT is still unclear. Whether the existence of antithyroid antibodies only represents an epiphenomenon in the setting of SREAT or whether they represent a pathogenic factor is still unknown. It could be speculated that an associated inflammatory response may result in perivascular nociceptor activation which might have led to a thunderclap headache in our patient. Because of the broad number of possible differential diagnosis, including subarachnoid hemorrhages, associated with sudden severe headache, a thorough medical clarification is of utmost importance.

There are reports of different MRI findings ranging from mild generalized cerebral atrophy, bilateral subcortical lacunar infarcts, generalized leukoencephalopathy, diffuse signal abnormality involving the white matter of both cerebral hemispheres, as well as cerebellar and cerebral peduncles in patients with SREAT [12]. Our patient had documented evolving MRI changes spanning 7 years of diffuse leukoencephalopathy, mild cortical atrophy, and increased T2/FLAIR white matter and sulcal hyperintensities as well as leptomeningeal enhancements (Figure 2) illustrating a wide range of MRI changes that can be seen in a single case of SREAT.

Table 1: Diagnostic criteria for SREAT [6, 14].

1.	Encephalopathy characterized by cognitive impairment, neuropsychiatric symptoms, myoclonus, partial or generalized tonic-clonic epileptic seizures, and focal neurological deficits
2.	Euthyroid, subclinical, or mild-to-moderate clinical hypothyroidism (with corresponding TSH levels)
3.	Normal brain MRI or with nonspecific abnormalities
4.	Presence of antithyroperoxidase antibody and possibly antithyroglobulin antibody and/or anti-thyroid-stimulating hormone receptor stimulating antibody
5.	Absence of well-characterized neuronal antibodies in serum and CSF
6.	No evidence of infectious, toxic, neoplastic, or (other than thyroid-associated) metabolic disease
7.	Complete or near complete remission with steroid therapy

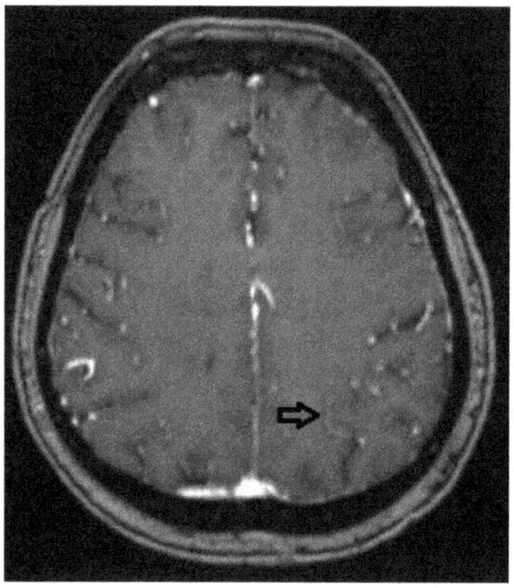

Figure 2: MRI from June 2012 showing hyperperfusion of the leptomeningeal arteries (black arrow).

The optimal dose of oral steroids is not known and is primarily based on the individual's response to treatment. Although steroid responsiveness represents a SREAT defining factor, more aggressive and long-term immunosuppressive therapy is needed in some cases [13]. In our patient, steroid therapy led to a complete remission of symptoms, and CSF results were normalized.

To conclude, the present case underlines that awareness for SREAT is important when evaluating patients with acute onset of high-intensity headache associated with neuropsychiatric symptoms, particularly because most patients respond very well to steroids.

Authors' Contributions

All authors have read and approved the case report before submission. N.Z., T.R., and L.W. drafted and revised the manuscript and interpretated clinical data. H.M. and B.J. revised the manuscript for important intellectual content.

References

[1] J. J. Craig and V. H. Patterson, "Headaches in the accident and emergency department," *British Journal of Hospital Medicine*, vol. 57, pp. 202–206, 1997.

[2] Headache Classification Committee of the International Headache Society (IHS), "The international classification of headache disorders, 3rd edition," *Cephalalgia*, vol. 33, pp. 629–808, 2013.

[3] E. Devenney, H. Neale, and R. B. Forbes, "A systematic review of causes of sudden and severe headache (thunderclap headache): should lists be evidence based?" *The Journal of Headache and Pain*, vol. 15, p. 49, 2014.

[4] A.-M. Landtblom, S. Fridriksson, J. Boivie, J. Hillman, G. Johansson, and I. Johansson, "Sudden onset headache: a prospective study of features, incidence and causes," *Cephalalgia*, vol. 22, no. 5, pp. 354–360, 2002.

[5] F. Ferracci, G. Bertiato, and G. Moretto, "Hashimoto's encephalopathy: epidemiologic data and pathogenetic considerations," *Journal of the Neurological Sciences*, vol. 217, no. 2, pp. 165–168, 2004.

[6] P. Castillo, B. Woodruff, R. Caselli et al., "Steroid-responsive encephalopathy associated with autoimmune thyroiditis," *Archives of Neurology*, vol. 63, no. 2, pp. 197–202, 2006.

[7] F. Graus, M. J. Titulaer, R. Balu et al., "A clinical approach to diagnosis of autoimmune encephalitis," *The Lancet Neurology*, vol. 15, no. 4, pp. 391–404, 2016.

[8] J. Y. Zhou, B. Xu, J. Lopes, J. Blamoun, and L. Li, "Hashimoto encephalopathy: literature review," *Acta Neurologica Scandinavica*, vol. 135, no. 3, pp. 285–290, 2017.

[9] I. Kothbauer-Margreiter, M. Sturzenegger, J. Komor, R. Baumgartner, and C. W. Hess, "Encephalopathy associated with Hashimoto thyroiditis: diagnosis and treatment," *Journal of Neurology*, vol. 243, no. 8, pp. 585–593, 1996.

[10] Y. Tang, Y. Xing, M. Lin, J. Zhang, and J. Jia, "Hashimoto's encephalopathy cases: Chinese experience," *BMC Neurology*, vol. 12, p. 60, 2012.

[11] G. A. Marshall and J. J. Doyle, "Long-term treatment of hashimoto's encephalopathy," *The Journal of Neuropsychiatry and Clinical Neurosciences*, vol. 18, no. 1, pp. 14–20, 2006.

[12] N. I. L. J. Bohnen, K. J. Parnell, and C. M. Harper, "Reversible MRI findings in a patient with hashimoto's encephalopathy," *Neurology*, vol. 49, no. 1, pp. 246-247, 1997.

[13] P. J. Shaw, T. J. Walls, P. K. Newman, P. G. Cleland, and N. E. F. Cartlidge, "Hashirnoto's encephalopathy: a steroid-responsive disorder associated with high anti-thyroid antibody titers--report of 5 cases," *Neurology*, vol. 41, no. 2, pp. 228–233, 1991.

[14] Dgn leitlinien, ll-32-2012-immunvermittelte erkrankungen der grauen zns substanz sowie neurosarkoidose (https://dgn.org/leitlinien/2396-ll-32-2012-immunvermittelte-erkrankungen-der-grauen-zns-substanz-sowie-neurosarkoidose?tmpl=component&page=) and NIH Genetic and Rare Diseases Information Center's Hashimoto's encephalitis guidelines (https://rarediseases.info.nih.gov/diseases/8570/hashimotos-encephalitis).

40

Posterior Reversible Leukoencephalopathy Syndrome in a Patient after Acute COVID-19 Infection

Ketino Kobaidze,[1] Yoo Mee Shin,[2] Mariam Japaridze,[3] Ioannis Karakis,[4] and Xin Wu[5]

[1]*Associate Professor of Medicine, Emory University School of Medicine, Division of Hospital Medicine 550 Peachtree Street, Atlanta, GA 30308, USA*
[2]*Division of Hospital Medicine, Emory University School of Medicine, Atlanta, GA 30308, USA*
[3]*Ross University School of Medicine, New Jersey, USA*
[4]*Department of Neurology, Emory University School of Medicine, Atlanta, GA 30308, USA*
[5]*Department of Radiology and Imaging Science, Emory University School of Medicine, Atlanta, GA 30308, USA*

Correspondence should be addressed to Ketino Kobaidze; kkobaid@emory.edu

Academic Editor: Isabella Laura Simone

The SARS-CoV-2 infection affects numerous organs, including the central nervous system. The neuroinvasive abilities and neuroinflammation may lead to short- and long-term neurological manifestations. Among neurological disorders associated with SARS-CoV-2 infection, posterior reversible encephalopathy syndrome (PRES) has been described in a few case-based observational studies during the acute phase of COVID-19 hospitalization. We present a case of a patient who developed seizures and PRES after recovering from an acute severe COVID-19 infection.

A 90-year-old African American female with multiple comorbidities and a severe COVID-19 infection was discharged home in stable condition after two weeks of hospitalization. A week later, she developed new-onset generalized tonic-clonic seizures requiring readmission to the hospital. The patient's clinical course and brain imaging supported PRES. Her mentation returned to baseline with supportive care and anticonvulsant treatment. Follow-up brain MRI four months later demonstrated resolution of FLAIR signal abnormalities confirming PRES. SARS-CoV-2 insult on the cerebrovascular endothelial cells likely continued and despite the clinical recovery eventually resulted in PRES. We believe that this is the first case describing the presentation of PRES after recovery from severe acute COVID-19 infection.

1. Introduction

Posterior reversible encephalopathy (PRES) is a neurological syndrome of cerebral dysautoregulation which can occur in multiple settings, including but not limited to acute migraine, occipital epilepsy, eclampsia/preeclampsia, hypertensive encephalopathy, and the use of cytotoxic and immunosuppressive medications [1]. While helpful in establishing the diagnosis, neuroimaging studies are unable to distinguish between the varying etiologies. Disruption of cerebral autoregulation combined with endothelial dysfunction appears to play important roles in the development of this clinical condition, which has been seen to be a result of transitional vasospasm, ischemic injury, or vasogenic edema, due to increased capillary permeability. Patients in all age groups are susceptible, though it has a slightly higher predilection for women.

The currently ongoing novel COVID-19 pandemic has affected millions of individuals across the globe, and there are over 539, 038 fatal cases reported in the United States alone [2]. Widespread dysregulation of pulmonary, renal, cardiac, and circulatory homeostasis contributes to morbidity and mortality in COVID-19 patients [3]. Knowledge about COVID-19's clinical presentation and disease progression is rapidly growing. However, less known are longer-term outcomes, especially for patients who are discharged from hospitals after severe acute COVID-19 infection.

There is already ample evidence that neurological complications of SARS-CoV-2 are common and may precede respiratory symptoms [4–8]. The expression of angiotensin-converting enzyme 2 (ACE-2) in brain vasculature creates an opportunity for the virus to enter into CNS cells, resulting in harm to neurological tissue [6, 9, 10]. It alters the blood-brain barrier permeability, which may result in brain autoregulation and vascular circulation disruption [11]. Several neurological complications of COVID-19 infection have been described in the literature. Patients may present with headache, acute encephalopathy, encephalitis, ischemic or hemorrhagic stroke, demyelinating neuropathy (Guillain–Barre syndrome), anosmia, ageusia, and seizures [3, 6, 7, 9].

Endothelial dysfunction in the setting of COVID-19 may contribute to PRES, as this complication has been described among hospitalized patients with COVID-19 [5]. Neurologic effects of SARS-CoV-2 may have long-term consequences. We present a case of an elderly patient who developed seizures and PRES after recovering from the acute phase of COVID-19 infection. We believe that this rare complication was associated with the recent SAR-CoV-2 virus infection affecting the nervous system.

2. Case Presentation

A 90-year-old African American female with a history of type 2 diabetes, essential hypertension, deep venous thrombosis, pulmonary embolism, and atrial flutter on chronic anticoagulation with apixaban presented for new-onset general tonic-clonic seizures, witnessed by her family. The patient had been bed-bound from arthritis in a nursing home, but her mental status had been intact. The patient had recently been hospitalized over 3 weeks ago for COVID-19 pneumonia and was discharged home with home hospice one week before readmission.

According to her family, the patient's mental status had severely declined during her previous hospitalization with COVID-19. She developed staring spells after discharge that culminated into generalized tonic-clonic seizures on the day of the current admission. The episode lasted two seconds. Per her hospice nurse, blood pressures and blood glucose were well controlled at home. The home medications were thoroughly reviewed and found not to have any typical pharmacologic culprits. When she presented to the emergency department, she had two more witnessed seizures. Her blood pressure during this episode was 227/95 mm Hg, her heart rate was 98 beats/min, the temperature was 36.7°C, her respiratory rate was 16 breaths/min, and oxygen saturation was 93% while she breathed room air. Intravenous labetalol, lorazepam, and levetiracetam were administered. Her blood pressure decreased to 160/70 mm Hg and remained well controlled during her hospitalization. Head CT and basic laboratory work (Table 1) were unremarkable. Her physical exam was notable for postictal confusion. She was alert and only oriented to person. An electroencephalogram (EEG) detected no evidence of seizure or epileptiform discharges, but generalized slowing with an intermittent focal slowing in the bilateral temporal regions was noticed (Table 1). Brain MRI demonstrated subcortical and cortical FLAIR signal abnormality involving the left greater than right parieto-occipital lobes and the left temporal lobe, in a pattern most compatible with posterior reversible encephalopathy syndrome (PRES) (Figures 1(a)–1(d)). There was no acute intracranial hemorrhage or infarction.

The patient had no further seizures after being treated with levetiracetam. Her mental state gradually returned to normal. She became more eager to participate in physical therapy and be more independent. She set a goal to walk without her walker and to cook for her family and friends. Her family was pleasantly surprised by this improvement in her mentation. She had no further seizure activity in the hospital and was discharged back home with home care services. She is doing well six months after discharge, is seizure-free, and follows her scheduled appointments. Follow-up MRI four months later after presentation showed complete or near resolution of the lesions (Figures 1(e)–1(h)).

No written consent has been obtained from the patient as there is no patient identifiable data included in the case report.

3. Discussion

The pathogenesis of PRES is controversial and not always clearly defined [10–15]. We speculate that the COVID-19 virus-associated endothelial dysfunction progressed after the acute phase of the disease and likely contributed to PRES in our patient.

PRES has been described in COVID-19 patients in a few case-based observational studies set during the acute phase of COVID-19 hospitalization [1, 16, 17]. We believe that this is the first case describing the presentation of PRES after discharge from initial COVID-19 hospitalization, which may reflect a delayed neurological sequela of SARS-CoV-2 requiring readmission. Our patient did not receive any specific medications for COVID-19 infection but was treated in a clinical trial known as the RESCUE trial with chest single low-dose radiation therapy for severe pneumonia [18].

Our patient's blood pressure during her presentation was elevated only on one occasion after grand mal seizure but was well controlled throughout both hospitalizations and at home. A list of home medications was thoroughly reviewed and found not to have any typical pharmacologic culprits. Her recovery from severe COVID-19 infection-associated pneumonia, acute renal failure, and seizure from PRES was remarkable given her age and multiple comorbidities. Treatment of PRES depends on identifying any potential triggers and removing them. Our patient was treated with supportive care and investigational single low-dose chest radiation during her initial hospitalization [19]. We guess that PRES could be a potential complication of severe COVID-19 infection and in appropriate clinical settings, and PRES diagnosis may prompt the clinician to consider a diagnosis of COVID-19 in the acute or reconvalescent phase.

Table 1: Clinical characteristics during initial hospitalization and readmission.

Variables	Initial admission	Readmission
Reason for admission	Fever	Seizure
Comorbidities	HTN, osteoarthritis, DM 2, VTE, CKD stage 2, atrial flutter, cataract, macular degeneration, right eye blindness, pressure ulcer stage II, mild dementia	HTN, osteoarthritis, DM 2, VTE, CKD stage 2, atrial flutter, cataract, macular degeneration, right eye blindness, pressure ulcer stage II, mild dementia
COVID-19 PCR	Positive At discharge: negative	Not tested
Symptoms of COVID-19	Fever and cough, acute, respiratory failure, altered mental status	NA
Hospital problem list	Acute respiratory failure, viral pneumonia, acute diffuse body pain, DM 2, HTN, acute renal failure, delirium, cystitis, hypokalemia	New-onset seizure, acute metabolic encephalopathy, cystitis, hypomagnesemia, hypokalemia
Risk factors for PRES	N/A	BP fluctuations, recent COVID-19 infection
The onset of PRES from diagnosing COVID-19	NA	31 days
LOS, total	22 days	6 days
LOS, ICU	2 days	0
LOS, floor	20 days	6 days
MAP, range	81–120	91–113
SBP, range	124–192	127–227
Medications	Acetaminophen, apixaban, ceftriaxone, insulin, labetalol, ondansetron, magnesium sulfate, potassium chloride, hydralazine, gabapentin, tramadol	Acetaminophen, apixaban, labetalol, ceftriaxone, insulin, levetiracetam, tramadol (stopped at admission)
Specific treatment for COVID-19	Enrolled in RESCUE trial: received single low-dose chest radiation	

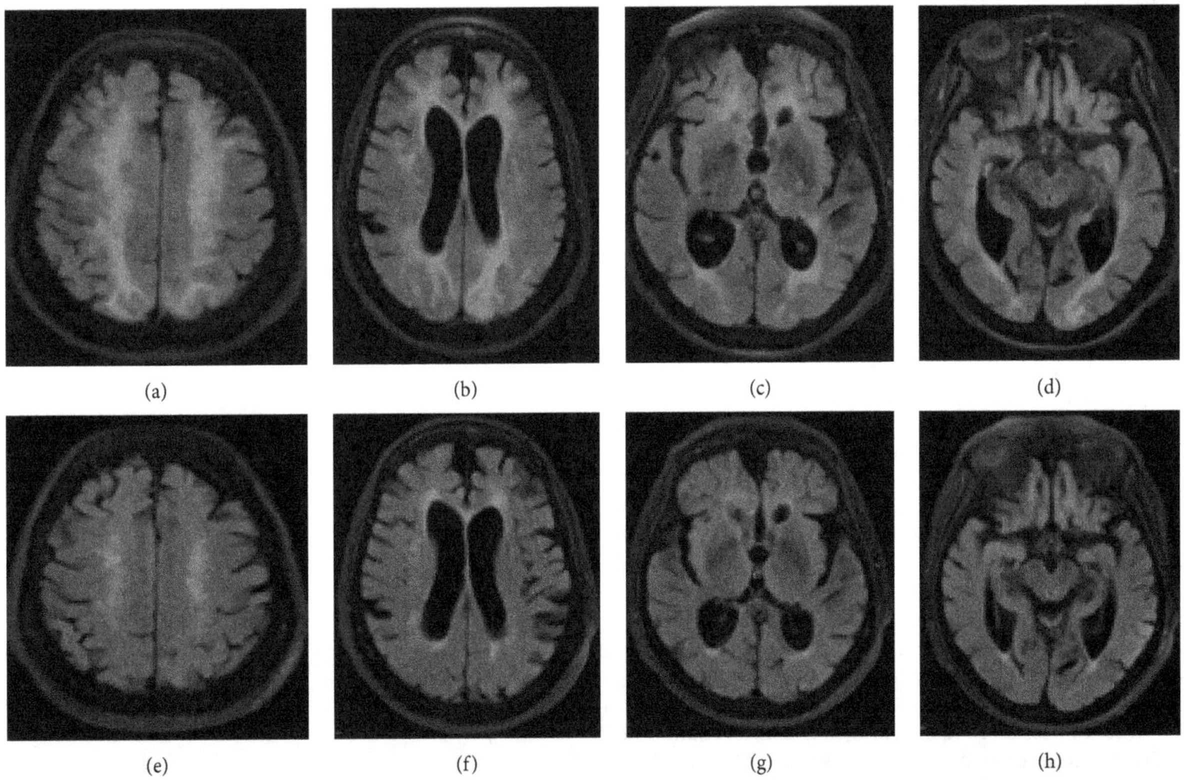

Figure 1: (a–d) Axial FLAIR images at multiple levels demonstrate cortical, subcortical, and periventricular signal hyperintensity and mild mass effect typical of PRES, predominantly involving the bilateral frontal, parietal, and occipital lobes on admission. Follow-up MRI (e–h) images four months after presentation showed resolution of the lesions.

References

[1] M. Fischer and E. Schmutzhard, "Posterior reversible encephalopathy syndrome," *Journal of Neurology*, vol. 264, no. 8, pp. 1608–1616, 2017.

[2] http://www.cdc.gov/covid-data-tracker/#cases.

[3] H. Li, S.-M. Liu, X.-H. Yu, S.-L. Tang, and C.-K. Tang, "Coronavirus disease 2019 (COVID-19): current status and future perspectives," *International Journal of Antimicrobial Agents*, vol. 55, no. 5, p. 105951, 2020.

[4] A. Whittaker, M. Anson, and A. Harky, "Neurological Manifestations of COVID-19: a systematic review and current update," *Acta Neurologica Scandinavica*, vol. 142, no. 1, pp. 14–22, 2020.

[5] L. Kishfy, M. Casasola, P. Banankhah et al., "Posterior reversible encephalopathy syndrome (PRES) as a neurological association in severe Covid-19," *Journal of the Neurological Sciences*, vol. 414, p. 116943, 2020.

[6] Y. Kaya, S. Kara, C. Akinci, and A. S. Kocaman, "Transient cortical blindness in COVID-19 pneumonia; a PRES-like syndrome: case report," *Journal of the Neurological Sciences*, vol. 413, p. 116858, 2020.

[7] R. Bridwell, B. Long, and M. Gottlieb, "Neurologic complications of COVID-19," *American Journal of Emergency Medicine*, vol. 38, no. 7, p. 1549, 2020.

[8] A. M. Baig, A. Khaleeq, U. Ali, and H. Syeda, "Evidence of the COVID-19 virus targeting the CNS: tissue distribution, host-virus interaction, and proposed neurotropic mechanisms," *ACS Chemical Neuroscience*, vol. 11, no. 7, pp. 995–998, 2020.

[9] I. Ahmad and F. A. Rathore, "Neurological manifestations and complications of COVID-19: a literature review," *Journal of Clinical Neuroscience*, vol. 77, pp. 8–12, 2020.

[10] A. Agarwal, M. Pinho, K. Raj et al., "Neurological emergencies associated with COVID-19: stroke and beyond," *Emergency Radiology*, vol. 27, no. 6, p. 747, 2020.

[11] T. Coolen, V. Lolli, N. Sadeghi et al., "Early postmortem brain MRI findings in COVID-19 non-survivors," *Neurology*, vol. 95, pp. e2016–e2027, 2020.

[12] I. Alquisiras-Burgos, I. Peralta-Arrieta, L. A. Alonso-Palomares, A. E. Zacapala-Gómez, E. G. Salmerón-Bárcenas, and P. Aguilera, "Neurological complications associated with the blood-brain barrier damage induced by the inflammatory response during SARS-CoV-2 infection," *Molecular Neurobiology*, vol. 58, no. 2, pp. 520–535, 2021.

[13] R. Garg, N. Kumar, and H. Malhotra, "Posterior reversible encephalopathy syndrome in eclampsia," *Neurology India*, vol. 66, no. 5, pp. 1316–1323, 2018.

[14] S. Deguchi, K. Mitsuya, Y. Nakasu et al., "Posterior reversible encephalopathy syndrome (PRES) induced by pazopanib, a multi-targeting tyrosine kinase inhibitor, in a patient with soft-tissue sarcoma: case report and review of the literature," *Investigational New Drugs*, vol. 36, no. 2, p. 346, 2018.

[15] J. Shankar and J. Banfield, "Posterior reversible encephalopathy syndrome: a review," *Canadian Association of Radiologists Journal*, vol. 68, no. 2, pp. 147–153, 2017.

[16] F. X. Doo, G. Kassim, D. R. Lefton, S. Patterson, H. Pham, and P. Belani, "Rare presentations of COVID19 PRES-like leukoencephalopathy and carotid thrombosis," *Clinical Imaging*, vol. 69, pp. 94–101, 2020.

[17] L. Princiotta Cariddi, P. Tabaee Damavandi, F. Carimati et al., "Reversible Encephalopathy Syndrome (PRES) in a COVID-19 patient," *Journal of Neurology*, vol. 267, pp. 3157–3160, 2020.

[18] S. C. Parauda, V. Gao, A. N. Gewirtz et al., "Posterior reversible encephalopathy syndrome in patients with COVID-19," *Journal of the Neurological Sciences*, vol. 416, p. 117019, 2020 Jul 9.

[19] C. B. Hess, Z. S. Buchwald, W. Stokes et al., "Low-dose whole-lung radiation for COVID-19 pneumonia: planned day 7 interim analysis of a registered clinical trial," *Cancer*, vol. 126, no. 23, pp. 5109–5113, 2020.

41

Protracted COVID-19 during Treatment of Facial Palsy

Mehrdad Hasibi,[1] **Maral Seyed Ahadi**,[2] **Hamed Abdollahi**,[3] **and Mehrdad Jafari**[4]

[1]*Professor of Infectious Diseases, Amiralam Hospital, Tehran University of Medical Sciences, South Saadi St., Tehran, Iran*
[2]*Assistant Professor of Neurology, Amiralam Hospita, Iranian Center of Neurological Research, Neuroscience Institute, Tehran University of Medical Sciences, South Saadi St., Tehran, Iran*
[3]*Assistant Professor, Department of Anesthesiology, Amiralam Hospital, Tehran University of Medical Sciences, South Saadi St., Tehran, Iran*
[4]*Assistant Professor, Department of Otolaryngology—Head and Neck Surgery, Imam Khomeini Hospital Complex, Tehran University of Medical Sciences, Valiasr hospital, Baqerkhan St., Tehran, Iran*

Correspondence should be addressed to Mehrdad Jafari; mehrdadj82@yahoo.com

Academic Editor: Peter Berlit

Neurologic manifestations are increasingly reported as the coronavirus disease 2019 (COVID-19) pandemic continues. This is a report of a COVID-19 patient with Bell's palsy. Case Summary. A 52-year-old man with fever and malaise was tested positive for COVID-19. After a week, he developed right-sided peripheral facial palsy and was treated with corticosteroids in conjunction with antiviral treatment which resulted in complete recovery. Discussion. Concomitant treatment of corticosteroids and antiviral treatment can decrease morbidity in patients with COVID-19-related Bell's palsy.

1. Introduction

The COVID-19 pandemic has been a major health issue affecting millions of people around the world. Although respiratory symptoms are the main clinical features, associated neurologic manifestations are increasingly recognized. Studies have been published describing diverse neurological manifestations from anosmia to life-threatening acute necrotizing encephalopathy. Peripheral facial palsy is one of the neurologic manifestations reported with COVID-19. There is not a consensus regarding facial palsy treatment during the COVID-19 era. This is a report of the successful treatment of a patient with COVID-19-associated facial palsy.

2. Case Report

On July 10, 2020, a 52-year-old man presented to our outpatient clinic in Amiralam Hospital, Tehran, with fever, malaise, and anorexia from 2 days before without any respiratory symptoms. His blood oxygen (O2) saturation was 95% while breathing room air. Other physical examinations were unremarkable. He was diagnosed with COVID-19 based on a positive RT-PCR test result of the nasopharyngeal sample. The patient did not have any risk factors except class 1 obesity; therefore, he was managed in an outpatient setting with capsule Arbidol 200 mg (an antiviral agent) TID and naproxen 250 mg BID for 7 days. Three days later, his fever subsided and other symptoms partially resolved; however, he complained from new-onset mild dry coughs. One week following symptom onset, the patient developed right-sided facial palsy. On physical examinations, he had a grade V House–Brackmann [1] lower motor neuron facial palsy without any other cranial nerve involvement, parotid swelling, or auditory canal lesions. Other neurologic examinations were unremarkable. The result of brain MRI without contrast was normal. He was initially put on 60 mg prednisolone (to be tapered from the sixth day of treatment) and favipiravir tablet 600 mg three times a day. After 5 days of treatment, the facial palsy recovered partially but he complained of increased dry cough and severe malaise. He underwent a spiral chest CT scan which showed multiple

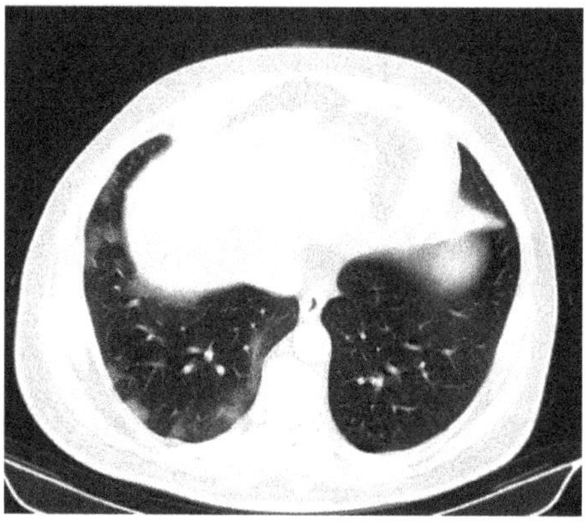

Figure 1: Spiral chest CT scan of the patient on day 12.

bilateral peripheral ground glass opacities with approximately 20% involvement of the lungs (Figure 1). He was admitted and received remdesivir (200 mg on the first day and continued with 100 mg daily from the 2nd to 5th day, afterwards). Oral prednisolone was changed to IV dexamethasone 4 mg BID. The treatment was continued for 5 days. The patient was discharged on the sixth day of admission without any antiviral agents or oral prednisolone tapering. On the discharge day, his facial palsy improved to the grade II/VI and he completely recovered from COVID-19 respiratory symptoms. After three months of follow-up, facial palsy improved completely. Written consent was obtained from the patient for reporting and publishing the results.

3. Discussion

This is a report of unilateral peripheral facial palsy in a COVID-19 patient with an excellent response to combination therapy of corticosteroids and remdesivir. Since the start of the pandemic, various antivirals have been administered off label with the succeeding articles justifying their use. A recent study by Beigel et al. has shown that remdesivir reduces the time to recovery in hospitalized COVID-19 patients [2]. Other studies have shown favapiravir to be effective as an oral agent in reducing viral clearance time [3, 4].

Bell's palsy has an annual incidence of 11.5–53.3 cases per 100,000 in a year in different populations [5]. However, there are increasing reports of Bell's palsy during the pandemic, either due to the viral infection or vaccination [6]. In a study by Codeluppi et al., there was an increased incidence of facial palsy during the COVID-19 pandemic and 21% of patients with Bell's palsy had a recent and active infection [7]. Prior evidence indicates that corticosteroids are effective in the treatment of Bell's palsy. However, there are debates on corticosteroid therapy during the COVID-19 pandemic, and it is reserved for serious cases. A recent consensus recommends treatment with short courses of corticosteroid therapy in grade V and VI Bell's palsy, in the absence of signs and symptoms suggestive of COVID-19 [8]. The concern about corticosteroid therapy is more in patients with COVID-19. Although corticosteroids are one of the mainstays of treatment in severe and critical COVID-19, it is not recommended in patients with mild and moderate symptoms due to potential disease exacerbation [9, 10]. It seems that facial palsy associated with COVID-19 should be treated based on each patient's medical condition, as worse motor function based on House–Brackmann decreases the probability of complete recovery [11, 12]. Goh et al. reported a case of facial palsy 6 days after disease onset. The patient had an isolated lower motor neuron left facial palsy, and he was treated with oral prednisone and valacyclovir and lopinavir/ritonavir to reduce viral replication. However, he did not report a significant improvement after a week of treatment [13]. In another case report, a 57-year-old woman developed an acute left-side facial palsy, a week after developing symptoms of COVID-19. She only received symptomatic treatment and was reported to have a complete recovery after a month [14]. Figueiredo et al. reported a pregnant woman presented with an isolated facial palsy. She had a positive RT-PCR test for SARS-Cov-2 and was treated with corticosteroid, but the outcome was not reported [15]. In a case series by Lima et al., eight patients with COVID-19 and Bell's palsy were evaluated for clinical presentation and outcome [16]. Their patients had mild respiratory and systemic manifestations and grade II-III House–Brackmann, and none required hospitalization; seven patients received steroids from which four patients had complete recovery and three patients had partial recovery. However, concomitant use of antiviral agents is not reported.

There are reports of Bell's palsy following COVID-19 vaccination. Repajic et al. reported the first case of Bell's palsy following the 2nd dose of Pfizer-BioNTech COVID-19 vaccination in a 57-year-old Caucasian female. She was treated with prednisone and an antiviral agent, and her symptoms started to improve from the 14th day [17]. Their choice of antiviral treatment is not reported. Colella et al. also reported a patient developing Bell's palsy after the first dose of Pfizer-BioNTech COVID-19 vaccination [6]. He had a grade V House–Brackmann and received corticosteroids without improvement after 23 days of follow-up.

In our patient, soon after starting corticosteroid treatment, the course of COVID-19 progressed despite oral favipiravir therapy. In our experience, short-term corticosteroid therapy in combination with remdesivir may prove beneficial in patients with severe facial palsy associated with COVID-19. We suggest conduction of future clinical trials on concomitant administration of a potent antiviral agent and corticosteroid therapy in patients with severe Bell's palsy associated with COVID-19 to prevent potential disease exacerbation.

References

[1] J. W. House, "Facial nerve grading systems," *The Laryngoscope*, vol. 93, no. 8, pp. 1056–1069, 1983.

[2] J. H. Beigel, K. M. Tomashek, L. E. Dodd et al., "Remdesivir for the treatment of covid-19 - final report," *New England Journal of Medicine*, vol. 383, no. 19, pp. 1813–1826, 2020.

[3] Q. Cai, M. Yang, D. Liu et al., "Experimental treatment with favipiravir for COVID-19: an open-label control study," *Engineering*, vol. 6, no. 10, pp. 1192–1198, 2020.
[4] A. A. Ivashchenko, K. A. Dmitriev, N. V. Vostokova et al., "AVIFAVIR for treatment of patients with moderate coronavirus disease 2019 (COVID-19): interim results of a phase II/III multicenter randomized clinical trial," *Clinical Infectious Diseases*, 2020.
[5] W. Zhang, L. Xu, T. Luo, F. Wu, B. Zhao, and X. Li, "The etiology of Bell's palsy: a review," *Journal of Neurology*, vol. 267, no. 7, pp. 1896–1905, 2020.
[6] G. Colella, M. Orlandi, and N. Cirillo, "Bell's palsy following COVID-19 vaccination," *Journal of Neurology*, vol. 21, 2021.
[7] L. Codeluppi, F. Venturelli, J. Rossi et al., "Facial palsy during the COVID-19 pandemic," *Brain and Behavior*, vol. 11, no. 1, Article ID e01939, 2021.
[8] P. Herman, C. Vincent, C. Parietti Winkler et al., "Consensus statement. Corticosteroid therapy in ENT in the context of the COVID-19 pandemic," *European Annals of Otorhinolaryngology, Head and Neck Diseases*, vol. 137, no. 4, pp. 315–317, 2020.
[9] R. M. Johnson and J. M. Vinetz, "Dexamethasone in the Management of Covid-19," *British Medical Journal Publishing Group*, vol. 370, 2020.
[10] Z. Yang, J. Liu, Y. Zhou, X. Zhao, Q. Zhao, and J. Liu, "The effect of corticosteroid treatment on patients with coronavirus infection: a systematic review and meta-analysis," *Journal of Infection*, vol. 81, no. 1, pp. e13–e20, 2020.
[11] E. Urban, G. F. Volk, K. Geißler et al., "Prognostic factors for the outcome of Bells' palsy: a cohort register-based study," *Clinical Otolaryngology*, vol. 45, no. 5, pp. 754–761, 2020.
[12] M. C. Yoo, Y. Soh, J. Chon et al., "Evaluation of factors associated with favorable outcomes in adults with Bell palsy," *JAMA Otolaryngology-Head and Neck Surgery*, vol. 146, no. 3, pp. 256–263, 2020.
[13] Y. Goh, D. L. L. Beh, A. Makmur, J. Somani, and A. C. Y. Chan, "Pearls and Oy-sters: facial nerve palsy in COVID-19 infection," *Neurology*, vol. 95, no. 8, pp. 364–367, 2020.
[14] C. Derollez, T. Alberto, I. Leroi, M.-A. Mackowiak, and Y. Chen, "Facial nerve palsy: an atypical clinical manifestation of COVID-19 infection in a family cluster," *European Journal of Neurology*, vol. 27, pp. 2670–2672, 2020.
[15] R. Figueiredo, V. Falcão, M. J. Pinto, and C. Ramalho, "Peripheral facial paralysis as presenting symptom of COVID-19 in a pregnant woman," *BMJ Case Reports*, vol. 13, Article ID e237146, 2020.
[16] M. A. Lima, M. T. T. Silva, C. N. Soares et al., "Peripheral facial nerve palsy associated with COVID-19," *Journal of NeuroVirology*, vol. 26, no. 6, pp. 941–944, 2020.
[17] M. Repajic, X. L. Lai, P. Xu, and A. Liu, "Bell's Palsy after second dose of Pfizer COVID-19 vaccination in a patient with history of recurrent Bell's palsy," *Brain, Behavior, and Immunity—Health*, vol. 13, Article ID 100217, 2021.

Efficacy of Tocilizumab in Limbic Encephalitis with Anti-CASPR2 Antibodies

Maurizio Benucci,[1] Luciana Tramacere,[2] Maria Infantino,[3] Mariangela Manfredi,[3] Valentina Grossi,[3] Arianna Damiani,[1] Francesca Li Gobbi,[1] Maristella Piccininni,[2] Gaetano Zaccara,[2] and Massimo Cincotta[2]

[1]*Rheumatology Unit, S. Giovanni di Dio Hospital, Florence, Italy*
[2]*Neurology Unit, S. Giovanni di Dio Hospital, Florence, Italy*
[3]*Immunology and Allergology Laboratory, S. Giovanni di Dio Hospital, Florence, Italy*

Correspondence should be addressed to Maurizio Benucci; maubenucci@tiscali.it

Academic Editor: Isabella Laura Simone

We report the case of a 64-year-old man who presented with subacute memory, balance impairment, behavioral and mood changes, and epileptic seizures. Magnetic resonance imaging (MRI) showed bilateral hippocampal abnormalities. Brain [^{18}F]-FDG fluorodeoxyglucose positron emission tomography (PET) revealed hypometabolism in both the temporal lobe as well as in the left insular and parietal regions. The clinical and neuroradiological picture and the detection of anti-CASPR2 antibodies in serum oriented the diagnosis towards autoimmune limbic encephalitis. Intravenous high-dose steroid and immunoglobulin treatments were ineffective. We did not use rituximab for the presence of antibodies to HbcAg positivity. Tocilizumab given intravenously 8 mg/kg once a month for six months and then subcutaneously 162 mg every week for six months resulted in clinical and neuroradiological improvement. These data support the efficacy of tocilizumab in autoimmune limbic encephalitis associated with anti-CASPR2 antibodies, which has been sporadically reported in the literature.

1. Introduction

Autoimmune etiology is increasingly recognized as a major cause of encephalitis [1–3]. The spectrum of autoimmune encephalitis (AE) is rapidly expanding with the continuous discovery of novel auto-antibodies [4]. Moreover, in other patients, clinical and magnetic resonance imaging (MRI) findings support the diagnosis of probable AE without demonstrated auto-antibody [5]. In a subset of patients, the outcomes following immunotherapies are good, regardless of the identification of auto-antibodies [6, 7]. For patients nonresponsive to first-line immunotherapy such as steroids and IVIg, second-line immunotherapies such as rituximab, which induces CD20+ B-cell destruction, may yield substantial benefit [8]. Tocilizumab is a humanized anti-interleukin (IL)-6 receptor monoclonal antibody, which blocks IL-6-mediated signal transduction [9]. Owing to the crucial role of IL-6 in stimulating both B and T cells in autoimmune processes [10–12], tocilizumab was established as efficient in various autoimmune diseases, including rheumatoid arthritis and systemic lupus erythematosus [13, 14]. Among the autoimmune central nervous system (CNS) disorders, a recent study reported a powerful disease modulation by tocilizumab in rituximab-refractory neuromyelitis optica (NMO) [15]. Regarding AE, successful treatment by tocilizumab was reported in several patients [16, 17], but in only one of these cases, contactin-associated protein-like 2 (CASPR2) antibodies were detected [16].

2. Case Report

A 64-year-old man was admitted to the neurology ward because of a disorder starting four months earlier with a one-week-long hypomanic episode. Subsequently, he had presented attention deficit, loss of recollection for recent events, and repetitive questioning, anxiety, loss of emotional control, balance disorder, and secondarily generalized seizures preceded by impaired language production.

The medical history consisted of hypertension, cervical spondylosis, and a previous, short episode of paroxysmal atrial fibrillation.

On admission, routine blood tests including erythrocyte sedimentation rate were normal. Also, blood serology for cytomegalovirus, herpes simplex 1 and 2, herpes zoster, human immunodeficiency (HIV) viruses, and Lyme disease were negative.

Anti-dsDNA antibodies, antiextractable nuclear antigens, antiphospholipid antibodies, and antineutrophil cytoplasmic antibodies were negative. Cerebrospinal fluid (CSF) examination showed slightly increased protein (0.57 g/l) and normal cellular content, as well as unremarkable IgG index. CSF oligoclonal bands were absent. No neurotrophic viruses neither mycobacterium tuberculosis were identified by CSF polymerase chain reaction analysis. Testing for anticontactin-associated protein 2 (CASPR2) auto-antibodies performed by indirect immunofluorescence on transfected cells and control-transfected cells (EU 90) at a starting dilution of 1 : 10 detected IgG against CASPR2 in serum (1 : 1000) (Euroimmun, Lübeck, Germany). We also evaluated the determination of anti-NMDA glutamate receptor antibodies, antileucine-rich glioma-inactivated 1 (LGI1), and antibody panels for paraneoplastic neurological syndromes with negative results. Antibody assessment was not performed in the cerebrospinal fluid. MRI showed slight bilateral hippocampal swelling, and mild FLAIR hyperintensity [^{18}F] fluorodeoxyglucose positron emission tomography ([^{18}F]-FDG PET) showed glucose metabolic alterations in both temporal lobes, mainly involving the mesial regions and in the left insular and parietal regions (Figure 1). Chest and abdomen CT scan, testicular ecography, and search for tumoral markers were negative. Clinical, neuroradiological, and laboratory investigations oriented the diagnosis towards anti-CASPR2 antibody-associated autoimmune limbic encephalitis. At the initiation of first-line immunotherapy, functional status assessed using the modified Rankin Scale (mRS) score was 3. High-dose steroid therapy (i.v. methylprednisolone 1 g daily for 5 days) and administration of IVIg 2 g/kg in 5 days were ineffective. Conversely, cognitive disturbances worsened and disinhibited behaviour appeared in spite of risperidone treatment. In addition, despite the intake of lacosamide 200 mg daily and levetiracetam 2000 mg daily, seizure frequency increased to 2-3 per month. We did not use rituximab for the presence of antibodies to HbcAg positivity (total Hb core positive) and anti-HBV antibodies 64.90 mU/ml. The patient presented a negative QuantiFERON (ESAT-6-CFP10 CD4/CD8). Flow cytometric analysis of lymphocyte profiles showed CD3+ 557 cells/mcl, CD4+ 386 cells/mcl, CD8+ 142 cells/mcl, CD56+ 111 cells/mcl, CD14HLADR+ 745 cells/mcl, CD28+ 35.9 cells/mc, CD28− 0.5 cells/mcl, CD19+ 184 cells/mcl, CD20+ 169 cells/mcl, CD38+ 8.4 cells/mcl, CD27+ naive 133 cells/mcl, and CD27+ memory 2 cells/mcl. The value of the circulating interleukin (IL)-6 was 23.9 pg/mL (human IL-6 instant enzyme-linked immunosorbent assay, eBioscience, Bender MedSystem GmbH, Vienna, Austria; normal value <3 pg/mL). We started tocilizumab 8 mg/kg once a month for six months i.v. and then 162 mg every week sc. This treatment determined cognitive, balance, and a significant improvement in metabolic uptake at [18F] fluorodeoxyglucose positron emission tomography ([18F]-FDG PET) (Figure 2). Findings of formal neuropsychological assessment before and after one month of tocilizumab treatment are shown in Table 1. Moreover, behavioral changes and seizures subsided. Also, the titer of anti-CASPR2 antibodies was also reduced to 1 : 100. After 4 months of therapy, functional status assessed using the mRS score was 0, and the patient was able to resume his work.

3. Discussion

In recent years, case reports and clinical series have been published in the use of tocilizumab in AE [17, 18]. Ninety-one patients with inadequate clinical response to first-line immunotherapy and following rituximab were retrospectively reviewed. Thirty (33.0%) patients were included in the tocilizumab group, 31 (34.0%) in the additional rituximab group, and 30 (33.0%) in the observation group. The tocilizumab group showed more frequent favorable mRS scores at 2 months from treatment initiation and at the last follow-up compared with those at the relevant time points of the remaining groups. The majority (89.5%) of the patients with clinical improvement at 1 month from tocilizumab treatment maintained a long-term favorable clinical response [17]. According to the auto-antibody tests of the patients' serum/CSF, 26 (28.6%) patients had anti-NMDA-R antibodies, 3 (3.3%) had antileucine-rich glioma-inactivated 1 antibodies, and 2 (2.2%) had antiamphiphysin antibodies. The remaining 60 (65.9%) patients showed negative results on the auto-antibody detection test, and no patient had anti-CASPR2 antibodies [17]. In another clinical series on 3 cases, tocilizumab has also been used successfully in pediatric forms [19]. Therefore, the drug was included as a third line of treatment even in the encephalitis forms of children [20]. Based on the review of the literature, this is the second case of autoimmune encephalitis with antipositive CASPR2 treated with tocilizumab [16]. In our patient, the therapy resulted in a titer reduction of anti-CASPR2 antibodies although this does not seem to correlate according to some reports with the prognostic trend [21]. The presence of CASPR2 antibodies is associated with a subgroup of autoimmune-mediated neurological disorders, including limbic encephalitis, neuromyotonia, and Morvan syndrome [22]. A previous study has revealed the efficacy of tocilizumab in rituximab-refractory NMO spectrum disorders [15]. The efficacy of tocilizumab can be explained by the extensive pathophysiologic mechanisms by which IL-6 induces and enhances autoimmunity [23, 24]. IL-6 not only induces B-cell differentiation and proliferation but also promotes the differentiation of a main inducer of autoimmune tissue damage, IL-17-producing T-helper cells, from naive T cells

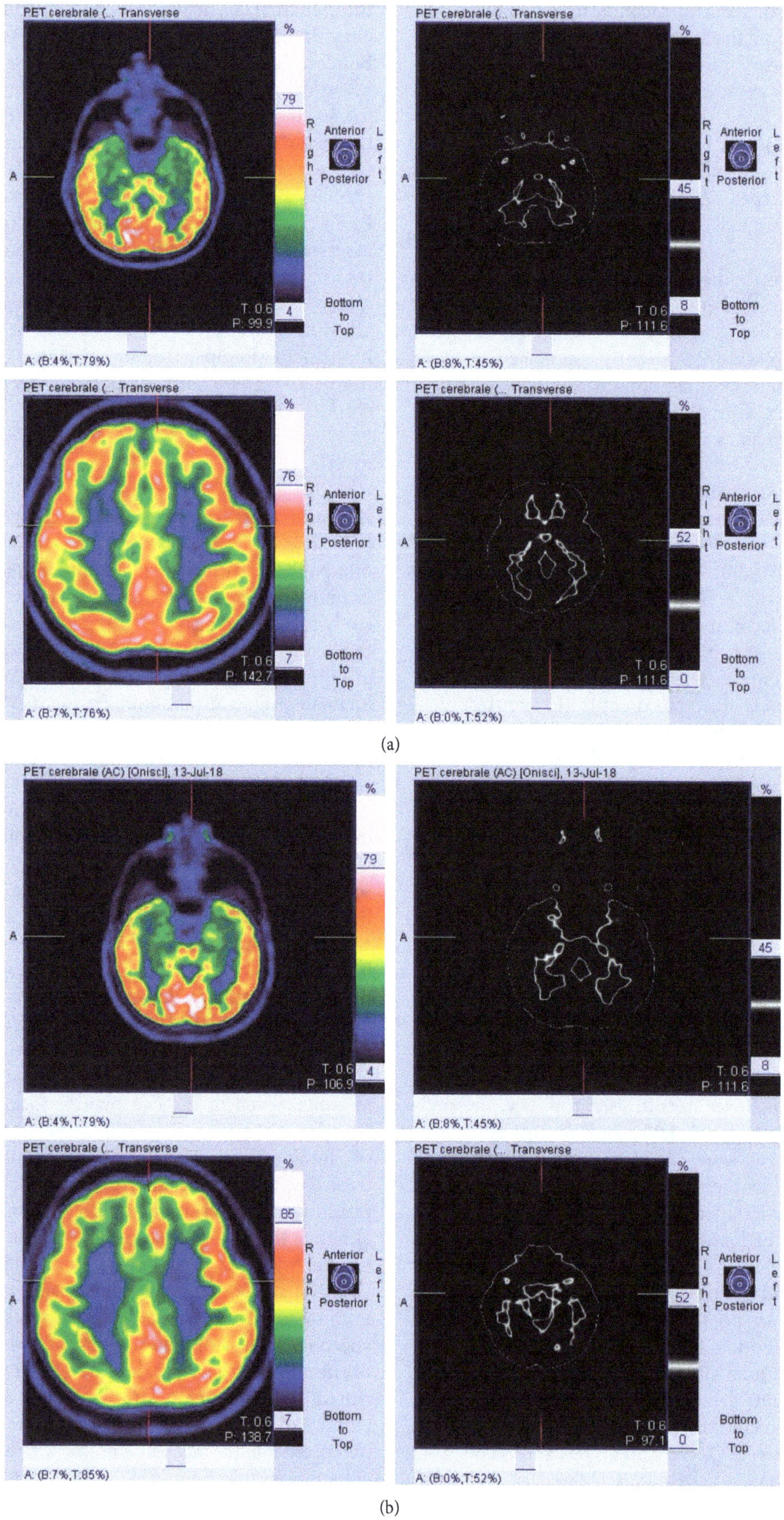

FIGURE 1: [18F] fluorodeoxyglucose positron emission tomography ([18F]-FDG PET) showed glucose metabolic alterations in both temporal lobes, mainly involving the mesial regions, and in the left insular and parietal regions.

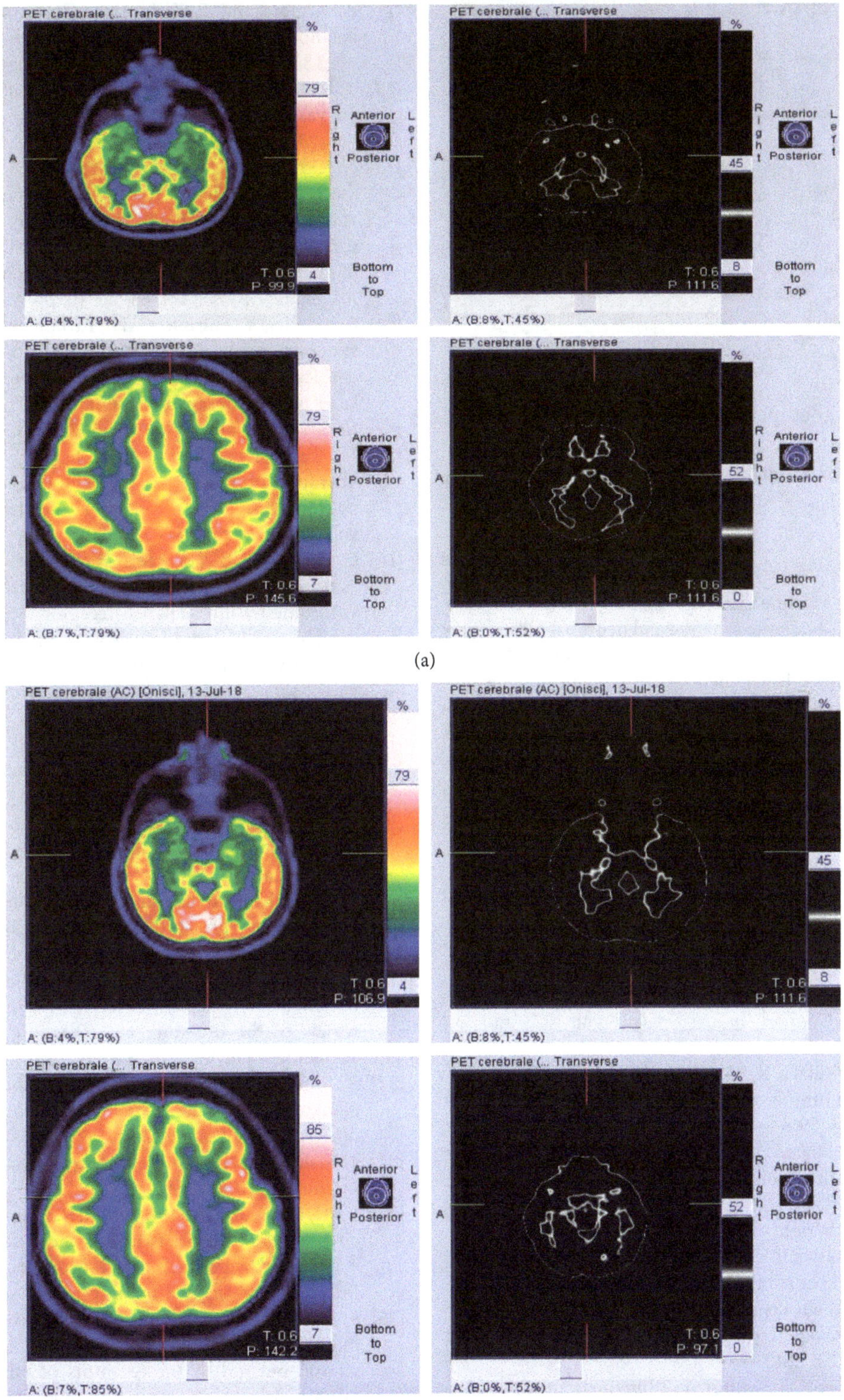

(a)

(b)

FIGURE 2: A significant improvement in metabolic uptake at [18F] fluorodeoxyglucose positron emission tomography ([18F]-FDG PET).

[24]. IL-6 inhibits regulatory T-cell differentiation, which is crucial in maintaining the balance against IL-17-producing T-helper cells in regulating autoimmune processes. Furthermore, IL-6 stimulates the differentiation of CD8+ cytotoxic T cells, which promote excitotoxicity-induced neuronal damage [25]. Recently, the safety of tocilizumab has also been observed in demyelinating pathologies and CNS complications in rheumatoid arthritis [26].

Our clinical case confirms that tocilizumab can improve the cases of autoimmune encephalitis with anti-CASPR2

Table 1: Evaluation of psychometric tests during tocilizumab treatment.

Psychometric tests	First evaluation score	Second evaluation score
Rey auditory verbal learning test	0	2
Babcock story recall test	4	4
Semantic verbal fluency test	4	4
Phonemic verbal fluency test	3	4
Attentive matrices test	2	4
Trail making test	0	2

antibodies, and this therapeutic strategy can be reserved for patients resistant or intolerant to other first- or second-line immunosuppressive therapy.

References

[1] E. Lancaster, E. Martinez-Hernandez, and J. Dalmau, "Encephalitis and antibodies to synaptic and neuronal cell surface proteins," *Neurology*, vol. 77, no. 2, pp. 179–189, 2011.

[2] L. Zuliani, F. Graus, B. Giometto, C. Bien, and A. Vincent, "Central nervous system neuronal surface antibody associated syndromes: review and guidelines for recognition," *Journal of Neurology, Neurosurgery & Psychiatry*, vol. 83, no. 6, pp. 638–645, 2012.

[3] M. S. Gable, H. Sheriff, J. Dalmau, D. H. Tilley, and C. A. Glaser, "The frequency of autoimmune N-methyl-D-aspartate receptor encephalitis surpasses that of individual viral etiologies in young individuals enrolled in the California Encephalitis Project," *Clinical Infectious Diseases*, vol. 54, no. 7, pp. 899–904, 2012.

[4] T. Armangue, F. Leypoldt, and J. Dalmau, "Autoimmune encephalitis as differential diagnosis of infectious encephalitis," *Current Opinion in Neurology*, vol. 27, no. 3, pp. 361–368, 2014.

[5] F. Graus, M. J. Titulaer, R. Balu et al., "A clinical approach to diagnosis of autoimmune encephalitis," *The Lancet Neurology*, vol. 15, no. 4, pp. 391–404, 2016.

[6] T. D. Singh, J. E. Fugate, and A. A. Rabinstein, "The spectrum of acute encephalitis: causes, management, and predictors of outcome," *Neurology*, vol. 84, no. 4, pp. 359–366, 2015.

[7] Y. Hacohen, S. Wright, P. Waters et al., "Paediatric autoimmune encephalopathies: clinical features, laboratory investigations and outcomes in patients with or without antibodies to known central nervous system autoantigens," *Journal of Neurology, Neurosurgery & Psychiatry*, vol. 84, no. 7, pp. 748–755, 2013.

[8] W.-J. Lee, S.-T. Lee, J.-I. Byun et al., "Rituximab treatment for autoimmune limbic encephalitis in an institutional cohort," *Neurology*, vol. 86, no. 18, pp. 1683–1691, 2016.

[9] T. Tanaka, M. Narazaki, and T. Kishimoto, "Anti-interleukin-6 receptor antibody, tocilizumab, for the treatment of autoimmune diseases," *FEBS Letters*, vol. 585, no. 23, pp. 3699–3709, 2011.

[10] M. Okada, M. Kitahara, S. Kishimoto, T. Matsuda, T. Hirano, and T. Kishimoto, "IL-6/BSF-2 functions as a killer helper factor in the in vitro induction of cytotoxic T cells," *Journal of Immunology*, vol. 141, no. 5, pp. 1543–1549, 1988.

[11] A. Kimura and T. Kishimoto, "IL-6: regulator of treg/Th17 balance," *European Journal of Immunology*, vol. 40, no. 7, pp. 1830–1835, 2010.

[12] T. Kishimoto, "Interleukin-6: from basic science to medicine-40 years in immunology," *Annual Review of Immunology*, vol. 23, no. 1, pp. 1–21, 2005.

[13] N. Nishimoto, N. Miyasaka, K. Yamamoto, S. Kawai, T. Takeuchi, and J. Azuma, "Long-term safety and efficacy of tocilizumab, an anti-IL-6 receptor monoclonal antibody, in monotherapy, in patients with rheumatoid arthritis (the STREAM study): evidence of safety and efficacy in a 5-year extension study," *Annals of the Rheumatic Diseases*, vol. 68, no. 10, pp. 1580–1584, 2009.

[14] G. G. Illei, Y. Shirota, C. H. Yarboro et al., "Tocilizumab in systemic lupus erythematosus: data on safety, preliminary efficacy, and impact on circulating plasma cells from an open-label phase I dosage-escalation study," *Arthritis & Rheumatism*, vol. 62, no. 2, pp. 542–552, 2010.

[15] M. Ringelstein, I. Ayzenberg, J. Harmel et al., "Long-term Therapy with interleukin 6 receptor blockade in highly active neuromyelitis optica spectrum disorder," *JAMA Neurology*, vol. 72, no. 7, pp. 756–763, 2015.

[16] C. Krogias, R. Hoepner, A. Müller, C. Schneider-Gold, A. Schröder, and R. Gold, "Successful treatment of anti-Caspr2 syndrome by interleukin 6 receptor blockade through tocilizumab," *JAMA Neurology*, vol. 70, no. 8, pp. 1056–1059, 2013.

[17] W.-J. Lee, S.-T. Lee, J. Moon et al., "Tocilizumab in autoimmune encephalitis refractory to rituximab: an institutional cohort study," *Neurotherapeutics*, vol. 13, no. 4, pp. 824–832, 2016.

[18] Y. W. Shin, S. T. Lee, K. I. Park et al., "Treatment strategies for autoimmune encephalitis," *Therapeutic Advances in Neurological Disorders*, vol. 11, p. 175628561772234, 2017.

[19] R. L. Randell, A. V. Adams, and H. Van Mater, "Tocilizumab in refractory autoimmune encephalitis: a series of pediatric cases," *Pediatric Neurology*, vol. 86, pp. 66–68, 2018.

[20] C. Stingl, K. Cardinale, and H. Van Mater, "An update on the treatment of pediatric autoimmune encephalitis," *Current Treatment Options in Rheumatology*, vol. 4, no. 1, pp. 14–28, 2018.

[21] C. G. Bien, "Value of autoantibodies for prediction of treatment response in patients with autoimmune epilepsy: review of the literature and suggestions for clinical management," *Epilepsia*, vol. 54, no. Suppl 2, pp. 48–55, 2013.

[22] R. Singh, P. Das, U. Kaur et al., "Morvan's syndrome-is a pathogen behind the curtain?" *Neurological Sciences*, vol. 39, no. 11, pp. 1965–1969, 2018.

[23] T. Kishimoto, "IL-6: from its discovery to clinical applications," *International Immunology*, vol. 22, no. 5, pp. 347–352, 2010.

[24] K.-M. Chavele, E. Merry, and M. R. Ehrenstein, "Cutting edge: circulating plasmablasts induce the differentiation of human T follicular helper cells via IL-6 production," *The Journal of Immunology*, vol. 194, no. 6, pp. 2482–2485, 2015.

[25] M. Mihara, K. Kasutani, M. Okazaki et al., "Tocilizumab inhibits signal transduction mediated by both mIL-6R and sIL-6R, but not by the receptors of other members of IL-6 cytokine family," *International Immunopharmacology*, vol. 5, no. 12, pp. 1731–1740, 2005.

[26] F. Atzeni, R. Talotta, I. F. Masala, M. C. Gerardi, R. Casale, and P. Sarzi-Puttini, "Central nervous system involvement in rheumatoid arthritis patients and the potential implications of using biological agents," *Best Practice & Research Clinical Rheumatology*, vol. 32, no. 4, pp. 500–510, 2018.

43

Rituximab for Autoimmune Encephalitis with Epilepsy

Mohankumar Kurukumbi,[1] **Rahul H. Dave,**[1] **Jose Castillo,**[2] **Tulsi Shah,**[2] **and Joanne Lau**[2]

[1]*Department of Neurology, Inova Fairfax Hospital, Falls Church, VA, USA*
[2]*Virginia Commonwealth University School of Medicine, Inova Campus, Falls Church, VA, USA*

Correspondence should be addressed to Mohankumar Kurukumbi; mohan311@gmail.com

Academic Editor: Dominic B. Fee

Intractable epilepsy remains a significant medical challenge, resulting in recurrent and prolonged intensive care unit (ICU) admissions. Autoimmune encephalitis is emerging as a treatable cause of intractable epilepsy. It is characterized by antibodies against cerebral antigens, such as potassium channels such as leucine-rich, glioma inactivated 1 (LGI1) and contactin-associated protein 2 (CASPR2), calcium channels such as the voltage-gated calcium channel (VGCC), or neurotransmitter receptors such as the α-amino-3-hydroxy-5-methyl-4-isoxazolepropionic acid receptor (AMPAR), gamma aminobutyric acid receptor (GABAR), and *N*-methyl-D-aspartate receptor (NMDAR). Diagnosis requires a syndrome consistent with an antibody identified in serum or cerebrospinal fluid (CSF) using methods that minimize risk of false-positives. Although there is no officially approved therapy for these disorders, typical approaches involve chronic high-dose steroids, intravenous immunoglobulin (IVIG), or plasma exchange. Rituximab is effective for antibody-associated disorders such as lupus, myasthenia gravis, and neuromyelitis optica. Here, we present three patients who were admitted with recalcitrant status epilepticus and demonstrated serum antibodies against NMDAR, LGI1, or VGCC using a cell-based assay. All patients demonstrated complete, long-term epilepsy control and improvement in symptoms with rituximab.

1. Introduction

Autoimmune encephalitis is now well recognized as a treatable cause of intractable epilepsy. Certain antibodies have been identified as likely culprits of these syndromes, and early diagnosis with prompt treatment is the mainstay understanding when combating these conditions. Therapy for these disorders include largely some form of immunosuppressants, with steroids, IVIG, or plasma exchange in some combination being the commonly used first line options. Rituximab has been shown to be a promising medication to administer in other autoimmune disorders when the first line immunosuppressive agents fail to control the condition, but its use for autoimmune encephalitis remains unconfirmed. In this case series, we will be presenting three cases that presented with epilepsy and were all found to subsequently have the respective antibodies known to be associated with a specific autoimmune encephalitis, and we demonstrated symptom control with the use of rituximab.

2. Case Presentations

2.1. Case 1. A 32-year-old female with no history of seizures presented with an acute onset of behavioral changes and witnessed seizure activity. Behavioral changes included uncontrolled laughter, screaming, signs of agitation, spitting on the floor, complete lack of appetite, and foreign accent syndrome. She had two seizures characterized by tongue biting with postictal confusion and agitation. Initial head computed tomography (CT), urine toxicology, and serum electrolytes were normal. She was discharged on 500 mg of levetiracetam by mouth twice a day and plans for magnetic resonance imaging (MRI) as an outpatient.

Several days later, the patient was readmitted to a neighboring hospital for continued symptoms. A brain MRI revealed bilateral (left more than right) temporal lobe fluid-attenuated inversion recovery (FLAIR) hyperintensity (Figure 1). A test of the CSF revealed 53 white blood cells

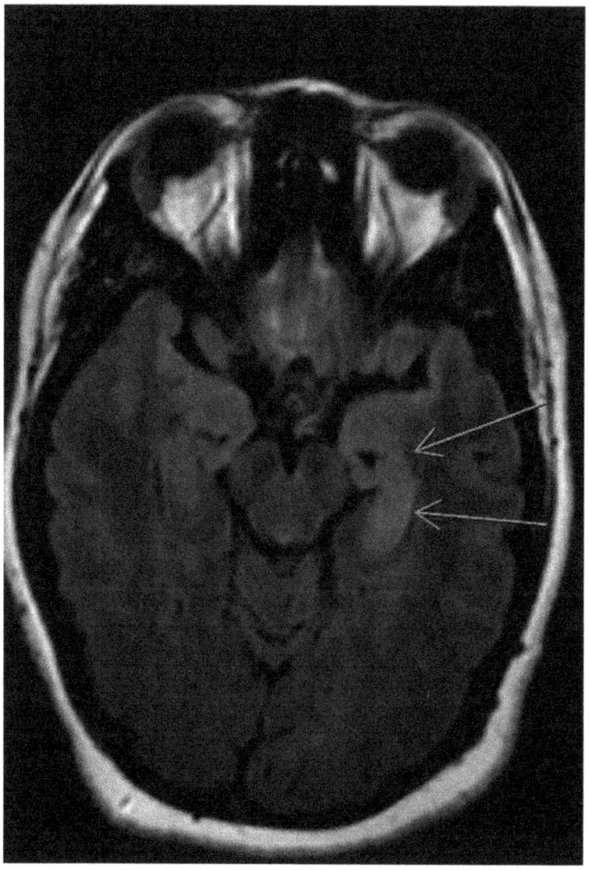

Figure 1: Brain MRI showing T2 flair hyperintensity in the medial temporal lobes with left lobe (pink arrows) revealing greater hyperintensity than right lobe.

(WBC) (98% lymphocytes) and 2 oligoclonal bands. An electroencephalogram (EEG) revealed status epilepticus characterized by onset of discharges from the left frontocentral and left fronto-temporal region, accompanied by delta brushes (Figure 2). A test for anti-NMDAR antibodies showed presence in the serum and CSF (1 : 64), consistent with a diagnosis of NMDAR encephalitis. Given the inflammatory CSF, the patient was given 1000 mg of methylprednisolone IV and 0.4 gm/kg of IVIG for 5 days. Antiepileptic drugs (AED) started included levetiracetam, lacosamide, and lamotrigine. She was also maintained on risperidone. However, the patient remained with frequent seizures, behavioral agitation, and psychotic symptoms. CT of the chest, abdomen, and pelvis showed no evidence of neoplasm and a transvaginal ultrasound was negative for ovarian teratoma or other tumors. Given her recalcitrant course and presence of antibodies, on day 27 of status, she was started on 375 mg/m^2 of rituximab weekly for 4 weeks. This resulted in clinical and electrographic improvement: normalized EEG and resolution of psychosis and agitation, with a return to baseline cognition and personality. Since then, she has remained on lacosamide 200 mg twice a day and rituximab 1000 mg IV every 6 months without recrudescence of symptoms.

2.2. Case 2. A 72-year-old female with a history of hypertension and anxiety presented after a motor vehicle collision with sudden loss of awareness while driving. The patient endorsed complete amnesia regarding the collision until her admission to the emergency department. The family also noted a recent three-month history of sporadic episodes of confusion lasting less than a minute in which the patient suddenly would become unaware of her surroundings, become pale with a blank stare, or display inappropriate behaviors such as getting up from her seat during dinner and spitting food into a vase, as well as a dystonic posturing of her right face and right upper limb concerning for faciobrachial seizures. She abruptly returned to baseline with no recollection of the event.

The patient continued to have seizures during the hospital course that was treated with levetiracetam. Initial EEG revealed background slowing suggesting mild encephalopathy, but no seizures were reported. The patient also exhibited cognitive decline with a Montreal Cognitive Assessment (MoCA) score of 18, with difficulty in areas of executive functioning, delayed recall, orientation, and abstraction. MRI revealed no acute process. She was discharged after a negative workup with recommendations for outpatient CSF studies and follow-up.

She was readmitted to the hospital several weeks later for rapid cognitive decline, and increased frequency of staring episodes, up to 28 times per day. The patient's outpatient CSF workup results revealed an elevated white blood cell count, 4 oligoclonal bands, and elevated 14-3-3 levels. The CSF also eventually returned positive for anti-LGI1. Note that 14-3-3 is a nonspecific marker of cerebral damage and is not specific for Creutzfeldt–Jakob disease. Repeat brain MRI revealed FLAIR hyperintensity in the bilateral hippocampi, right mesial temporal lobe, and mild diffusion restriction in the right insular cortex without contrast enhancement or hemorrhage (Figure 3). On re-review of the first EEG, it was found to have left temporal discharges likely responsible for the seizures (Figure 4). A repeat EEG during this hospitalization was done and found to be abnormal, demonstrating a slower background than the prior EEG and overall having a generalized intermittent rhythmic slowing consistent with an encephalopathic picture. The left temporal originating epileptiform discharges and electrographic seizures were not seen on the repeat EEG.

Given the lack of response to AED and inflammatory-appearing CSF, autoimmune encephalitis was deemed to be the diagnosis. 1000 mg of methylprednisolone IV was started and continued for 5 days, resulting in improvements in the faciobrachial seizures and marked improvements in cognitive function to near-baseline. She was discharged on chronic prednisone that was tapered over 1 year. The CSF tested during her second hospital admission eventually returned positive for antibodies against LGI1.

Once the prednisone was discontinued, she had recrudescent cognitive decline and agitation requiring inpatient care. Repeat CSF revealed the presence of anti-LGI1 antibodies. She was treated acutely with 1000 mg methylprednisolone IV and 0.4 gm/kg IVIG for 5 days, which resulted in partial improvement. However, she had persistent

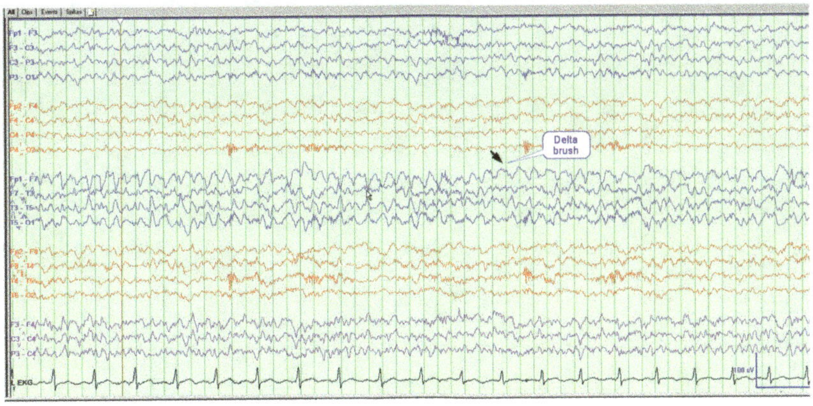

FIGURE 2: EEG showing electroclinical seizures exhibiting delta brushes.

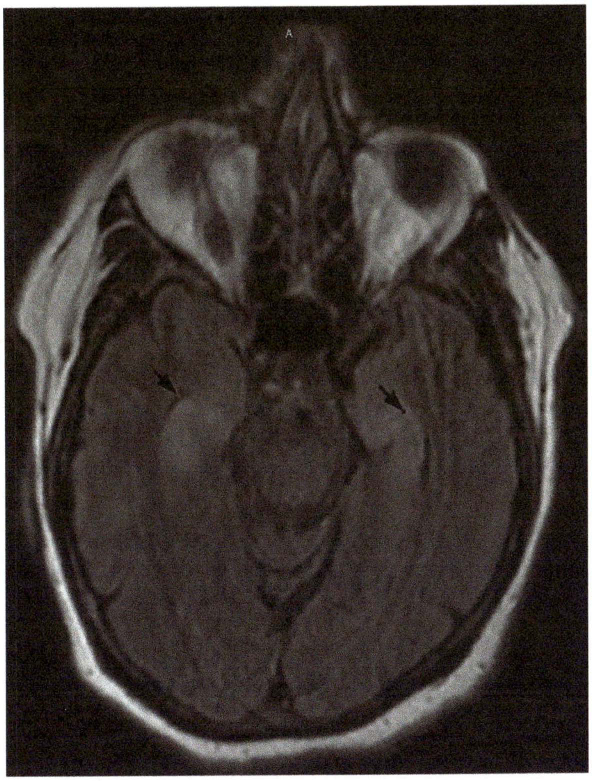

FIGURE 3: Brain MRI revealing symmetric signal abnormality, swelling of the hippocampus and right mesial temporal lobe, and a T2 FLAIR signal abnormality.

expressive aphasia and impaired 5-minute recall. She was then given 1000 mg of rituximab IV resulting in an electrographic and clinical seizure freedom with return of premorbid cognitive function. The patient is currently maintained on 1000 mg of rituximab IV every 6 months.

2.3. Case 3. A 19-year-old male presented with high-grade fever, malaise, and complex partial seizures characterized by facial twitches, staring spells, and rigidity followed by brief unresponsiveness with amnesia. Over a few days, the syndrome progressed to status epilepticus recalcitrant to pharmacotherapy. His workup for infectious etiology was found to be negative. Initial MRI was unremarkable (Figure 5), and the CSF revealed 18 WBC (91% lymphocytes). His EEG showed left fronto-temporal sharp waves with intermittent slowing (Figure 6). Given the inflammatory CSF findings, he was treated with 0.4 gm/kg of IVIG and 1000 mg of methylprednisolone IV for 5 days with minimal clinical response and was subsequently administered 1000 mg of rituximab IV with abrogation of seizures and return to baseline functioning. Autoimmune encephalitis testing was negative in the CSF, but serum was found positive for N-type anti-VGCC antibodies, with titer levels at 0.28 (normal <0.02), obtained via send-out to Mayo Clinic Labs.

He has since demonstrated a full recovery and remains asymptomatic on 1000 mg of rituximab IV every 6 months. Antibodies to the voltage-gated N-type calcium channel are classically associated with Lambert–Eaton syndrome, a paraneoplastic neuromuscular disorder resulting from non-small-cell lung carcinoma. Our patient underwent a CT chest, and it was found to be negative.

3. Discussion

Intractable epilepsy remains a significant medical challenge, causing recurrent and prolonged hospitalizations and ICU stays. Autoimmune epilepsy is emerging as a treatable cause of intractable epilepsy [1]. It remains controversial whether the antibodies are directly pathogenic or markers of the disease. Common antigens include LGI1, CASPR2, AMPAR, GABAR, and NMDAR.

These antibodies are variably associated with cancer, in which case they are termed paraneoplastic. Autoimmune paraneoplastic syndromes are hypothesized to be due to cross-reactivity of antitumor antibodies binding to structurally similar but unrelated native neuronal antigens [2].

The incidence of autoimmune encephalitis has increased recently—from 0.4/100,000 to 1.2/100,00 person-years over the last 20 years—mostly due to increased awareness of autoimmune encephalitis and improved access to antibody-detection methodologies.

As illustrated by our series, the presentation of autoimmune encephalitis can mimic epilepsy due to other

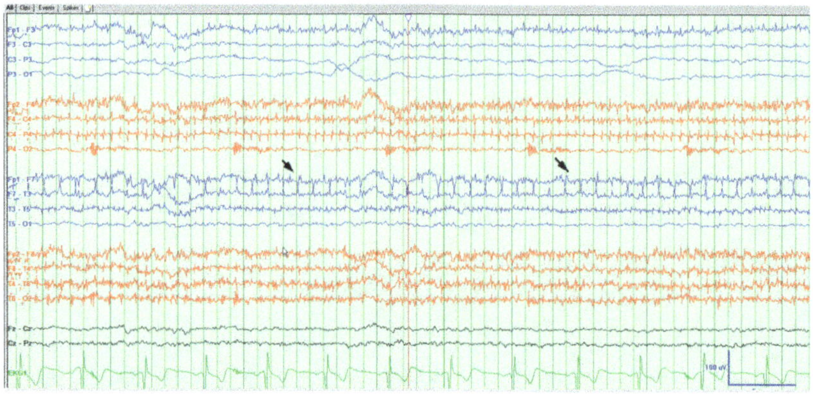

Figure 4: EEG showing background slowing and generalized slowing compatible with diffuse cortical dysfunction. EEG Also showing temporal lobe discharges.

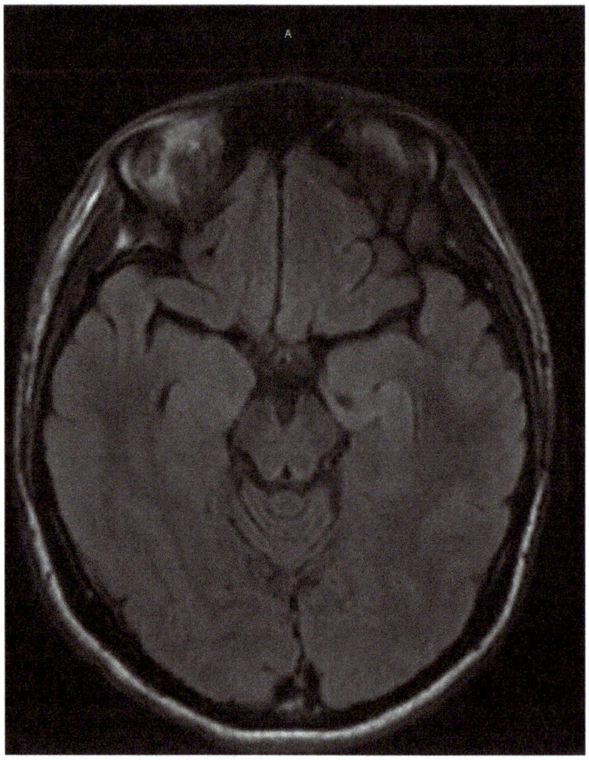

Figure 5: Normal brain MRI.

causes. Historical clues include a subacute decline in memory, cognition, seizures, and alterations of consciousness. Another hallmark is the presence of psychiatric or limbic symptoms such as psychosis, aggression, paranoia, or inappropriate sexual behavior in the absence of a psychiatric disorder. However, a diagnosis of autoimmune encephalitis cannot be made on the basis of semiology alone.

Each antibody correlates with specific clinical and electrographic features [3]. For instance, anti-NMDAR encephalitis is frequently associated with psychosis and delta brush on EEG [4]. Anti-LGI1 encephalitis is frequently associated with faciobrachial dystonic seizures, but the electrographic appearance can be variable depending upon the brain region involved (typically cortex, basal ganglia, and hippocampus) [5].

Delay in diagnosis and treatment has been associated with a worse prognosis and increased risk of relapse [6]. To reduce the risk of false-positive antibody results, we suggest the use of cell-based assays, as this methodology offers increased sensitivity and specificity compared to ELISA, RIA, or Western blot methods. In our patient with VGCC encephalitis, our titer of 0.28 is comparable to that of other reports of N-type VGCC encephalitis [6–9]. Therefore, this antibody is likely truly present and associated with our patient's syndrome. The question of pathogenicity may be raised, but this cannot be answered without mechanistic studies. The history of antibody-associated disease—whether SLE, NMO, MOG, or RA—is characterized by identification of antibody association years or decades prior to determining whether a given antibody is pathogenic and identifying the mechanism of pathogenesis. The focus of our report is purely clinical and we cannot make conclusions about the pathogenesis of any of the antibodies based upon our data. Ultimately, an accurate diagnosis requires the identification of an inflammatory syndrome and the correlation of any identified antibodies with its described clinical syndrome.

Typically, autoimmune encephalitis responds to immunomodulation or immunosuppression [5]. A single-center prospective study of 220 patients with anti-NMDAR encephalitis was done in which 99.5% received immunosuppressants including glucocorticoids, IVIG, and plasmapheresis (either individually or combined) and 7.3% received rituximab or cyclophosphamide (either individually or combined). In the first 12 months, 94.1% of patients improved, 2.3% died, and 17.3% had a relapse [10]. A case series of 5 patients with anti-LGI1 encephalitis showed that rituximab was efficacious and well tolerated as a treatment option [11]. Prior case studies of anti-VGCC associated with autoimmune encephalitis have shown that treatment with high-dose IV steroids combined with IVIG or plasmapheresis resulted in marked improvement of symptoms and resolution of seizures [12, 13]. Treatment response should be evaluated clinically since antibody titers do not correlate with disease activity [11].

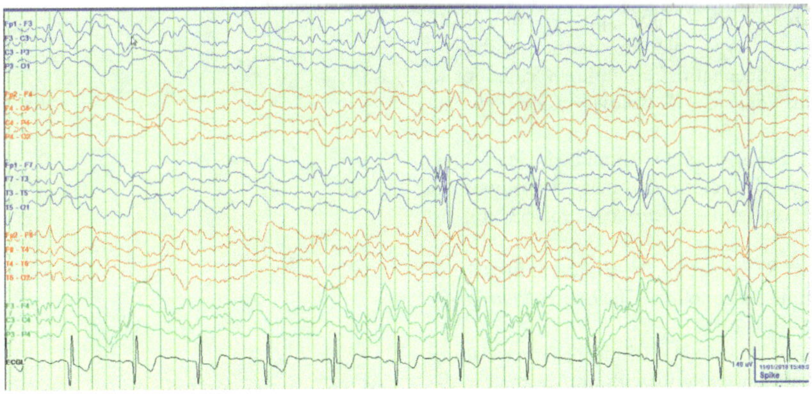

Figure 6: EEG showing left fronto-temporal sharp waves with intermittent slowing.

All patients in this series met diagnostic criteria for autoimmune encephalitis and required immunosuppressive therapy for seizure control [12, 14–16]. Besides rituximab, options include IVIG, plasma exchange, chronic glucocorticoid therapy, azathioprine, mycophenolate mofetil, and cyclophosphamide. All three patients described are clinically normal on AED and rituximab only. None of our patients have developed serious infusion reactions, life-threatening infections, or cancer. Following treatment, behavioral disturbances and seizure activity ceased in all three patients and progression of the disease as well as permanent impairment of executive function was prevented.

4. Conclusion

We suggest that off-label use of rituximab may be an option in the acute and long-term management of intransigent autoimmune epilepsy. Early initiation of aggressive therapy can lead to normalization of clinical function. Randomized trials are required to establish the safety and efficacy of rituximab in this setting.

Abbreviations

ICU: Intensive care unit
FLAIR: Fluid-attenuated inversion recovery
WBC: White blood cells
AED: Antiepileptic drugs
CSF: Cerebrospinal fluid
CT: Computed tomography
EEG: Electroencephalogram
MRI: Magnetic resonance imaging
LP: Lumbar puncture
NMDAR: *N*-methyl-D-aspartate receptor
IV: Intravenous
IVIG: Intravenous immunoglobulin
LGI1: Leucine-rich, glioma inactivated 1
CASPR2: Contactin-associated protein 2
VGCC: Voltage-gated calcium channel
AMPAR: α-Amino-3-hydroxy-5-methyl-4-isoxazolepropionic acid receptor
GABAR: Gamma aminobutyric acid receptor
MoCA: Montreal Cognitive Assessment.

References

[1] G. Zaccara, G. Giannasi, R. Oggioni, E. Rosati, L. Tramacere, and P. Palumbo, "Challenges in the treatment of convulsive status epilepticus," *Seizure*, vol. 47, pp. 17–24, 2017.

[2] B. P. Kelley, S. C. Patel, H. L. Marin, J. J. Corrigan, P. D. Mitsias, and B. Griffith, "Autoimmune encephalitis: pathophysiology and imaging review of an overlooked diagnosis," *American Journal of Neuroradiology*, vol. 38, no. 6, pp. 1070–1078, 2017.

[3] E. Lancaster, "The diagnosis and treatment of autoimmune encephalitis," *Journal of Clinical Neurology*, vol. 12, no. 1, pp. 1–13, 2016.

[4] M. J. Titulaer, L. McCracken, I. Gabilondo et al., "Treatment and prognostic factors for long-term outcome in patients with anti-NMDA receptor encephalitis: an observational cohort study," *The Lancet Neurology*, vol. 12, no. 2, pp. 157–165, 2013.

[5] M. Spatola and J. Dalmau, "Seizures and risk of epilepsy in autoimmune and other inflammatory encephalitis," *Current Opinion in Neurology*, vol. 30, no. 3, pp. 345–353, 2017.

[6] J. Dalmau, F. Taha, and E. Segal, "Clinical presentation and outcome in autoimmune encephalitis associated with N-type voltage-gated calcium channels in children," *Journal of Child Neurology*, vol. 34, no. 9, pp. 499–505, 2019.

[7] J. Frey and A. Murray, "Autoimmune encephalitis with elevated N-type calcium channel antibodies as a multiple sclerosis mimic," *Multiple Sclerosis and Related Disorders*, vol. 26, pp. 201–203, 2018.

[8] D. Dubey, M. Devine, K. Blackburn, and W. Warnack, "Relapsing-remitting chronic lymphocytic inflammation with pontine perivascular enhancement responsive to steroids syndrome in association with P/Q-type voltage-gated calcium channel antibody," *Journal of Postgraduate Medicine*, vol. 62, no. 4, pp. 269-270, 2016.

[9] C. Kamiya-Matsuoka, D. Blas-Boria, M. D. Williams, P. Garciarena, S. Tummala, and I. W. Tremont-Lukats, "N-type calcium channel antibody-mediated paraneoplastic limbic encephalitis: a diagnostic challenge," *Journal of the Neurological Sciences*, vol. 338, no. 1-2, pp. 188–190, 2014.

[10] X. Xu, Q. Lu, Y. Huang et al., "Anti-NMDAR encephalitis: a single-center, longitudinal study in China," *Neurol Neuroimmunol Neuroinflamm*, vol. 7, no. 1, 2019.

[11] S. R. Irani, J. M. Gelfand, B. M. Bettcher, N. S. Singhal, and M. D. Geschwind, "Effect of rituximab in patients with leucine-rich, glioma-inactivated 1 antibody-associated enceph-

alopathy," *JAMA Neurology*, vol. 71, no. 7, pp. 896–900, 2014.
[12] L. Finkel and S. Koh, "N-type calcium channel antibody-mediated autoimmune encephalitis: an unlikely cause of a common presentation," *Epilepsy & Behavior Case Reports*, vol. 1, pp. 92–96, 2013.
[13] A. Alwaki, A. Lugo, C. Goshgarian, O. Ahmad, H. Hefzy, and P. Mitsias, "Voltage gated calcium channels antibody-associated autoimmune encephalitis," *Neurology*, vol. 82, no. 10 Supplement, 2014.
[14] F. Graus, M. J. Titulaer, R. Balu et al., "A clinical approach to diagnosis of autoimmune encephalitis," *The Lancet Neurology*, vol. 15, no. 4, pp. 391–404, 2016.
[15] L. Zhang, M.-Q. Wu, Z.-L. Hao et al., "Clinical characteristics, treatments, and outcomes of patients with anti-N-methyl-d-aspartate receptor encephalitis: a systematic review of reported cases," *Epilepsy & Behavior*, vol. 68, pp. 57–65, 2017.
[16] W. Li, S. Wu, Q. Meng et al., "Clinical characteristics and short-term prognosis of LGI1 antibody encephalitis: a retrospective case study," *BMC Neurology*, vol. 18, no. 1, p. 96, 2018.

44

Susac Syndrome and Pregnancy

Yazan Al-Hasan, Justin L. Hoskin, John C. Wolf, and Kamala Saha

Barrow Neurological Institute, 350 W Thomas Rd, Phoenix, AZ 85013, USA

Correspondence should be addressed to Kamala Saha; kamala.saha@dignityhealth.org

Academic Editor: Isabella Laura Simone

Susac syndrome (SuS) is a rare poorly characterised disorder that affects the brain, retina, and cochlea. Here, we present a case of a 31-year-old pregnant female with a new diagnosis of SuS that was successfully managed to 36 weeks of gestation with minimal disease burden to both the mother and newborn. She was treated initially using intravenous methylprednisolone followed by oral prednisone, and intravenous immunoglobulin (IVIg). We stress the importance of a multidisciplinary approach, involving both neurology and maternal-fetal medicine, and provide guidance in navigating the various options for immunosuppressive therapy during pregnancy.

1. Introduction

Susac syndrome (SuS) is a rare poorly characterised microangiopathy that causes small infarcts in the brain, cochlea, and retina [1]. Classically, it presents with the clinical triad of visual loss caused by branch retinal artery occlusions (BRAO), sensorineural hearing loss, and subacute encephalopathy [2, 3]. Previous reviews of SuS identified 300–405 cases reported in the literature [4, 5], while a recent estimation of SuS patients in Austria estimates a five-year period prevalence of the disease at 0.148/100,000 and an annual incidence of 0.024/100,000 [6]. Here, we discuss a female pregnant patient with a new diagnosis of SuS.

2. Case Presentation

This patient was a 31-year-old right-handed G3P0020 twenty-week pregnant female with a past medical history of idiopathic intracranial hypertension who presented to the emergency department with 4 days of vertigo and worsening vision. At the onset of symptoms, she experienced sudden nonpositional vertigo with severe nausea as well as decreased hearing in the left ear. She also noted nystagmus when looking in the mirror. Her symptoms improved mildly over the course of the day, so she did not seek immediate medical advice.

Two days following the initial onset, her symptoms returned, at which point she was evaluated at an outside emergency department. She was diagnosed with vertigo and discharged with prescriptions for meclizine and metoclopramide. Her symptoms then progressed to involve peripheral vision loss bilaterally, for which she was examined by an ophthalmologist. On dilated ophthalmic exam, she was found to have multiple areas of retinal ischemia and she was referred to our emergency department for further evaluation.

On magnetic resonance imaging (MRI) brain without contrast, nonspecific diffuse white matter signal abnormality was observed (Figures 1(a) and 1(b)), which was considered markedly abnormal for the patient's age. A bedside lumbar puncture was performed, and cerebral spinal fluid analysis showed glucose 58 mg/dL, protein 48 mg/dL, nucleated count 2 per uL, oligoclonal bands negative, and myelin basic protein 8.92 ng/mL. In addition, the patient had an MRI brain with and without contrast performed a year earlier that mentioned white matter lesions in the corpus callosum (Figure 1(c)). She also had with her an audiogram from a year earlier showing low frequency sensorineural hearing loss in the right ear (Figure 2). Given the constellation of

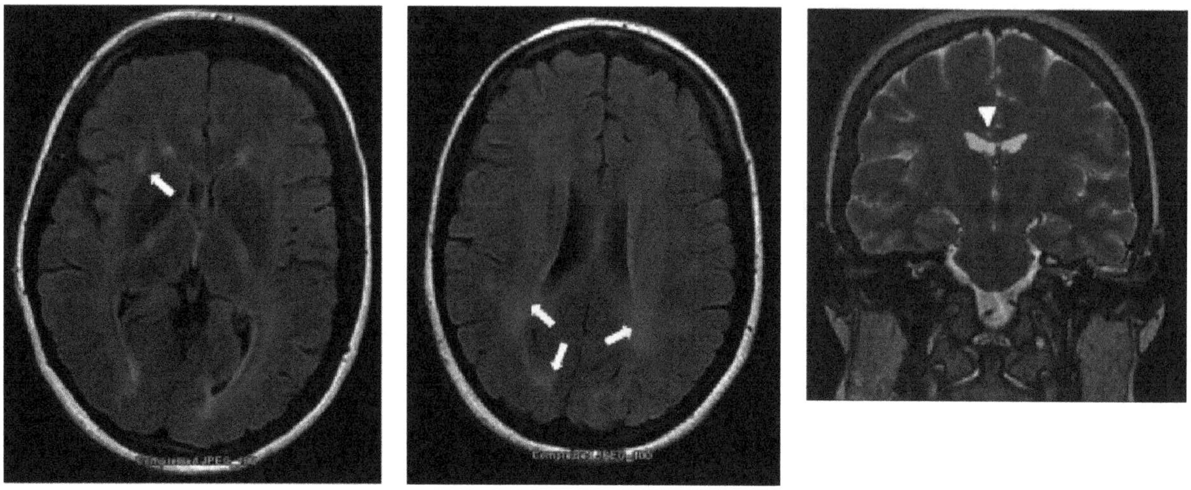

(a) (b) (c)

Figure 1: (a) and (b) Axial MRI brain without contrast demonstrating patchy and confluent FLAIR hyperintensity throughout the white matter, markedly abnormal for age (arrows). (c) Coronal MRI brain FLAIR sequence demonstrating a lesion in the corpus callosum (arrowhead), performed prior to her presentation to our facility.

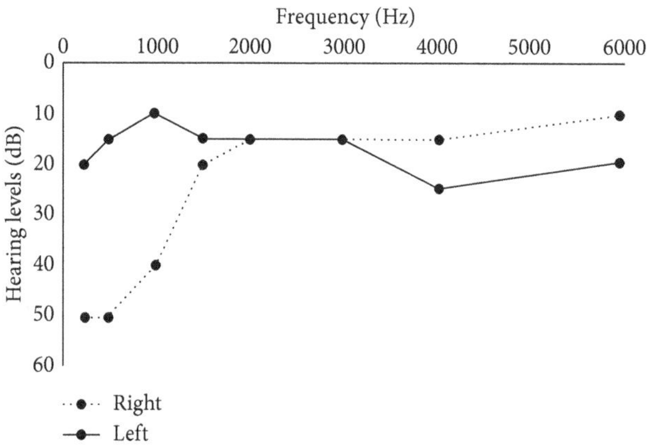

Figure 2: Audiogram results demonstrating low-frequency sensorineural hearing loss in the right ear (dotted line) with her left ear (solid line) unaffected.

symptoms (vertigo, hearing loss, and visual disturbances) in conjunction with her MRI changes, eye exam findings, and audiometric testing results, a diagnosis of SuS was established.

She was treated with methylprednisolone 1 gm IV for 3 days followed by oral prednisone 50 mg daily. Additionally, she was started on intravenous immunoglobulin (IVIg) 0.5 gm/kg for 4 days for a total of 2 gm/kg. During admission, she noted improvement, with near resolution of her vertiginous symptoms as well as some improvement in her hearing. In conjunction with her maternal-fetal medicine physician and her obstetrician, the plan at discharge was to continue prednisone 50 mg daily and maintenance IVIg 0.5 gm/kg for 2 days every 3 weeks. The decision to start steroid sparing immunosuppressants was delayed per patient preference given her pregnancy status.

After discharge, she returned to the hospital three weeks later for one additional round of IVIg and continued on oral prednisone for the duration of her pregnancy. A cesarean section was performed at 36 weeks without complications of SuS to the mother and child. She continued to follow up with neurology for serial imaging and initiation of steroid sparing immunotherapy, namely, rituximab.

3. Discussion

3.1. Pathophysiology. SuS is a rare condition whose definitive etiology remains unknown [3, 7]. At this time, it is classified as an immune-mediated, occlusive microvascular endotheliopathy and/or basement membranopathy that results in endothelium-induced microvascular occlusion in the central nerve system, inner ear, and retina [2, 4]. It has also been termed small infarctions of cochlear, retinal and encephalic tissue (SICRET syndrome), and retinocochleocerebral vasculopathy [8, 9]. As mentioned in the introduction to this paper, SuS is a rare condition and the prevalence is likely underreported. Women seem to be more commonly affected than men at a rate of 3 : 1, and most cases involve Caucasian individuals, though this may be related to medical discrepancies [4]. The estimated mean age of onset is approximately 31.6 years, ranging from 8 to 65 [2, 4, 10–12].

Previous theories regarding pathophysiology suggested that the syndrome is an autoimmune vasculitis that affects the endothelium likely mediated by antiendothelial cell antibodies (AECAs) [13, 14]. AECAs were thought to cause activation of the complement system leading to subsequent deposition of C4d, basement membrane thickening, and endothelial necrosis [10]. Evidence supporting this etiology included SuS patients with high serum AECA, elevated factor VIII (released by damaged endothelium), and tissue pathology with endothelial cell necrosis, basement membrane thickening, and C3d and C4d deposition in vessel walls [10]. However, a recent study showed that only 30% of patients with a definite SuS had elevated serum AECA, suggesting that AECA may represent an epiphenomenon [15]. Interestingly, data presented by Gross et al. strongly implicate cytotoxic T-lymphocyte adhesion to

CNS microvessels leading to endotheliopathy in both pathological specimens and a mouse model of SuS [16]. Furthermore, they also report the use of natalizumab, an inhibitor of T-cell adhesion, ameliorated symptoms in four SuS patients.

3.2. Disease Course. The syndrome typically presents as a clinical triad of encephalopathy, sensorineural hearing loss, and visual disturbances secondary to BRAO [1, 3]. There is a large variability on initial presentation; some estimates suggest that at the time of initial evaluation, less than 20% of patients exhibit the full clinical triad, while other reports suggest that 81% of cases have the complete triad at onset [2–4]. However, estimates suggest that during the clinical course, 70–98% of patients will develop the full triad of symptoms [3, 4]. At presentation, CNS involvement was the most frequent manifestation (80%), followed by ocular involvement (50%) and finally auditory involvement (30%) [3, 4, 9].

Classically, encephalopathy was described as cognitive impairment or psychosis, often leading to patients undergoing psychiatric evaluation [1]. However, more recent articles have discussed encephalopathy as "brain involvement," widening the symptom inclusion criteria to headache, motor and sensory deficiencies, aphasia, cognitive impairment, emotional disturbances, apathy, psychosis, urinary insufficiency, and others [4, 17].

For the criterion of vestibulocochlear involvement, the patient should have at least one of the following symptoms: hearing loss, tinnitus, or vertigo [17–19]. By far, hearing loss is the most common vestibulocochlear disorder identified; one review identified hearing loss in 93% of patients [19]. The hearing loss can be either unilateral or bilateral and is often described as low-frequency sensorineural hearing loss [2, 19, 20].

The manifestations of BRAO vary greatly from subtle to expansive, unilateral, or bilateral [3]. The most common complaints are segmental loss of vision in one or both eyes as well as visual scintillating scotomas [21]. More recently, Gass plaques (retinal arterial wall plaques) have been described in fluorescein staining of retinal arterioles which can help confirm the diagnosis of SuS [18]. In addition to the classic triad of symptoms, a plethora of other symptoms have been found to occur frequently in these patients including headache, myalgia, and dermatological signs [4, 22]. Headache is often present on disease onset and resembles migraine headache [17]. While SuS is a rare condition, it is an important differential diagnosis for several neurologic, psychiatric, otolaryngologic, and ophthalmologic conditions [23].

Similar to the variability in the initial presentation, the disease course can be volatile as well. At one end of the spectrum, patients may present with mild and brief (less than a year) disease. These patients may experience full reversible ischemia in the brain, retina, and cochlea [2]. Occasionally, these patients acquire little to no residual disability. In contrast, patients with severe SuS experience a prolonged disease course that lasts for years and can lead to permanent ischemic damage [2]. The primary organs impacted by SuS, the brain, retina, and cochlea, are highly susceptible to ischemic damage. In addition to the variability in severity, the disease can vary in its remission status. Some suggest that SuS can be monocyclic, polycyclic, and chronic-continuous, with a time frame of 2 years being used to separate the monocyclic course from the other forms [4, 21, 24]. It is likely that there is no pathological difference between these forms of SuS and that this represents a relapsing-remitting course [5]. Separating them into different entities may be more deleterious for patients and confusing for providers. Of note, there are reports of recurrence of SuS after years of remission [25, 26].

3.3. Diagnosis. There are several diagnostic modalities that help confirm the diagnosis SuS. Arguably the most important diagnostic procedures are MRI of the brain, audiometric testing, and retinal fluorescein angiography [27]. Classically, the corpus callosum has been found to have T2 hyperintensities that resemble "snow balls" [28]. These lesions are thought to occur as a result of infarction of tiny arterioles in the central part of the corpus callosum. T2-weighted images may demonstrate small multifocal hyperintensities in the periventricular regions and centrum semiovale. These SuS lesions tend to be more punctate than the large ovoid lesions often identified with multiple sclerosis (MS) lesions [28]. Audiogram testing can show bilateral sensorineural hearing loss predominantly in the low frequencies [2]. Funduscopy and fluorescein retinal angiography may demonstrate unilateral or bilateral distal BRAO [12]. Some estimates suggest that BRAOs are detected in 99% of patients [4].

Laboratory studies including specific serological markers for SuS do not currently exist. As discussed, AECA titers have been shown to be elevated in only 26% of patients. Moderate elevation of protein was the most common CSF finding in SuS, observed in 84% of cases with available CSF data [4, 15, 29]. While the presence of oligoclonal bands or elevation in IgG in the CSF does not exclude SuS, their absence can help differentiate this disease from MS [4, 20]. Additional diagnostic tests including comprehensive screening for autoantibodies, blood clotting abnormalities, CSF analysis, EEG, cerebral catheter angiography, and leptomeningeal biopsy have not proven to provide clinically relevant information [4]. Interestingly, our patient had both vestibular as well as cochlear involvement and therefore not only was an audiogram performed but videonystagmography (VNG) as well. This demonstrated a significant unilateral vestibulopathy that appeared partially compensated, reflecting her recent onset of improving vertigo. We recommend performing a VNG in all patients with vestibular symptoms and also recommend using this test to monitor patients over time who may present with vertigo upon relapse.

3.4. Treatment. Due to the rarity of SuS, the great variability of disease presentation and severity, and the lack of adequate objective biomarkers of disease activity, the development of a treatment guideline with a randomized control trial has been challenging [2]. Based on the current understanding of pathogenesis, the primary target in treatment is the immune system, often with immunosuppression [12, 24]. The most recent guidelines are dependent on the symptoms at presentation. For example, a patient with severe encephalopathy

Table 1: Summary of several medications that are used in the treatment of Susac syndrome and their risk categories established by the United States Food and Drug Administration.

Agent	Pregnancy category	Comments
Corticosteroids		
Prednisone	C/D	Maternal and fetal risks include hyperglycemia, hypertension, and adrenal axis suppression
Methylprednisolone	C	Fetal risk of cleft lip and low birth weight
IVIg	C	Limited data. Crosses the placenta, and it is used to treat some neonatal conditions
Infliximab	Low-to-moderate risk [43]	Crosses the placenta. Report of agranulocytosis in infants [44]
Cyclophosphamide	D	If exposed in the first trimester, reports of skeletal malformations, leukopenia, anemia, pancytopenia, severe bone marrow hypoplasia, and gastroenteritis
Azathioprine	D	Reports of congenital anomalies, immunosuppression, lymphopenia, pancytopenia, and intrauterine growth retardation
Mycophenolate mofetil	D	Associated with congenital malformations and first-trimester pregnancy loss
Rituximab	C	Limited data available; transient B-cell lymphocytopenia
Plasmapheresis	Unknown	Potential maternal risk during plasmapheresis does not seem to increase as a result of pregnancy
Aspirin	D	Likely safer in low doses Increased perinatal mortality, delayed closure of ductus arteriosus, and intrauterine growth retardation
Gadolinium (IV)	C	Crosses the placenta. May be an increased risk for rheumatological, inflammatory, or infiltrative skin conditions
Cyclosporine	C	May result in low birth weight and premature births
Methotrexate	X	Can cause teratogenic effects, embryotoxicity, abortion, and fetal defects. Contraindicated during pregnancy

A = controlled studies show no fetal risk. B = animal studies do not demonstrate risk. There is no evidence of risk in humans. C = animal studies show adverse reaction on the fetus, no studies in humans. D = positive evidence of human fetal risk. X = contraindicated in pregnancy.

may require more aggressive and prolonged treatment than a patient who has mild-moderate hearing loss or BRAO [2].

While treatment must be tailored to the individual patient, the mainstays have included corticosteroids, IVIg, and rituximab, plus one or two additional immunomodulating drugs (methotrexate, mycophenolate, tacrolimus, infliximab, or cyclophosphamide) [30]. Corticosteroids can be given intravenously in the emergent setting with methylprednisolone 1 g/day before switching to an oral prednisone taper based on symptom severity [2, 18]. IVIg is commonly started at 2 g/kg given over several days, with maintenance IVIg then given every 2–4 weeks, for a total of 6 months. From there, the most common medication choices tend to be rituximab and mycophenolate, with one report suggesting initiation of these medications at the onset of symptoms and another recommending reserving these medications for breakthrough symptoms only [2, 18]. The ability to distinguish between a diagnosis of MS and SuS is important as some MS treatments may worsen SuS [31]. Eventually, these medications may be tapered off if symptoms improve or stabilize and the MRI remains inactive. Of note, patients with primary retinal disease may have difficulty tapering off IVIg as this medication has been found to be quite effective at preventing retinal relapses [18].

3.5. Susac and Pregnancy. Reported cases of SuS during pregnancy are rare with an estimate of 5% of cases occurring in association with pregnancy [4, 13, 22, 26, 27, 32–39]. Of the reported cases, the behavior of SuS during pregnancy has been heterogeneous and no statistically significant characteristics have been established [13]. The pathophysiology of disease onset remains unclear; however, it is reasonable to propose that hormonal and immunological changes associated with pregnancy as well as a transient hypercoagulable state may unmask the disease or induce a flare [3, 30, 31]. Recurrence of SuS is also reported in patients undergoing hormone replacement therapy [25], further emphasizing the hormonal contribution to SuS pathophysiology. This complex relationship between autoimmune disease and pregnancy is not unusual and is also seen in other autoimmune diseases including rheumatoid arthritis, thyroid disease, and others [40, 41]. In the postpartum period, there are reports of worsening encephalopathy as well as a reported case of SuS exacerbation occurring after an aborted pregnancy [30]. Despite the increased risk of SuS associated with pregnancy, it is possible for patients in remission to have a safe pregnancy without flare [42]. The pathophysiology behind this relationship is unknown, but we hypothesize that there may be a hormonal influence on the patient's immunity.

As discussed, treatment guidelines for SuS are suggested, but these guidelines have potential limitations with pregnant patients. Careful discussion with the patient and maternal-fetal medicine specialists is warranted. A list of possible treatment options and their risk in pregnancy are discussed below (Table 1) [37, 45–50]. Our patient was started on IVIg in the acute setting and received one maintenance IVIg dose [2]. She showed nearly immediate improvement with her first doses of IVIg. She was also maintained on prednisone 50 mg daily for a long duration (14 weeks) to aid with symptom control. While there is no treatment guideline for

SuS in pregnancy, other cases have demonstrated a positive response to IVIG as well [13]. The overall prognosis of SuS and pregnancy remains unknown.

4. Conclusion

SuS is a rare neurologic disease with a variable course. Treatment regimens have been suggested, but it is unclear what treatment options are best for pregnant patients with SuS. For our patient, she had an initial positive response to IVIg and required a maintenance dose 3 weeks after her initial dose. There was a discussion with the patient regarding addition of rituximab to her regimen, but she decided to forego that treatment until after delivery. She underwent an elective cesarean section at week 36 of pregnancy without complications. As discussed, there may be an exquisite response to IVIg in SuS. We recommend that patients be started quickly on IVIg and that it be continued throughout their pregnancy with maintenance dosing every 2–4 weeks based on the patient's clinical course. Intravenous methylprednisolone with maintenance oral prednisone is also relatively safe and is a rapid bridge to IVIg therapy. Additional steroid sparing immunosuppressants such as rituximab can be considered, though this discussion should involve a multidisciplinary approach.

Abbreviations

SuS: Susac syndrome
BRAO: Branch retinal artery occlusion
AECA: Antiendothelial cell antibody
IVIG: Intravenous immunoglobulin
MS: Multiple sclerosis
MRI: Magnetic resonance imaging
VNG: Videonystagmography.

References

[1] J. O. Susac, J. M. Hardman, and J. B. Selhorst, "Microangiopathy of the brain and retina," *Neurology*, vol. 29, no. 3, pp. 313–316, 1979.

[2] R. M. Rennebohm, N. Asdaghi, S. Srivastava, and E. Gertner, "Guidelines for treatment of Susac syndrome—an update," *International Journal of Stroke*, vol. 15, no. 5, pp. 484–494, 2018.

[3] V. Vishnevskia-Dai, J. Chapman, R. Sheinfeld et al., "Susac syndrome," *Medicine*, vol. 95, no. 43, p. e5223, 2016.

[4] J. Dörr, S. Krautwald, B. Wildemann et al., "Characteristics of Susac syndrome: a review of all reported cases," *Nature Reviews Neurology*, vol. 9, no. 6, pp. 307–316, 2013.

[5] I. Vodopivec and S. Prasad, "Short follow-up bias confounds estimates of the "typical" clinical course of susac syndrome," *Journal of Neuro-Ophthalmology*, vol. 37, no. 2, pp. 149–153, 2017.

[6] T. Seifert-Held, B. J. Langner-Wegscheider, M. Komposch et al., "Susac's syndrome: clinical course and epidemiology in a Central European population," *International Journal of Neuroscience*, vol. 127, no. 9, pp. 776–780, 2017.

[7] J. Schwitter, R. Agosti, P. Ott, A. Kalman, and W. Waespe, "Small infarctions of cochlear, retinal, and encephalic tissue in young women," *Stroke*, vol. 23, no. 6, pp. 903–907, 1992.

[8] P. Kalisa, G. Constantinides, M. Bodson-Halleux, and J. J. De Laey, "Small infarctions of cochlear, retinal and encephalic tissue (SICRET syndrome)," *Bulletin de la Société belge d'ophtalmologie*, vol. 282, pp. 5–12, 2001.

[9] G. W. Petty, A. G. Engel, B. R. Younge et al., "Retinocochleocerebral vasculopathy," *Medicine*, vol. 77, no. 1, pp. 12–40, 1998.

[10] J. O. Susac, R. A. Egan, R. M. Rennebohm, and M. Lubow, "Susac's syndrome: 1975–2005 microangiopathy/autoimmune endotheliopathy," *Journal of the Neurological Sciences*, vol. 257, no. 1-2, pp. 270–272, 2007.

[11] J. O. Susac, F. R. Murtagh, R. A. Egan et al., "MRI findings in Susac's syndrome," *Neurology*, vol. 61, no. 12, pp. 1783–1787, 2003.

[12] T. Papo, V. Biousse, P. Lehoang et al., "Susac syndrome," *Medicine*, vol. 77, no. 1, pp. 3–11, 1998.

[13] E. Gomez-Figueroa, S. Garcia-Trejo, R. A. Garcia-Santos, G. Quiñones-Pesqueira, and J. M. Calleja-Castillo, "Exquisite response to intravenous immunoglobulin in Susac syndrome during pregnancy," *eNeurologicalSci*, vol. 10, pp. 1–4, 2018.

[14] C. M. Magro, J. C. Poe, M. Lubow, and J. O. Susac, "Susac syndrome: an organ-specific autoimmune endotheliopathy syndrome associated with anti-endothelial cell antibodies," *American Journal of Clinical Pathology*, vol. 136, no. 6, pp. 903–912, 2011.

[15] S. Jarius, I. Kleffner, J. M. Dörr et al., "Clinical, paraclinical and serological findings in Susac syndrome: an international multicenter study," *Journal of Neuroinflammation*, vol. 11, p. 46, 2014.

[16] C. C. Gross, C. Meyer, U. Bhatia et al., "CD8+ T cell-mediated endotheliopathy is a targetable mechanism of neuro-inflammation in Susac syndrome," *Nature Communications*, vol. 10, no. 1, p. 5779, 2019.

[17] I. Kleffner, J. Dörr, M. Ringelstein et al., "Diagnostic criteria for Susac syndrome," *Journal of Neurology, Neurosurgery & Psychiatry*, vol. 87, no. 12, pp. 1287–1295, 2016.

[18] R. A. Egan, "Diagnostic criteria and treatment algorithm for susac syndrome," *Journal of Neuro-Ophthalmology*, vol. 39, no. 1, p. 60, 2019.

[19] T. A. Hardy, R. L. Taylor, J. Qiu et al., "The neuro-otology of Susac syndrome," *Journal of Neurology*, vol. 267, no. 12, pp. 3711–3722, 2020.

[20] D. Ayache, I. Plouin-Gaudon, P. Bakouche, P. Elbaz, and O. Gout, "Microangiopathy of the inner ear, retina, and brain (susac syndrome)," *Archives of Otolaryngology-Head & Neck Surgery*, vol. 126, no. 1, pp. 82–84, 2000.

[21] T. H. Do, C. Fisch, and F. Evoy, "Susac syndrome: report of four cases and review of the literature," *American Journal of Neuroradiology*, vol. 25, no. 3, pp. 382–388, 2004.

[22] M. Engeholm, B. Leo-Kottler, H. Rempp et al., "Encephalopathic Susac's syndrome associated with livedo racemosa in a young woman before the completion of family planning," *BMC Neurology*, vol. 13, p. 185, 2013.

[23] J. D. Triplett, K. A. Buzzard, M. Lubomski et al., "Immune-mediated conditions affecting the brain, eye and ear (BEE syndromes)," *Journal of Neurology, Neurosurgery & Psychiatry*, vol. 90, no. 8, pp. 882–894, 2019.

[24] R. M. Rennebohm, R. A. Egan, and J. O. Susac, "Treatment of Susac's syndrome," *Current Treatment Options in Neurology*, vol. 10, no. 1, pp. 67–74, 2008.

[25] G. W. Petty, E. L. Matteson, B. R. Younge, T. J. McDonald, and C. P. Wood, "Recurrence of Susac syndrome (retinocochleocerebral vasculopathy) after remission of 18 years," *Mayo Clinic Proceedings*, vol. 76, no. 9, pp. 958–960, 2001.

[26] A. Feresiadou, U. Eriksson, H.-C. Larsen, R. Raininko, I. Nygren, and A. Melberg, "Recurrence of susac syndrome following 23 years of remission," *Case Reports in Neurology*, vol. 6, no. 2, pp. 171–175, 2014.

[27] R. Antulov, I. Holjar Erlic, O. Perkovic, D. Miletic, and I. Antoncic, "Susac's syndrome during pregnancy—the first Croatian case," *Journal of the Neurological Sciences*, vol. 341, no. 1-2, pp. 162–164, 2014.

[28] K. A. Buzzard, S. W. Reddel, C. Yiannikas, D. Sean Riminton, M. H. Barnett, and T. A. Hardy, "Distinguishing Susac's syndrome from multiple sclerosis," *Journal of Neurology*, vol. 262, no. 7, pp. 1613–1621, 2015.

[29] S. Jarius, B. Neumayer, K. P. Wandinger, M. Hartmann, and B. Wildemann, "Anti-endothelial serum antibodies in a patient with Susac's syndrome," *Journal of the Neurological Sciences*, vol. 285, no. 1-2, pp. 259–261, 2009.

[30] T. A. Hardy, R. J. Garsia, and G. M. Halmagyi, "Tumour necrosis factor (TNF) inhibitor therapy in Susac's syndrome," *Journal of the Neurological Sciences*, vol. 302, no. 1-2, pp. 126–128, 2011.

[31] P. W. Laird, N. J. Newman, and S. Yeh, "Exacerbation of Susac syndrome retinopathy by interferon Beta-1a," *Archives of Ophthalmology*, vol. 130, no. 6, pp. 804–806, 2012.

[32] F. J. Mateen, A. Y. Zubkov, R. Muralidharan et al., "Susac syndrome: clinical characteristics and treatment in 29 new cases," *European Journal of Neurology*, vol. 19, no. 6, pp. 800–811, 2012.

[33] D. J. MacFadyen, R. J. Schneider, and I. A. Chisholm, "A syndrome of brain, inner ear and retinal microangiopathy," *Canadian Journal of Neurological Sciences*, vol. 14, no. 3, pp. 315–318, 1987.

[34] D. L. Gordon, S. S. Hayreh, and H. P. Adams Jr., "Microangiopathy of the brain, retina, and ear: improvement without immunosuppressive therapy," *Stroke*, vol. 22, no. 7, pp. 933–937, 1991.

[35] L. H. Hua, S. L. Donlon, and D. T. Okuda, "A case of Susac syndrome with cervical spinal cord involvement on MRI," *Journal of the Neurological Sciences*, vol. 337, no. 1-2, pp. 228–231, 2014.

[36] Z. A. Ioannides, C. Airey, N. Fagermo, S. Blum, P. A. McCombe, and R. J. Henderson, "Susac syndrome and multifocal motor neuropathy first manifesting in pregnancy," *Australian and New Zealand Journal of Obstetrics and Gynaecology*, vol. 53, no. 3, pp. 314–317, 2013.

[37] K. D. Deane, K. N. Tyler, D. W. Johnson et al., "Susac syndrome and pregnancy: disease management," *Journal of Clinical Rheumatology*, vol. 17, no. 2, pp. 83–88, 2011.

[38] Z. M. Grinspan, J. Z. Willey, M. J. Tullman, and M. S. V. Elkind, "Clinical Reasoning: a 28-year-old pregnant woman with encephalopathy," *Neurology*, vol. 73, no. 15, pp. e74–e79, 2009.

[39] L. Ramos-Ruperto, N. Martínez-Sánchez, J. L. Bartha-Rasero, and Á. Robles-Marhuenda, "Susac syndrome and pregnancy: a relationship to clarify. About two cases and review of the literature," *The Journal of Maternal-Fetal & Neonatal Medicine*, pp. 1–6, 2020.

[40] Y. A. de Man, R. J. E. M. Dolhain, F. E. van de Geijn, S. P. Willemsen, and J. M. W. Hazes, "Disease activity of rheumatoid arthritis during pregnancy: results from a nationwide prospective study," *Arthritis & Rheumatism*, vol. 59, no. 9, pp. 1241–1248, 2008.

[41] A. P. Weetman, "Immunity, thyroid function and pregnancy: molecular mechanisms," *Nature Reviews Endocrinology*, vol. 6, no. 6, pp. 311–318, 2010.

[42] J. Qiu, D. S. Riminton, S. W. Reddel, and T. A. Hardy, "Pregnancy without relapse following treated Susac syndrome," *Multiple Sclerosis and Related Disorders*, vol. 45, Article ID 102357, 2020.

[43] ACOG Committee Opinion No. 776, "Immune modulating therapies in pregnancy and lactation," *Obstetrics and Gynecology*, vol. 133, no. 4, pp. e287–e295, 2019.

[44] T. Guiddir, M.-L. Fremond, T. B. Triki et al., "Anti-TNF- therapy may cause neonatal neutropenia," *Pediatrics*, vol. 134, no. 4, pp. e1189–e1193, 2014.

[45] US Food And Drug Administration, "Consumer medication guides," *Journal of Pain & Palliative Care Pharmacotherapy*, vol. 24, no. 3, pp. 298–301, 2010.

[46] L. Colla, D. Diena, M. Rossetti et al., "Immunosuppression in pregnant women with renal disease: review of the latest evidence in the biologics era," *Journal of Nephrology*, vol. 31, no. 3, pp. 361–383, 2018.

[47] J. L. Cox, S. A. Koepsell, and S. M. Shunkwiler, "Therapeutic plasma exchange and pregnancy: a case report and guidelines for performing plasma exchange in a pregnant patient," *Journal of Clinical Apheresis*, vol. 32, no. 3, pp. 191–195, 2017.

[48] S. C. Kim and S. Hernandez-Diaz, "Editorial: safety of immunosuppressive drugs in pregnant women with systemic inflammatory diseases," *Arthritis & Rheumatology*, vol. 66, no. 2, pp. 246–249, 2014.

[49] R. Ramsey-Goldman and E. Schilling, "Immunosuppressive drug use during pregnancy," *Rheumatic Disease Clinics of North America*, vol. 23, no. 1, pp. 149–167, 1997.

[50] F. Z. Ghandour, T. C. Knauss, and D. E. Hricik, "Immunosuppressive drugs in pregnancy," *Advances in Renal Replacement Therapy*, vol. 5, no. 1, pp. 31–37, 1998.

Permissions

All chapters in this book were first published by Hindawi Publishing Corporation; hereby published with permission under the Creative Commons Attribution License or equivalent. Every chapter published in this book has been scrutinized by our experts. Their significance has been extensively debated. The topics covered herein carry significant findings which will fuel the growth of the discipline. They may even be implemented as practical applications or may be referred to as a beginning point for another development.

The contributors of this book come from diverse backgrounds, making this book a truly international effort. This book will bring forth new frontiers with its revolutionizing research information and detailed analysis of the nascent developments around the world.

We would like to thank all the contributing authors for lending their expertise to make the book truly unique. They have played a crucial role in the development of this book. Without their invaluable contributions this book wouldn't have been possible. They have made vital efforts to compile up to date information on the varied aspects of this subject to make this book a valuable addition to the collection of many professionals and students.

This book was conceptualized with the vision of imparting up-to-date information and advanced data in this field. To ensure the same, a matchless editorial board was set up. Every individual on the board went through rigorous rounds of assessment to prove their worth. After which they invested a large part of their time researching and compiling the most relevant data for our readers.

The editorial board has been involved in producing this book since its inception. They have spent rigorous hours researching and exploring the diverse topics which have resulted in the successful publishing of this book. They have passed on their knowledge of decades through this book. To expedite this challenging task, the publisher supported the team at every step. A small team of assistant editors was also appointed to further simplify the editing procedure and attain best results for the readers.

Apart from the editorial board, the designing team has also invested a significant amount of their time in understanding the subject and creating the most relevant covers. They scrutinized every image to scout for the most suitable representation of the subject and create an appropriate cover for the book.

The publishing team has been an ardent support to the editorial, designing and production team. Their endless efforts to recruit the best for this project, has resulted in the accomplishment of this book. They are a veteran in the field of academics and their pool of knowledge is as vast as their experience in printing. Their expertise and guidance has proved useful at every step. Their uncompromising quality standards have made this book an exceptional effort. Their encouragement from time to time has been an inspiration for everyone.

The publisher and the editorial board hope that this book will prove to be a valuable piece of knowledge for researchers, students, practitioners and scholars across the globe.

List of Contributors

Nitya Prabhakaran, Douglas C. Miller and Shellaine R. Frazier
Department of Pathology and Anatomical Sciences, University of Missouri School of Medicine, Columbia, MO 65212, USA

N. Scott Litofsky
Division of Neurological Surgery, Department of Surgery, University of Missouri School of Medicine, Columbia, MO 65212, USA

Osmond C. Wu, Berje H. Shammassian, Arunit J. S. Chugh and Manish K. Kasliwal
Department of Neurological Surgery, University Hospitals Cleveland Medical Center, Cleveland, OH, USA

Aparna Harbhajanka
Department of Pathology, University Hospitals Cleveland Medical Center, Cleveland, OH, USA

Carmine Franco Muccio
Neuroradiology Unit, Neuroscience Department, "G. Rummo" Hospital, Benevento, Italy

Luca De Lipsis and Rossella Belmonte
Anesthesia Department, "Sacred Heart of Jesus" Hospital, Benevento, Italy

Alfonso Cerase
Neuroimaging and Neurointervention Unit, NHS and University Hospital "Saint Mary alle Scotte", Siena, Italy

Lauren Miller, Robert L. Archer and Nidhi Kapoor
Department of Neurology, University of Arkansas for Medical Sciences, Little Rock, AR, USA

Yu Na Choi
Department of Anesthesiology and Pain Medicine, Bucheon ST.Mary's Hospital, College of Medicine, The Catholic University of Korea, Bucheon 14647, Republic of Korea

Sang Ji Kang, Jin Deok Joo, Yu Mi Kim, Jang Hyeok In and Yoo Jung Park
Department of Anesthesiology and Pain Medicine, Saint Vincent's Hospital, College of Medicine, The Catholic University of Korea, Suwon 16247, Republic of Korea

Zhao-Quan Liu
Department of Neurosurgery, Cathay General Hospital, Taipei City, Taiwan

Jen-Hsien Liao
Department of Anesthesiology, Cathay General Hospital, Taipei City, Taiwan

Chih-Ju Chang
Department of Neurosurgery, Cathay General Hospital, Taipei City, Taiwan
Department of Medicine, School of Medicine, Fu Jen Catholic University, New Taipei City, Taiwan
Department of Mechanical Engineering, National Central University, Taoyuan City, Taiwan

D. Tsiptsios
Neurophysiology Department, Sunderland Royal Hospital, South Tyneside & Sunderland NHS Foundation Trust, Sunderland, UK

D. Daud and A. Cassidy
Neurology Department, Sunderland Royal Hospital, South Tyneside & Sunderland NHS Foundation Trust, Sunderland, UK

K. Tsamakis and E. Rizos
Second Department of Psychiatry, University General Hospital "Attikon", School of Medicine, Athens, Greece

A. Anastadiadis
First Department of Urology, Aristotle University of Thessaloniki, School of Medicine, Thessaloniki, Greece

Imalke Kankananarachchi
Department of Paediatrics, Faculty of Medicine, University of Ruhuna, Matara, Sri Lanka

Eresha Jasinge
Lady Ridgeway Hospital, Colombo, Sri Lanka

Gemunu Hewawitharana
Teaching Hospital Karapitiya, University of Ruhana, Matara, Sri Lanka

Taha Nisar, Abdul R. Alchaki and Erin Feinstein
Rutgers New Jersey Medical School, Newark, USA

Miyuki Miyamoto, Nobuyuki Ishii, Hitoshi Mochizuki, Kazutaka Shiomi and Masamitsu Nakazato
Division of Neurology, Respirology, Endocrinology and Metabolism, Department of Internal Medicine, University of Miyazaki, Miyazaki, Japan

Tomoko Kaida
Miyata Eye Hospital, Miyakonojo, Miyazaki, Japan

Hideki Chuman
Department of Ophthalmology, University of Miyazaki, Miyazaki, Japan

Yuwa Oka, Kenichi Komatsu, Soichiro Abe and Sadayuki Matsumoto
Department of Neurology, Kitano Hospital, Tazuke Kofukai Medical Research Institute, Osaka, Japan

Naoya Yoshimoto and Junya Taki
Department of Neurosurgery, Kitano Hospital, Tazuke Kofukai Medical Research Institute, Osaka, Japan

Eunyoung Chae and Soomin Jeong
Medical School, Jeonbuk National University, Jeonju, Republic of Korea

Chan-Hyuk Lee
Department of Neurology, Asan Medical Center, Seoul, Republic of Korea

Andy Y. Wang, Joseph N. Tingen and Ron I. Riesenburger
Department of Neurosurgery, Tufts Medical Center, Boston, MA, USA

Eric J. Mahoney
Department of Surgery, Tufts Medical Center, Boston, MA, USA

Alan Tesson
Inova Neuroscience Service Line, Inova Health System, 8081 Innovation Park Dr, Fairfax, VA 22031, USA

Peter Kranz
Department of Radiology, Duke University Medical Center, 2301 Erwin Rd, Durham, NC 27710, USA

Ali Zomorodi
Department of Neurosurgery, Duke University Medical Center, 2301 Erwin Rd, Durham, NC 27710, USA

Joel Morgenlander
Department of Neurology, Duke University Medical Center, 2301 Erwin Rd, Durham, NC 27710, USA

Ritsuo Hashimoto, Tomoko Ogawa and Hiroyuki Kato
Department of Neurology, International University of Health and Welfare Hospital, Japan

Asako Tagawa
Department of Neurology, Hiratsuka City Hospital, Japan

Noriyo Komori
Department of Language and Hearing Sciences, International University of Health and Welfare, Japan

Tulsi S. Shah, Jose A. Castillo, Rahul U. Nayak and Jahnnavi Madiraju
Virginia Commonwealth University School of Medicine, Inova Campus, Falls Church VA, USA

Heela Azizi, Alexander Kilpatrick, Maleeha Ahmad, Alexa Kahn, Dina Rimawi, Shantale Williams, Sinthuja Jayaraj, Sherina Langdon, Mirna Iskander, Ali Chohan, Deepa Nuthalapati and Geetha Vyas
American University of Antigua College of Medicine, Department of Psychiatry, Interfaith Medical Center, Brooklyn, New York, USA

Ayotomide Oyelakin, Kodjovi Kodjo, Chiedozie Ojimba, Oluwole Jegede, Carolina Nisenoff and Ayodeji Jolayemi
Department of Psychiatry, Interfaith Medical Center, Brooklyn, New York, USA

Tasmia Khan and Ulunma Umesi
Medical University of the Americas, Department of Psychiatry, Interfaith Medical Center, Brooklyn, New York, USA

Ivan Leung
Saba University School of Medicine, Department of Psychiatry, Interfaith Medical Center, Brooklyn, New York, USA

Arun Rajaratnam, Kishan Dissanayake, Kiertie Kularatne and Sunil Bowattage
Teaching Hospital Kandy, Kandy, Sri Lanka

Dhanashree Peddawad and Manoj K. Singh
Department of Neurology, Continental Hospital, Nanakrumguda, Financial District, 500032 Hyderabad, India

Birte Eikeland
Primary Health Clinic, A. Bergs vei 31, 5089 Bergen, Norway

Divine C. Nwafor
Department of Neuroscience, School of Medicine, West Virginia University, Morgantown, WV, USA

Ashley B. Petrone
Department of Pathology, Anatomy and Laboratory Medicine, School of Medicine, West Virginia University, School of Medicine, Morgantown, WV, USA

Joseph M. Collins
Department of Radiology, Mayo Clinic Arizona, Scottsdale, AZ, USA

Amelia K. Adcock
Department of Neurology, School of Medicine, West Virginia University, Morgantown, WV, USA

Justine Chan, Paarth Shah and Guillermo Moguel-Cobos
Department of Neurology, Barrow Neurological Institute, St. Joseph's Hospital and Medical Center, Phoenix, AZ, USA

Yao Christian Hugues Dokponou, Mamoune El Mostarchid, Housni Abderrahmane, Niamien Patrice Koffi, Miloudi Gazzaz and Brahim El Mostarchid
Department of Neurosurgery, Mohammed V Military Teaching Hospital, Faculty of Medicine and Pharmacy Rabat, Rabat, Morocco

Miral H. Gharib, Mohamed Awni AlKahlout, Hani Malallah AlEssa and Samar AlEmadi
Rheumatology, Department of Medicine, Hamad Medical Corporation, Doha, Qatar

Beatriz Garcia Canibano and Dirk Theophiel Deleu
Neurology, Department of Medicine, Hamad General Hospital, Doha, Qatar

Vijay Renga
Department of Neurology, Dartmouth Hitchcock Medical Center, Geisel School of Medicine at Dartmouth, One Medical Center Drive, Lebanon, NH 03756, USA

Kevin Ha, Kathryn Lewis, Vandan Patel and Jennifer Grinceri
University of California, Riverside, School of Medicine, USA

Aayesha Jalaluddin Soni and Edward Bernard Lee-Pan
Department of Neurology, University of Cape Town, Cape Town, South Africa

Marija Bender and Nataša Pejanović-Škobić
University Hospital Mostar, Department of Neurology, Mostar, Bosnia and Herzegovina

Gojko Bogdan and Dorijan Radančevič
University Hospital Mostar, Department of Radiology, Mostar, Bosnia and Herzegovina

Chiara Mozzini and Mauro Pagani
Department of Medicine, ASST Mantova, C. Poma Hospital Strada Lago Paiolo, Mantova 104600, Italy

Raffaele Ghirardi
Department of Medicine, ASST Mantova, Presidio di Pieve, Via Bugatte, Borgo Mantovano, Mantova 146036, Italy

Abinayaa Ravichandran and Hussam A. Yacoub
Lehigh Valley Physician Group - Neurology, Lehigh Valley Health Network, Allentown, PA, USA

Kareem S. Elsayed
Morsani College of Medicine, University of South Florida, Tampa, FL, USA

Samantha Novotny and Kenneth Serrano
Renaissance School of Medicine at Stony Brook University, 101 Nicolls Road, Stony Brook, New York 11794, USA

Danielle Bazer and Louis Manganas
Department of Neurology at Stony Brook University Hospital, 101 Nicolls Road Stony Brook, New York 11794, USA

Lindsey Dalka
Eastern Maine Medical Center, Department of Family Medicine, Bangor, USA

Antoine Harb
Eastern Maine Medical Center, Department of Hematology and Oncology, Bangor, USA

Kael Mikesell
Eastern Maine Medical Center, Department of Patient Blood Management, Bangor, USA

Gillian Gordon Perue
Eastern Maine Medical Center, Department of Neurology, Bangor, USA

Stacey Ho
Ross University School of Medicine, Department of Neurology, California Hospital Medical Center, Los Angeles, California, USA

Lawrence Chau
Department of Neurology, Adventist Health White Memorial, USA

Antonio Liu
Department of Neurology, Adventist Health White Memorial, USA
Ross University School of Medicine, Department of Neurology, California Hospital Medical Center, Los Angeles, California, USA

Sidonie Ibrikji, Tarek El Halabi and Bassem Yamout
American University of Beirut Medical Center, Department of Neurology, Beirut, Lebanon

Carlo Fornaini
Micoralis Laboratory EA7354, Faculty of Dentistry, University of Nice Sophia Antipolis, 24 Avenue des Diables Bleus, Nice 06357, France
Group of Applied ElectroMagnetics, Department of Engineering and Architecture, University of Parma, Viale G. P. Usberti 181/A, Parma 43124, Italy
Department of Stomatology, 2nd Hospital, Gonguong Road 425, Shijiazhuang, Hebei, China

Zhao Meng
Department of Stomatology, 2nd Hospital, Gonguong Road 425, Shijiazhuang, Hebei, China

Elisabetta Merigo
Micoralis Laboratory EA7354, Faculty of Dentistry, University of Nice Sophia Antipolis, 24 Avenue des Diables Bleus, Nice 06357, France

Jean-Paul Rocca
Micoralis Laboratory EA7354, Faculty of Dentistry, University of Nice Sophia Antipolis, 24 Avenue des Diables Bleus, Nice 06357, France
Department of Stomatology, 2nd Hospital, Gonguong Road 425, Shijiazhuang, Hebei, China

Maria das Dores Medina-Lopes
The Secretariat of Health of the Federal District and the Ministry of Health, Brasília, DF, Brazil

Luiz Augusto Casulari
The University Hospital of Bras´ılia and Clinic of Endocrinology and Neurology (CLINEN), Brasília, DF, Brazil

Raman Sohal, Vishal Phogat, Abha Harish, Basel Abuzuaiter and Nia Jagroop
Department of Medicine, SUNY Upstate Medical University Hospital, 750 E Adams St., Syracuse, NY 13210, USA

Steven H. Adams, Michael P. A. Williams and Kamal K. Khurana
Department of Pathology, SUNY Upstate Medical University Hospital, 750 E Adams St., Syracuse, NY 13210, USA

Carlos Ynigo D. Lopez and Bhavya Narapureddy
Department of Neurology, SUNY Upstate Medical University Hospital, 750 E Adams St., Syracuse, NY 13210, USA

Naman Zala, Lena Wirth, Berit Jordan and Timolaos Rizos
Department of Neurology, Heidelberg University Hospital, Im Neuenheimer Feld 400, Heidelberg 69120, Germany

Hagen Meredig
Department of Neuroradiology, Heidelberg University Hospital, Im Neuenheimer Feld 400, Heidelberg 69120, Germany

Ketino Kobaidze
Associate Professor of Medicine, Emory University School of Medicine, Division of Hospital Medicine 550 Peachtree Street, Atlanta, GA 30308, USA

Yoo Mee Shin
Division of Hospital Medicine, Emory University School of Medicine, Atlanta, GA 30308, USA

Mariam Japaridze
Ross University School of Medicine, New Jersey, USA

Ioannis Karakis
Department of Neurology, Emory University School of Medicine, Atlanta, GA 30308, USA

Xin Wu
Department of Radiology and Imaging Science, Emory University School of Medicine, Atlanta, GA 30308, USA

Mehrdad Hasibi
Professor of Infectious Diseases, Amiralam Hospital, Tehran University of Medical Sciences, South Saadi St., Tehran, Iran

Maral Seyed Ahadi
Assistant Professor of Neurology, Amiralam Hospita, Iranian Center of Neurological Research, Neuroscience Institute, Tehran University of Medical Sciences, South Saadi St., Tehran, Iran

Hamed Abdollahi
Assistant Professor, Department of Anesthesiology, Amiralam Hospital, Tehran University of Medical Sciences, South Saadi St., Tehran, Iran

Mehrdad Jafari
Assistant Professor, Department of Otolaryngology—Head and Neck Surgery, Imam Khomeini Hospital Complex, Tehran University of Medical Sciences, Valiasr hospital, Baqerkhan St., Tehran, Iran

Maurizio Benucci, Arianna Damiani and Francesca Li Gobbi
Rheumatology Unit, S. Giovanni di Dio Hospital, Florence, Italy

Luciana Tramacere, Maristella Piccininni, Gaetano Zaccara and Massimo Cincotta
Neurology Unit, S. Giovanni di Dio Hospital, Florence, Italy

Maria Infantino, Mariangela Manfredi and Valentina Grossi
Immunology and Allergology Laboratory, S. Giovanni di Dio Hospital, Florence, Italy

Mohankumar Kurukumbi and Rahul H. Dave
Department of Neurology, Inova Fairfax Hospital, Falls Church, VA, USA

Jose Castillo, Tulsi Shah and Joanne Lau
Virginia Commonwealth University School of Medicine, Inova Campus, Falls Church, VA, USA

Yazan Al-Hasan, Justin L. Hoskin, John C. Wolf and Kamala Saha
Barrow Neurological Institute, 350 W Thomas Rd, Phoenix, AZ 85013, USA

Index

www.ingramcontent.com/pod-product-compliance
Lightning Source LLC
LaVergne TN
LVHW082231200926
848484LV00008B/2334
9798887406084